Quick Guidebook
to Canine and Feline
Ophthalmology

Javier Esteban Martín

Second edition

Plaza Antonio Beltrán Martínez, n.° 1, planta 8 - letra I
(Centro empresarial El Trovador)
50002 Zaragoza - Spain

Second edition of *Quick Guidebook to Canine and Feline Ophtalmology*
(2017, ISBN: 978-84-16818-98-3)

First printing: September 2019

This book was originally published in Spanish under the title:
Guía rápida de oftalmología canina y felina
© 2009 Grupo Asís Biomedia, SL
ISBN Spanish edition: 978-84-92569-14-4

Translation:
Lori Newman

ISBN: 978-84-17640-87-3
DL: Z 1491-2019

Design, layout and printing:
Servet editorial - Grupo Asís Biomedia, SL
www.grupoasis.com
info@grupoasis.com

GRUPO asis

Servet is the publishing house of Grupo Asís

Warning:

Veterinary science is constantly evolving, as are pharmacology and the other sciences. Inevitably, it is therefore the responsibility of the veterinary surgeon to determine and verify the dosage, the method of administration, the duration of treatment and any possible contraindications to the treatments given to each individual patient, based on his or her professional experience. Neither the publisher nor the author can be held liable for any damage or harm caused to people, animals or properties resulting from the correct or incorrect application of the information contained in this book.

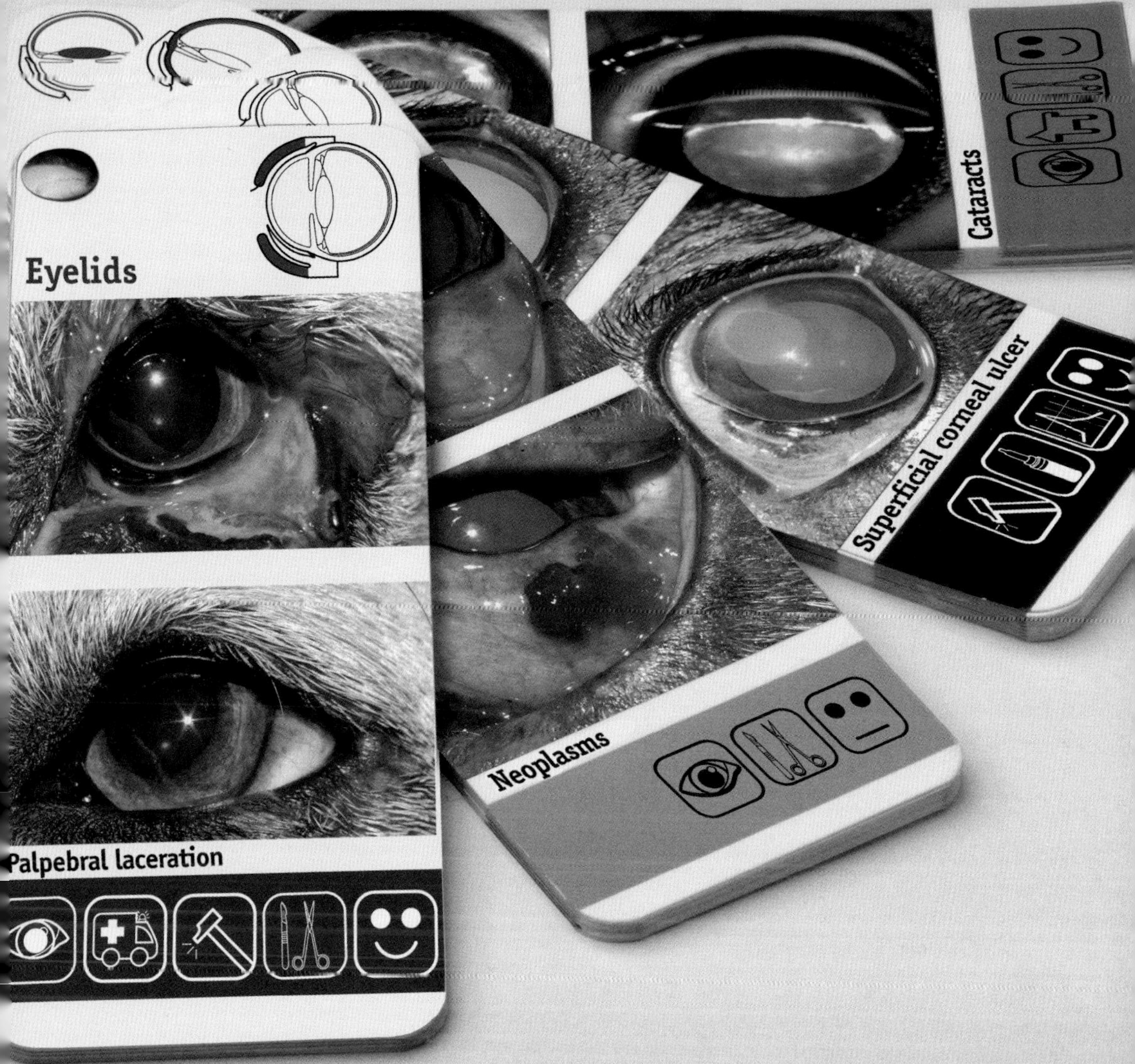

Quick Guidebook
to Canine and Feline
Ophthalmology

Second edition

Javier Esteban Martín

SERVET

To MARINA, my wife and my life, with all of my love.

In memory of “Yako”, my pet.

Author

Javier Esteban Martín

Degree in Veterinary Medicine.
Diplomate in Veterinary Ophthalmology.
Ocaña Veterinary Clinic.
Madrid, Spain.

Collaborating

Cristina Fernández Algarra

Degree in Veterinary Medicine.
Veterinary diagnostic cytology service.
Madrid, Spain.

Jaume Altimira Palau

PhD in Veterinary Medicine.
Veterinary diagnostic histopathology service.
HISTOVET.
Barcelona, Spain.

Elena Alonso Fernández-Aceytuno

PhD in Veterinary Medicine.
Veterinary Cytology and Pathology Laboratory.
Madrid.

Andrés Calvo Ibbitson

Veterinary pathologist.
CITOPATH.
Madrid, Spain.

Valentina Lorenzo Fernández

Diplomate ECVN.
Director of the Neurología Veterinaria neurology referral centre.
Madrid, Spain.

Mª Carmen Tovar Sahuquillo

Professor of Medicine and Clinical Surgery, professor of Ophthalmology, Murcia Veterinary School.
Diploma in Ophthalmology from the Autonomous University of Barcelona.
Certificate in Advanced Ophthalmology, Toulouse Veterinary School.
Member of the Latin American College of Veterinary Ophthalmology (CLOVE).
Multiple top awards in ophthalmology from AVEPA (Spanish Small Animal Veterinary Association).

Speaker at several scientific conferences and meetings, as well as director of several classes, seminars, and conferences on veterinary ophthalmology.

Foreword

Veterinary ophthalmology enjoys a rich history, and abundant information exists on the subject. The first papers in this discipline date back from the Antiquity, and since then numerous books on veterinary ophthalmology have been written, mainly by American and European authors. Many of these books have been translated into Spanish; however, Javier Esteban Martín, my friend Javier, was the first Spanish veterinary surgeon to write a book on veterinary ophthalmology.

When I met him several years ago at an ophthalmology conference, we were both starting our careers. He seemed to be a lovely person, slightly timid, with an exquisite manner. He was at once serious and rigourous in his work and tremendously generous. I realised over time that Javier is special. He is one of a kind. I thank him for giving me this opportunity to express my feelings about him because we do not often get the chance to do this. We tend to focus more on people's flaws than on their talents.

This is his second book and I am convinced readers will like it. It is educational, practical, useful, simple, and great to have around, just like Javier. The author is a guarantee of the book's quality, but his first book also provides a strong recommendation.

Javier, I am certain this book will be successful, and I encourage you to continue to pursue your other worthwhile endeavours.

Warmly,

Mª Carmen Tovar Sahuquillo

Acknowledgements

Behind such a small book is a great effort as well as enormous satisfaction.

This book would not exist without the support and work of every collaborator.

Thanks to SERVET for giving me the chance to convey my passion for veterinary ophthalmology. Thanks to the entire team for their excellent work and strong editorial efforts.

Thanks to HISTOVET, to Dr Elena Alonso Fernández-Aceytuno, to CITOPATH and to Cristina Fernández Algarra for giving me the histopathology and cytology pictures that are included in the guidebook. The high quality of these pictures reflects the high standards of professionalism of each contributor.

Thanks to my friend and colleague Valentina Lorenzo, a consummate professional and an even better person, for the magnificent veterinary magnetic resonance and cerebrospinal fluid cytology images.

MANY THANKS to all of the veterinary clinics who trusted in me year after year. Your cases have fuelled my professional curiosity and helped me improve every day.

Thanks to my colleagues at Ocaña Veterinary Clinic. To María for helping create the alphabetical index and for being a VET "in capitals". To Mario and Patricia for being great anaesthaetists. To Gustavo for being who you are (never change). To Pili and Mamen for your good work and patience. But above all... THANKS for your friendship.

Thanks to my vet friends who are also excited about ophthalmology: Marc, Mª Carmen, José Mª, Eduardo, Eva, Alfonso, Clinio, Elisa, Fernando, Victoria, Jorge... For the good times we shared and for your encouragement.

I would especially like to thank my family for your support and love. You are vital to me.

Finally, thanks to my wife MARINA, with her infinite patience, the long waits, and unconditional support. Each and every page of this book is dedicated to her. THANK YOU FOR EXISTING.

Javier Esteban

Introduction

The goal of this guidebook is to provide both veterinary surgeons and students with a quick reference to easily recognise the most common ophthalmological conditions seen in daily practice.

The intention is not to provide detailed anatomy or aetiopathogenesis, or to exhaustively list all possible diagnostic and treatment options in tables and graphics. This photographic guide is intended to familiarise general practice veterinary surgeons with ocular pathology sufficiently for them to be able to easily diagnose diseases and identify the affected area of the globe or associated structures.

All pictures are accompanied by a definition of the ocular disease, detailing the aspects most important to locate it. The book also provides interesting notes on the disease severity, the degree of urgency, diagnosis, treatment, breed predispositions, etc.

All pictures in this guidebook are taken from real cases; thus, some are straightforward to interpret, while others require more effort to identify the problem.

I hope this guidebook will answer some of your ophthalmology questions to empower you to help your patients.

Enjoy!

Javier Esteban

Table of contents

Nictitating membrane

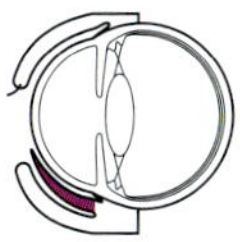

Conjunctiva

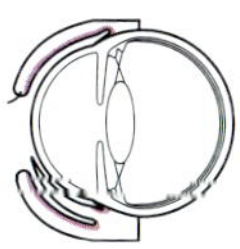

Cornea and sclera

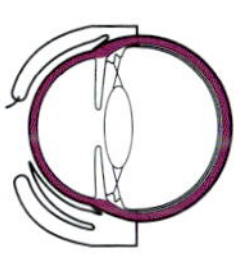

Quick Guidebook to Canine and Feline **Ophthalmology**

How to use this guidebook

The objective of this guidebook is to provide a practical, informative, and rapid visual reference for the veterinary surgeon during ophthalmology consultations. To this end, each page includes pictures of the condition with a brief explanation in the caption, as well as different sections in which the definition, clinical signs, therapy, prognosis, and other relevant information on the condition are provided.

The following example illustrates the basic structure of this guidebook. The next page defines the colour codes associated with each ocular structure, and the key to the symbols used in the book is at the bottom of the page.

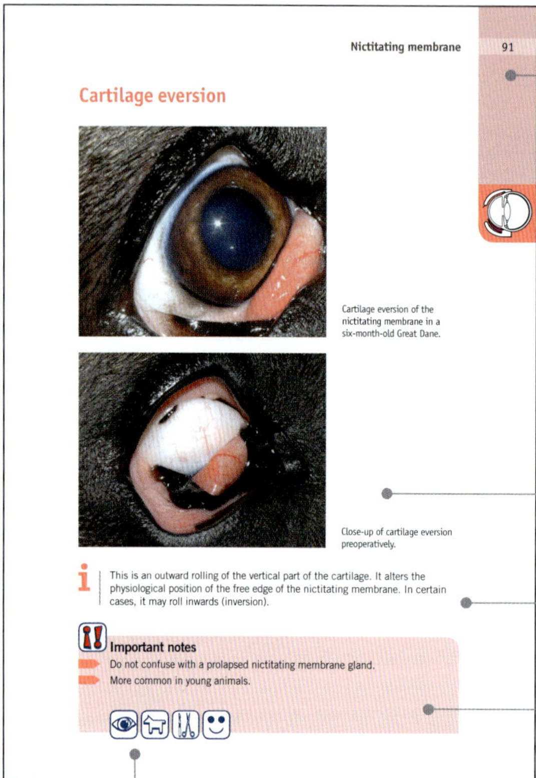

Nictitating membrane 91

Cartilage eversion

Cartilage eversion of the nictitating membrane in a six-month-old Great Dane.

Close-up of cartilage eversion preoperatively.

This is an outward rolling of the vertical part of the cartilage. It alters the physiological position of the free edge of the nictitating membrane. In certain cases, it may roll inwards (inversion).

Important notes

- Do not confuse with a prolapsed nictitating membrane gland.
- More common in young animals.

The coloured band on the right or left upper margin of the page and the small anatomical diagram underneath the band help quickly localise the lesion or the chapter of interest.

Each picture includes the signalment of the patient and the condition presented.

The "Information" section contains definitions and data to help identify each disease entity.

Symbols to help identify the lesion, understand its aetiology, and choose a medical or surgical treatment appear at the bottom of the page. These symbols also clarify whether the condition is an emergency, whether the treatment includes specific indications or contraindications, whether the presentation is acute or chronic, and the prognosis.

The lower part of the page, separated by a coloured box specific to the ocular structure, contains important points to remember in practice: species predispositions, treatments, contraindications, etc.

Key for the *Quick Guidebook to Canine and Feline Ophthalmology*

Anatomical structures

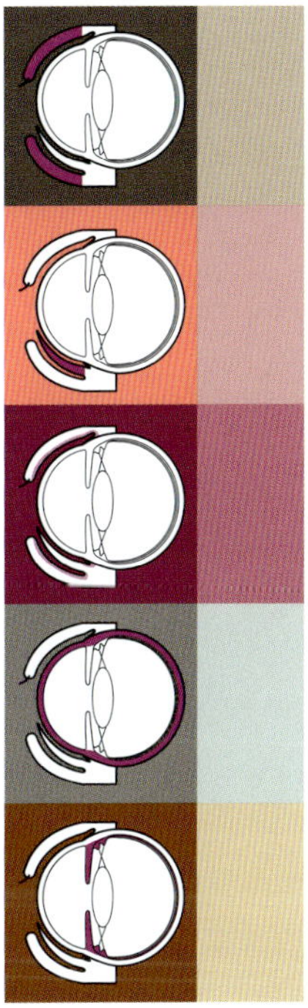

Eyelids

Nictitating membrane

Conjunctiva

Cornea and sclera

Uvea

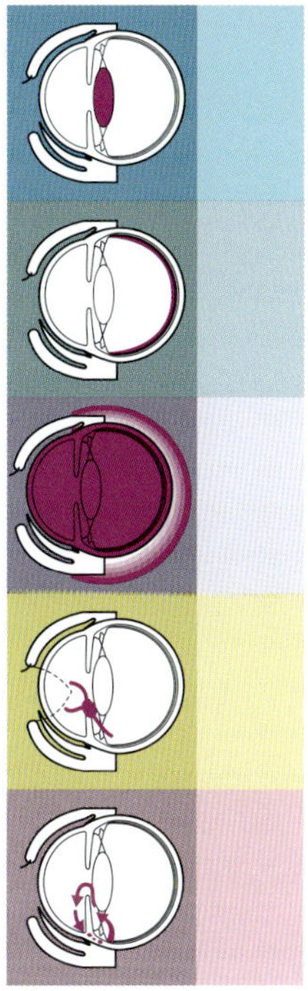

Lens

Ocular fundus

Globe and orbit

Lacrimal apparatus

Glaucoma

Symbols

- Feline patient
- Canine patient
- EMERGENCY
- Canine breed predisposition
- Feline breed predisposition
- Traumatic cause
- Infectious cause
- Immune cause
- Systemic process
- CONTRAINDICATED
- Medical treatment
- Surgical treatment
- Acute presentation
- Chronic process
- IMPORTANT
- Favourable prognosis
- Guarded prognosis
- Poor prognosis

Eye and adnexa

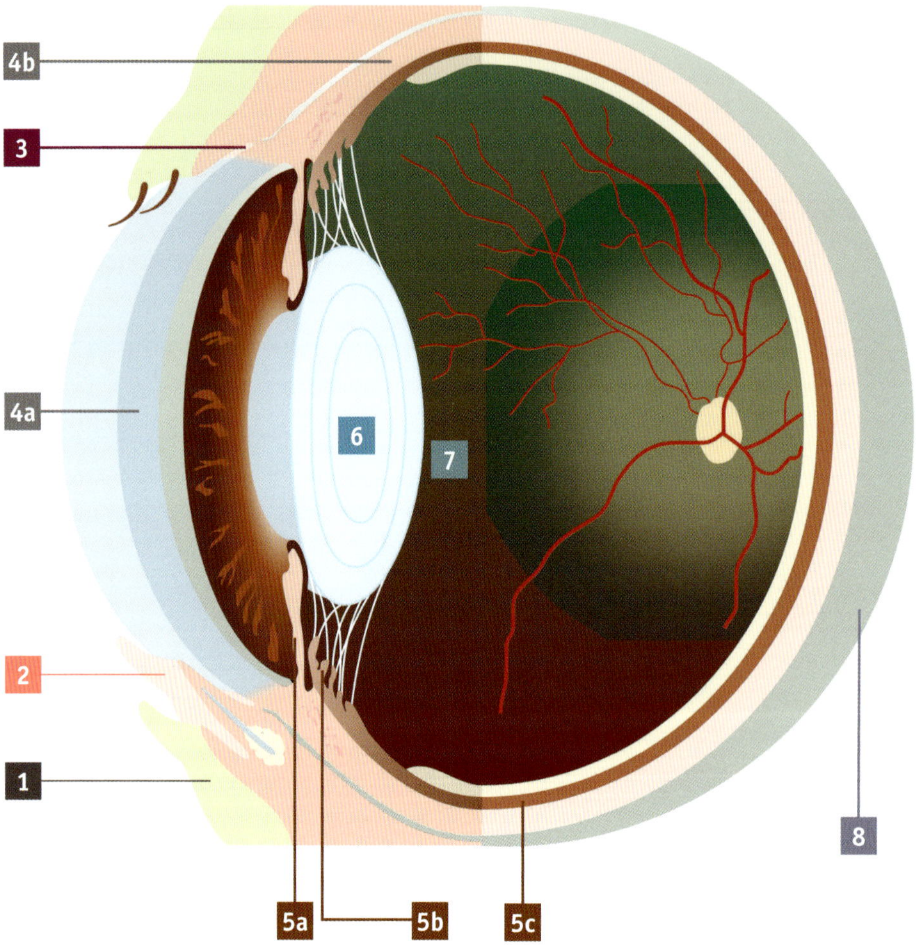

Anatomical structures

1	Eyelids	4b	Sclera	6	Lens
2	Nictitating membrane	5a	Iris	7	Ocular fundus
3	Conjunctiva	5b	Ciliary body	8	Globe and orbit
4a	Cornea	5c	Choroid		

Lacrimal apparatus

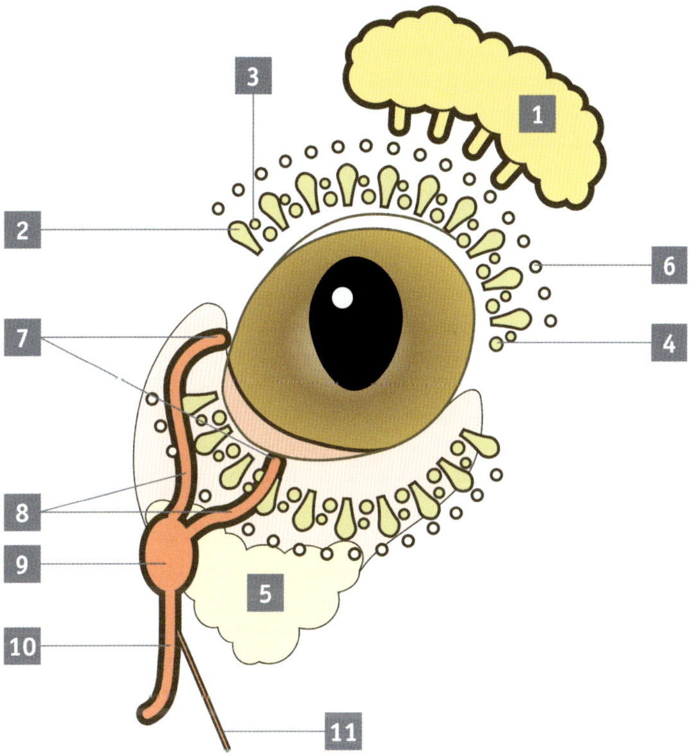

1 Lacrimal gland
2 Meibomian glands (lipid)
3 Glands of Zeis (lipid)
4 Glands of Moll (lipid)
5 Nictitating membrane gland (aqueous)
6 Conjunctival goblet cells (mucinous)
7 Lacrimal puncta
8 Lacrimal canaliculi
9 Lacrimal sac
10 Nasolacrimal duct
11 Accessory duct

Eyelids

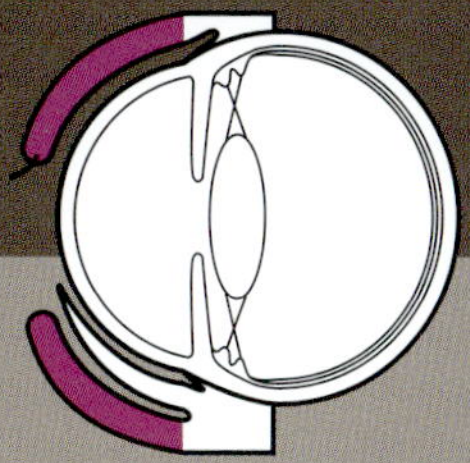

Palpebral agenesis

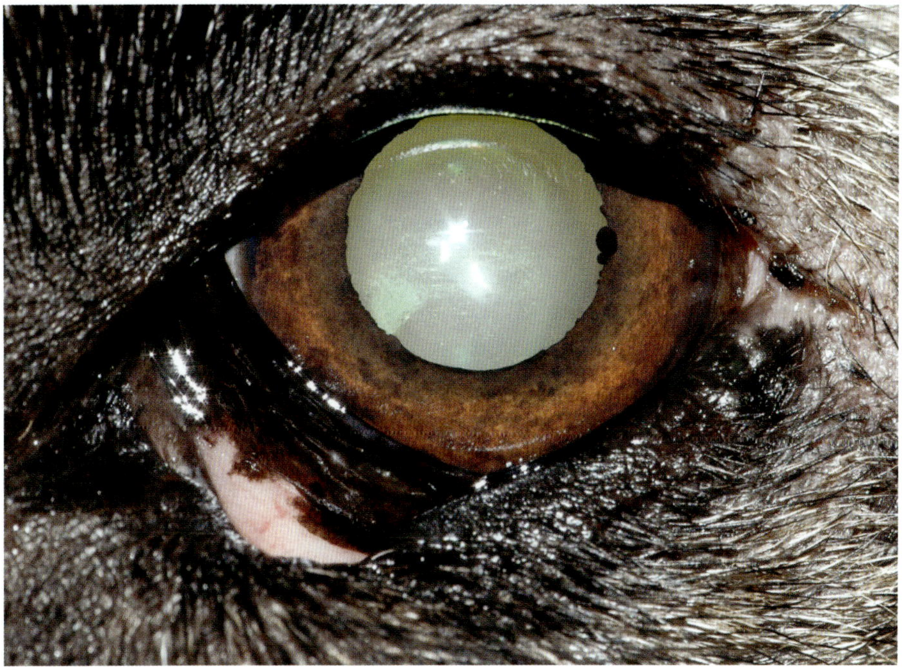

Nine-year-old German Shepherd presenting with a coloboma (partial agenesis) of the lower left eyelid.

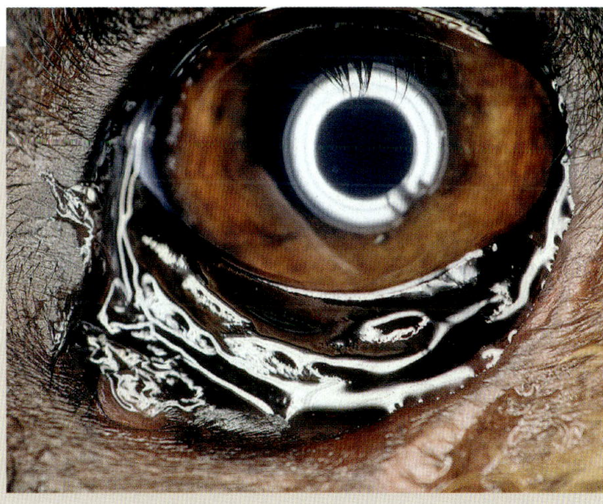

One-year-old German Shepherd with agenesis (complete absence) of the lower left eyelid.

Interesting notes

- Present from birth (congenital).
- In cats it is more common in the temporal area of the upper eyelid.
- Surgical reconstruction requires blepharoplasty.

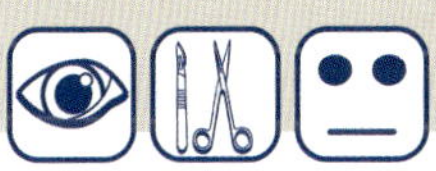

Palpebral dermoid

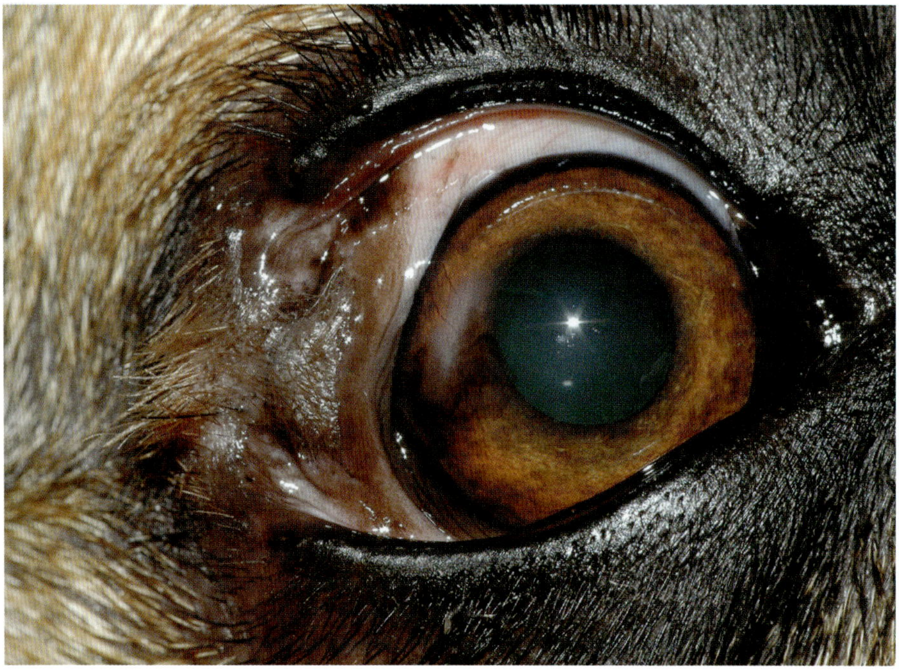

Ten-month-old German Shepherd with a conjunctival-palpebral dermoid. Note also the coloboma on the upper eyelid.

i | These form from ectopic islets of haired skin of embryonic origin. They are also known as choristomas (congenital benign tumours).

Breed predispositions

German Shepherd, Poodle, Saint Bernard, Dalmatian, Dachshund, French Bulldog and Pug.

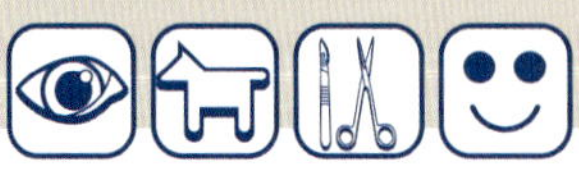

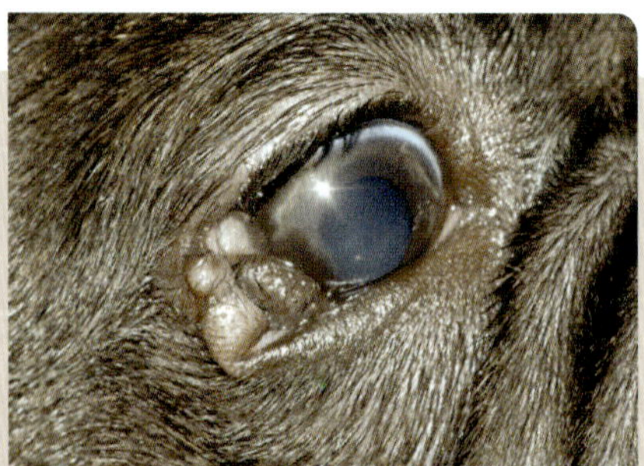

One-month-old Pug with a palpebral dermoid. Pigmentary keratitis can result from the rubbing of the hairs growing from the dermoid.

Palpebral dermoid

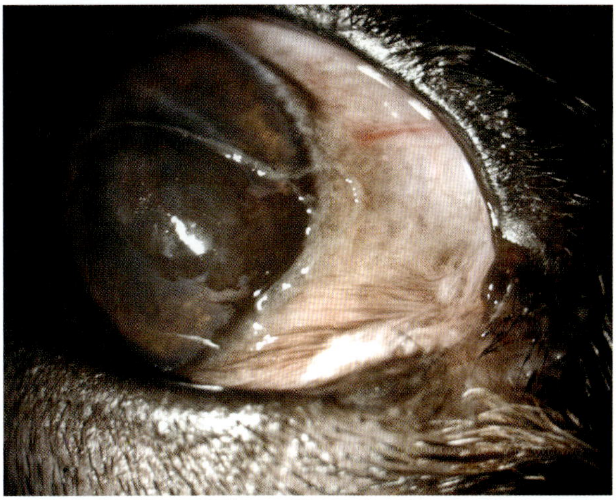

Dermoid on the upper left eyelid of a two-year-old Pug. Note the chronic corneal damage (pigment) caused by the rubbing of the hairs.

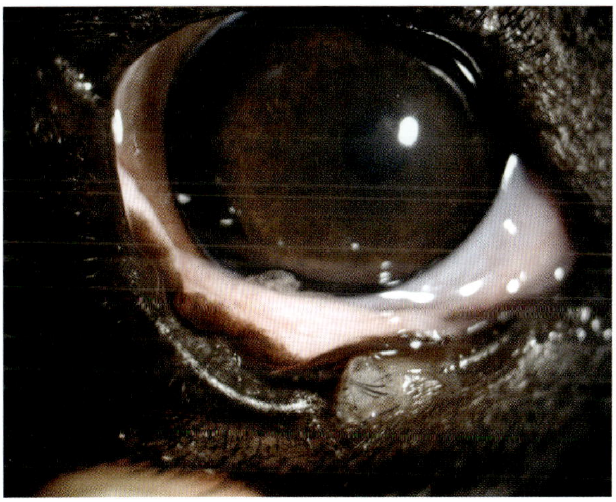

One-year-old French Bulldog with a dermoid on the lower palpebral margin of the right eye.

Important notes

- Congenital disease.
- Unilateral or bilateral presentation and may be associated with a coloboma.
- Surgical treatment: excision and blepharoplasty.

Entropion in a Shar Pei

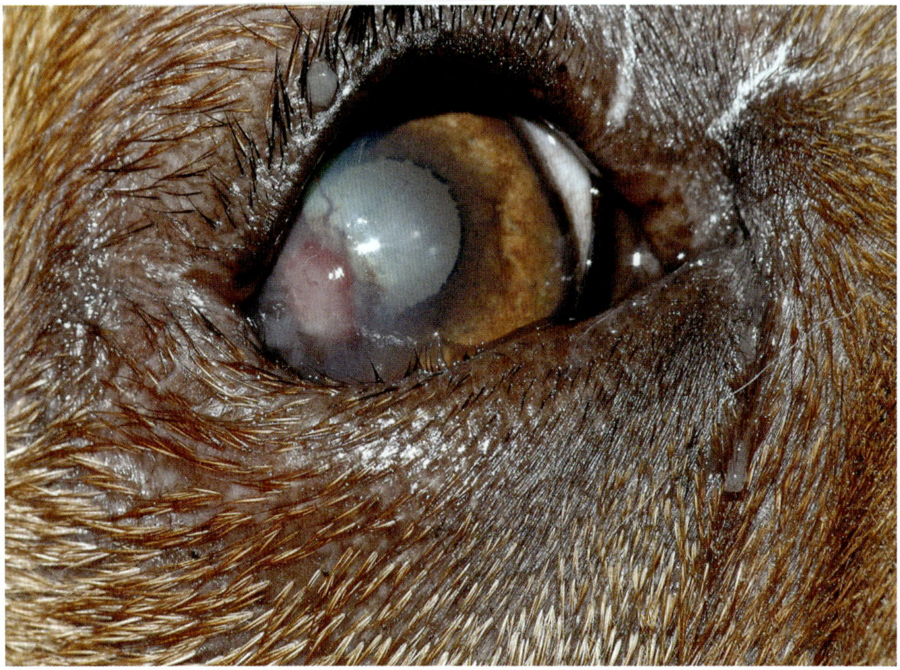

Lateral entropion of the lower eyelid in an 11-month-old Shar Pei. Close-up of the inversion and corneal damage caused by the hairs.

i Inversion of the palpebral margin. It may be unilateral or bilateral and affect any area of the palpebral margin (medial, central and/or temporal).

Clinical signs

- Epiphora (excessive lacrimation).
- Blepharospasm (pronounced blinking caused by ocular irritation).
- Photophobia (ocular disturbance due to bright light).

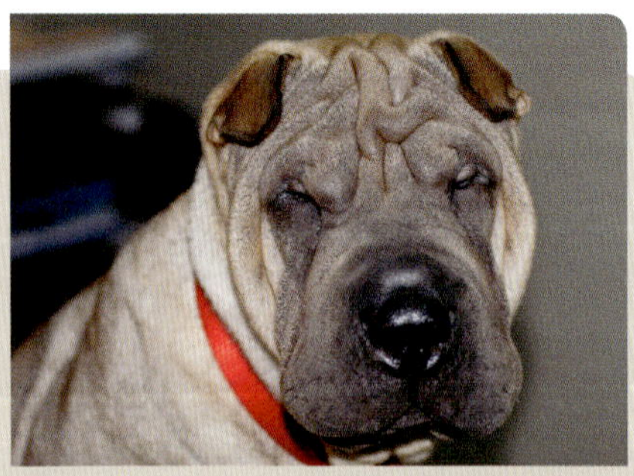

One-year-old Shar Pei with bilateral entropion. Rubbing of the hairs causes blepharospasm and epiphora.

Entropion in a Shar Pei

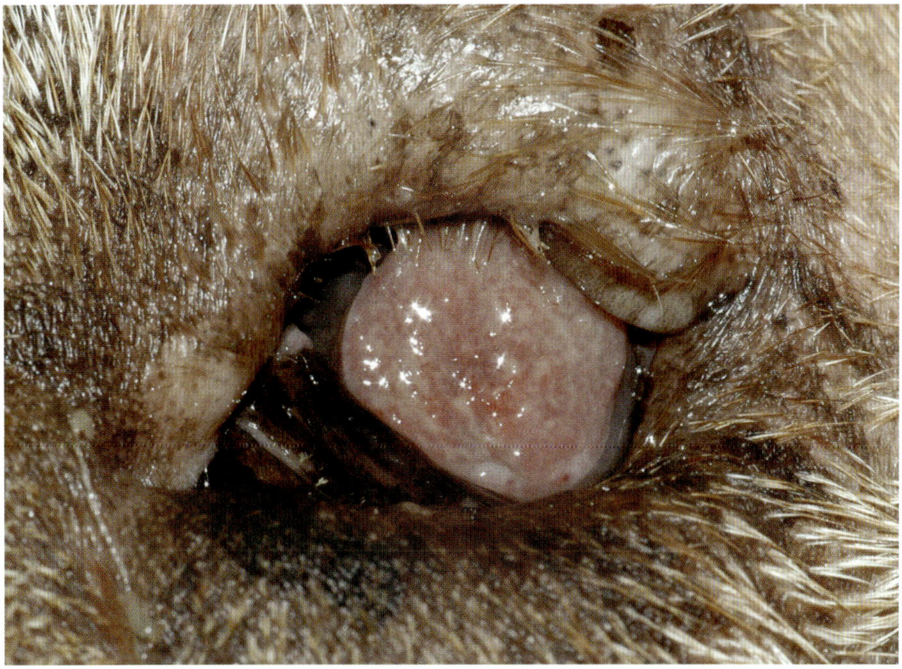

Aspect of the cornea of the patient pictured below as a result of the chronicity of the lesion.

Important notes

- Entropion surgery in an adult Shar Pei should be performed early to avoid spastic entropion and severe corneal damage.
- Cycloplegics (atropine or tropicamide) are used to alleviate blepharospasm.

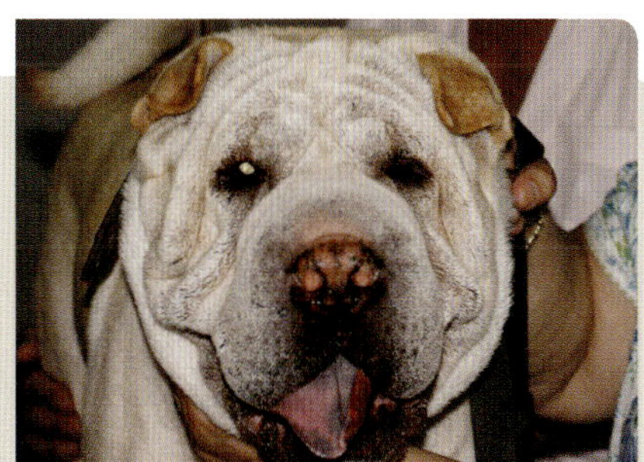

Five-year-old Shar Pei with bilateral entropion that is more severe in the left eye.

Entropion in a Shar Pei

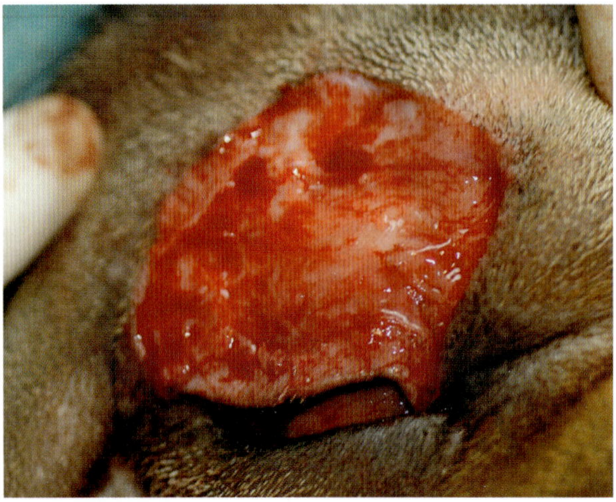

Stades technique for surgical correction of entropion in the Shar Pei.

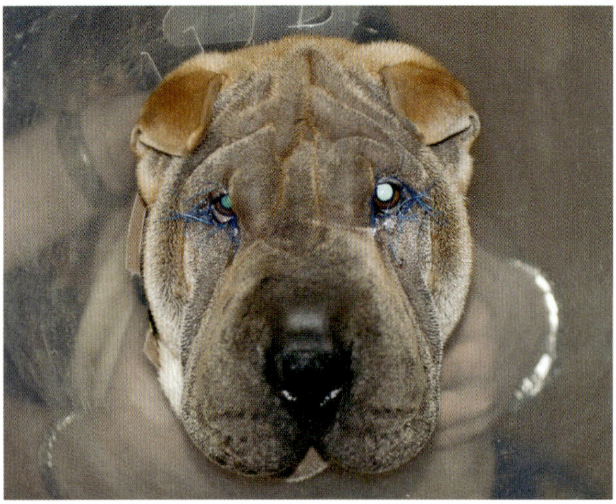

Patient seven days postoperatively.

Surgical technique: Stades technique

- Skin incision in the upper lid shaped like a “clown’s eyebrow”.
- Partial excision of orbicularis oculi muscle fibres from the eyelid.
- Sutures 4 mm from the palpebral margin (long ends).

Entropion in a Shar Pei

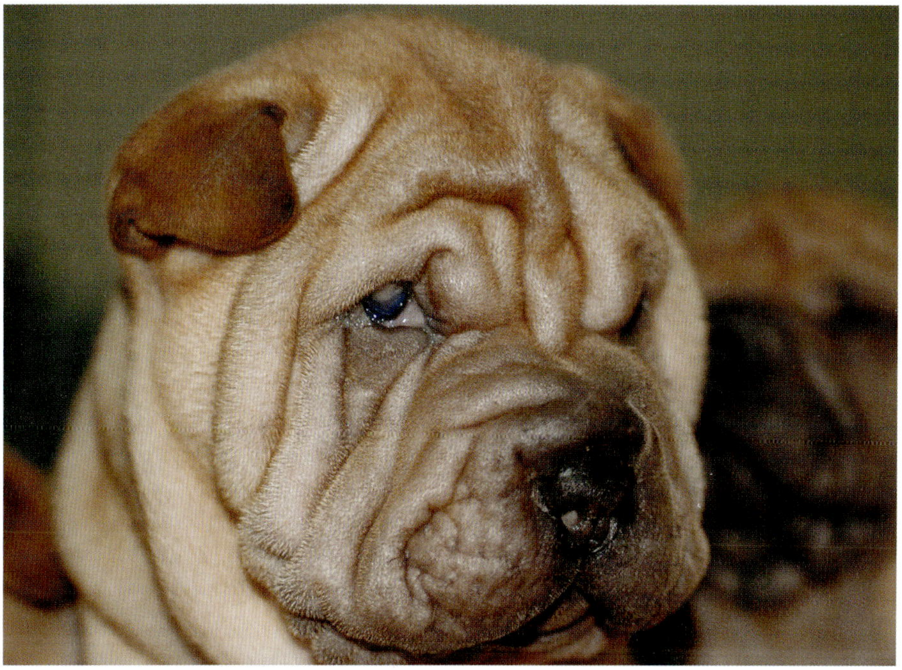

One-month-old Shar Pei puppy. Close-up of entropion and corneal damage.

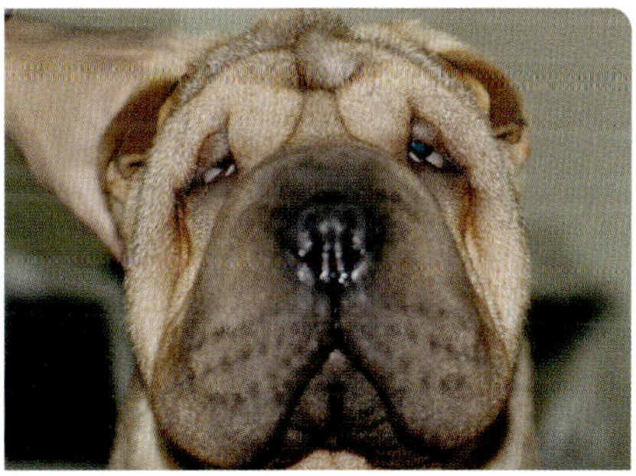

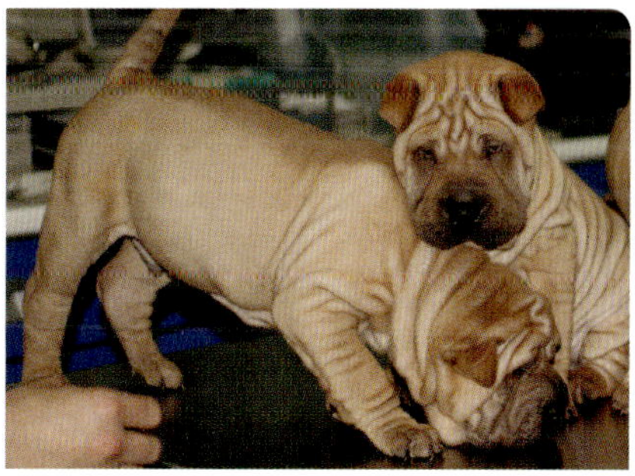

Entropion can also cause visual deficits in these patients.

i Excess skin and numerous skin folds are the main risk factors in the Shar Pei. Consider selective breeding.

Entropion in a Shar Pei

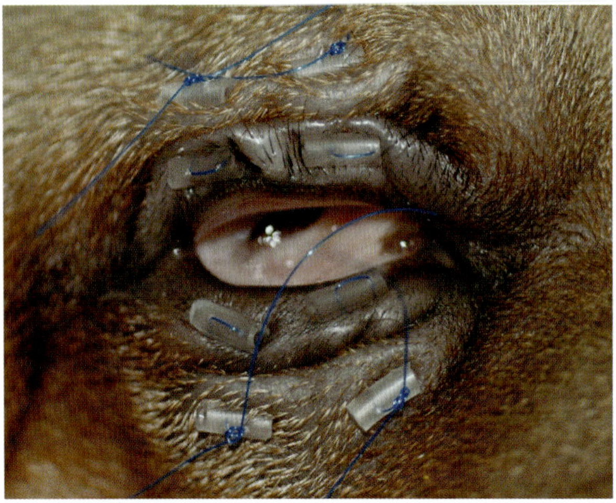

Eversion sutures in the palpebral margin of a three-month-old Shar Pei puppy.

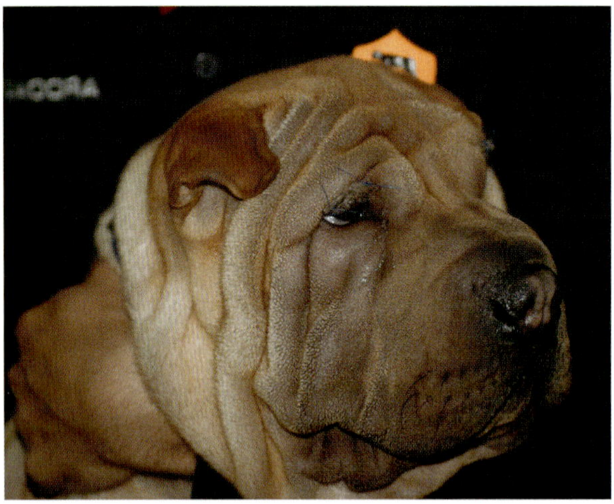

Tacking in a Shar Pei puppy.

Tacking

- This eversion of the palpebral margin is critical to prevent corneal damage in puppies.
- It should remain in place until the patient is 6–8 months old, at which point the aforementioned surgical intervention is performed.

Entropion in a Chow Chow

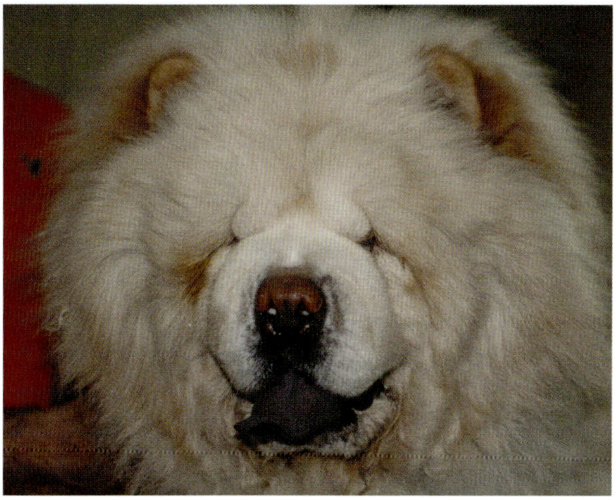

One-year-old Chow Chow with entropion. These patients may lose vision due to the inversion of the palpebral margin and the abundance of skin.

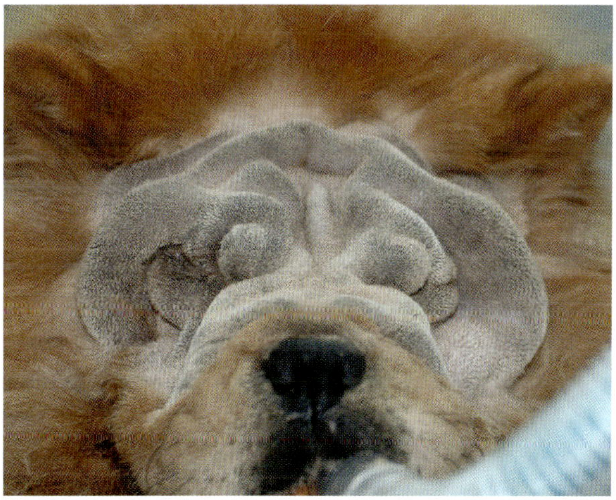

Close-up of the skin folds in an 11-month-old Chow Chow prior to entropion surgery.

Considerations

The skin thickness and lateral facial folds of some individuals of this breed can complicate surgery.

Entropion in a Chow Chow

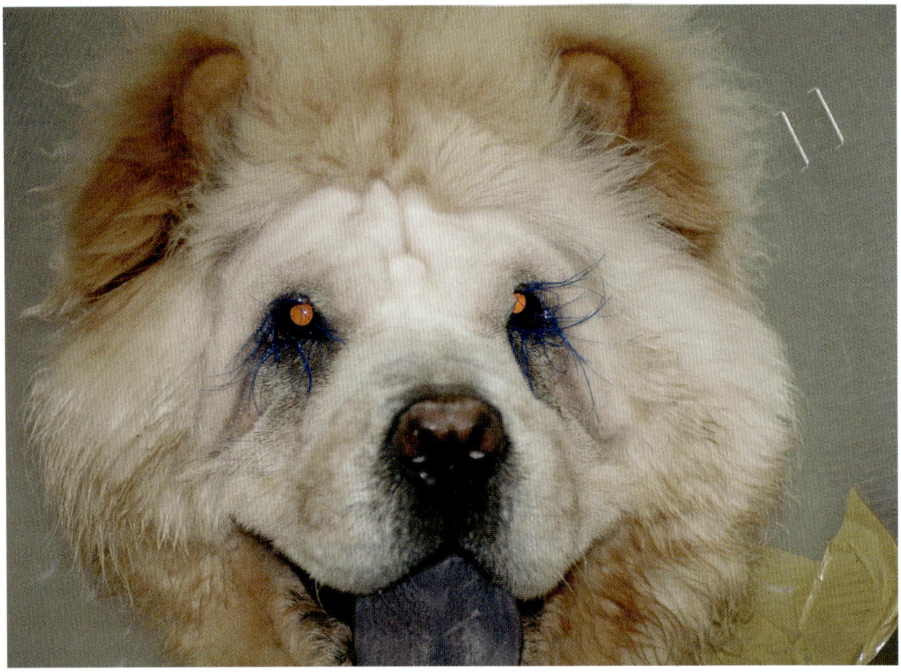

Chow Chow treated for entropion. Ten days postoperatively.

Interesting notes

In this breed, several genes predispose to entropion (polygenic trait), including those that control skull conformation, the amount and weight of skin on the head, and eyelid position.

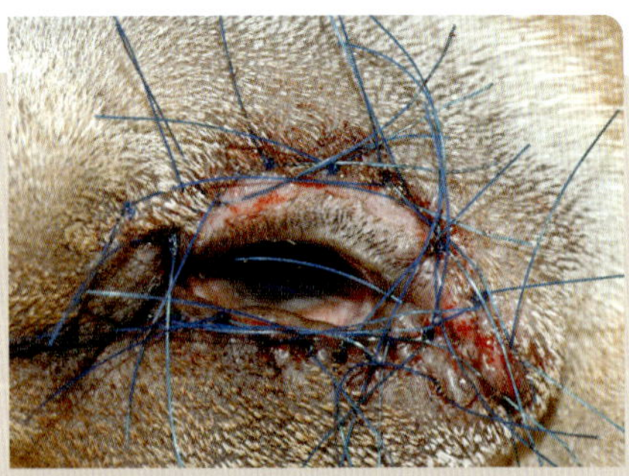

Stades technique on the upper eyelid and Hotz–Celsus technique on the lower eyelid in entropion surgery.

Entropion

Surgical techniques

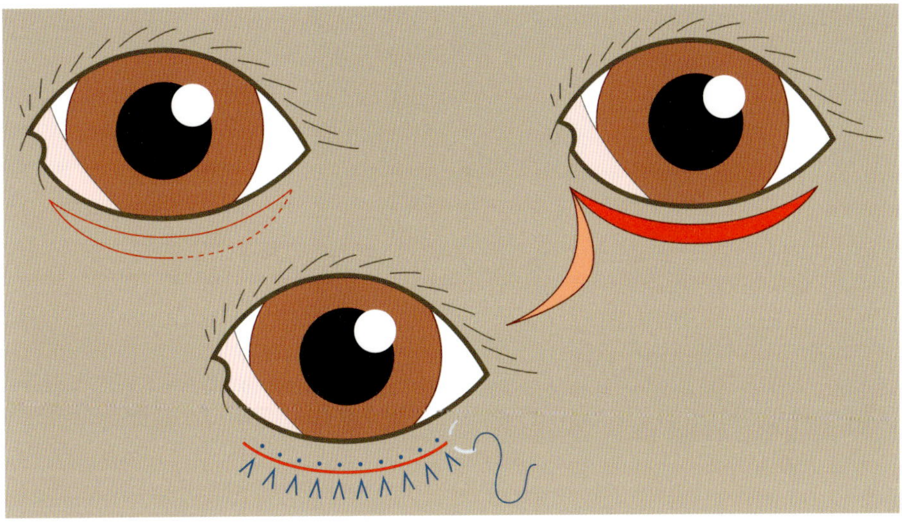

Hotz–Celsus technique.

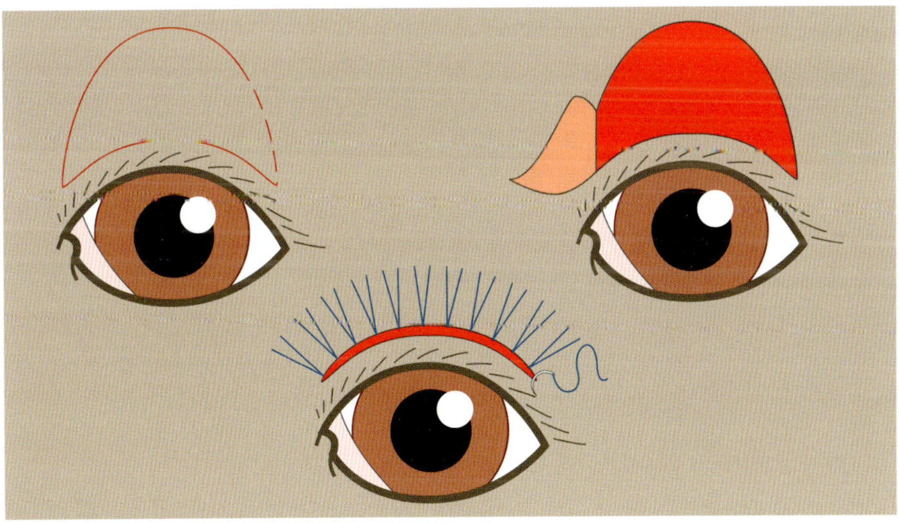

Stades technique.

The Stades technique, originally described for correcting upper eyelid entropion in the Shar Pei, is also quite useful in the Chow Chow.

The Hotz–Celsus technique is the most common technique used in entropion surgery and can generally be applied to both the upper and lower eyelids.

Medial entropion

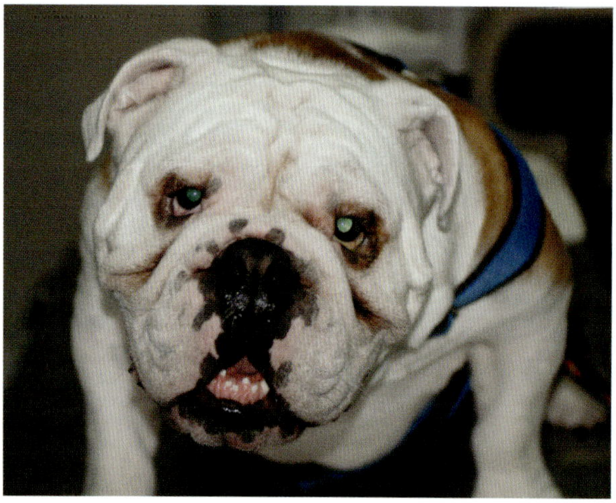

English Bulldog with epiphora secondary to medial entropion of the lower eyelids.

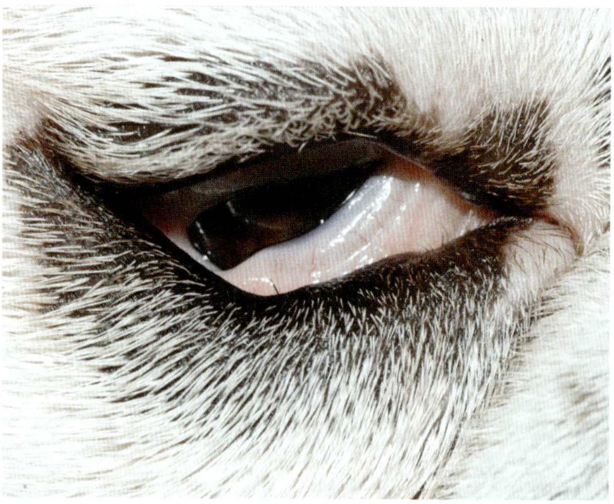

Close-up of the medial entropion in the patient pictured above.

Breed predisposition

The breeds most predisposed to medial entropion are the English Bulldog, Pug, Poodle, Shih-Tzu and Pekingese.

Medial entropion

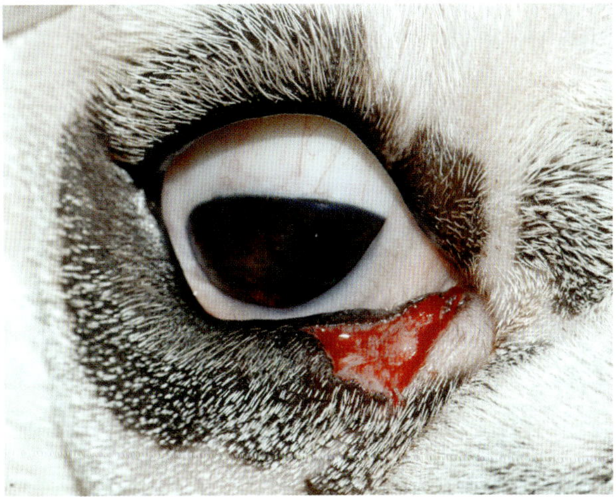

Hotz–Celsus technique for medial entropion. Close-up of the skin incision.

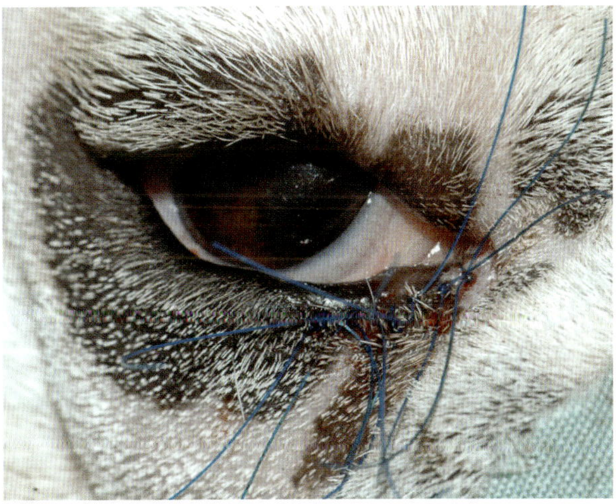

Closure of the surgical defect with 4-0 nylon. Note the normal position of the palpebral margin.

Important notes

- During surgery, do not damage the nearby lower lacrimal canaliculus.
- This surgery often alleviates nasal fold dermatitis by decreasing moisture in the skin folds.

Medial entropion

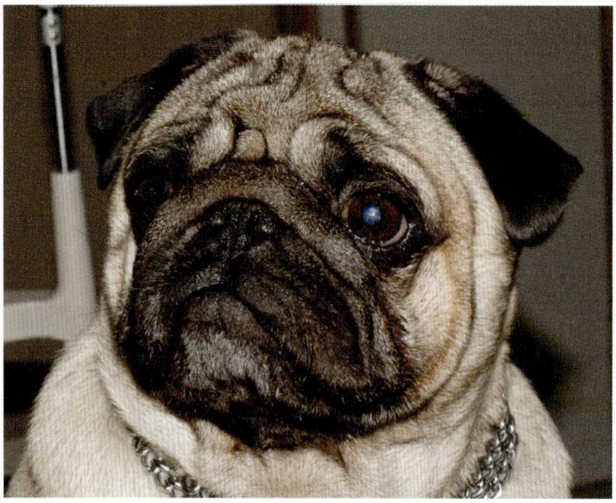

Pug with bilateral lower medial entropion.

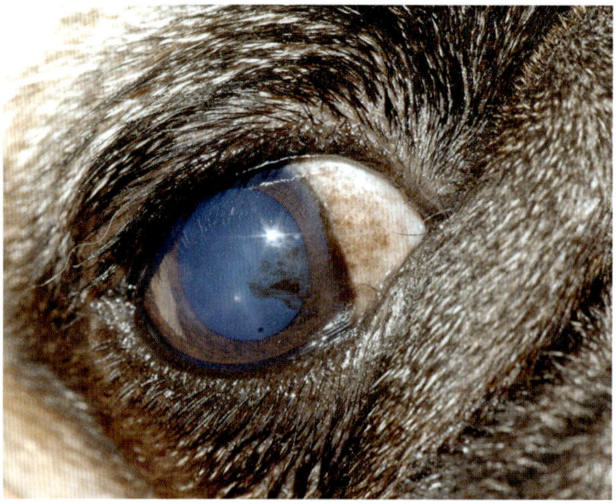

Note the inversion of the lower palpebral margin and the way the facial hairs rub on the cornea in the nasal region.

Important notes

In these patients, pigmentary keratitis may be exacerbated by medial entropion.

Medial entropion

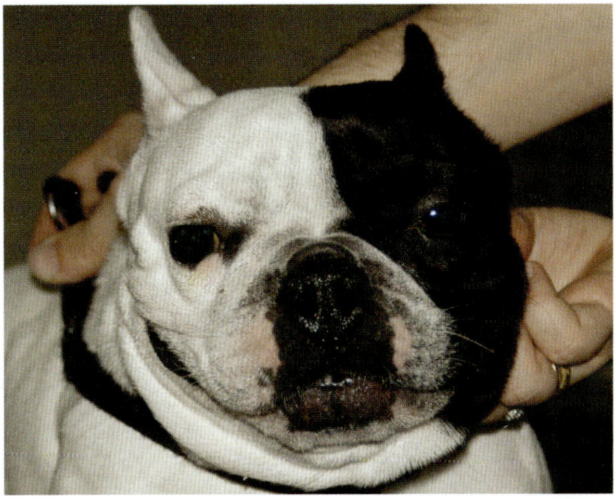

Medial canthoplasty in a French Bulldog to correct medial entropion and euryblepharon (Roberts-Jensen technique, see page 191).

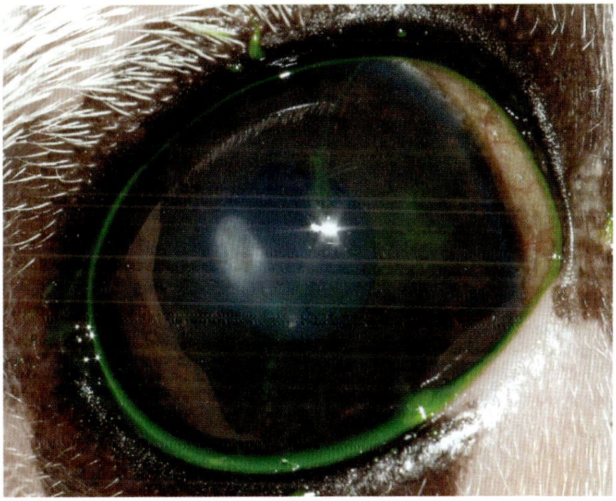

French Bulldog treated for medial entropion. Note the correct position of the palpebral fissure.

Important notes

In a medial canthoplasty using the Roberts-Jensen technique, the upper lacrimal punctum is sacrificed, but carefully avoid damaging the lower lacrimal punctum and canaliculus.

Lateral entropion

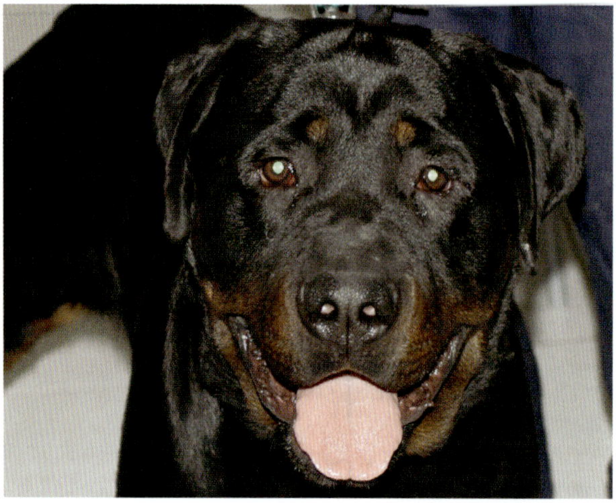

Eleven-month-old Rottweiler with bilateral lateral entropion of the lower eyelids.

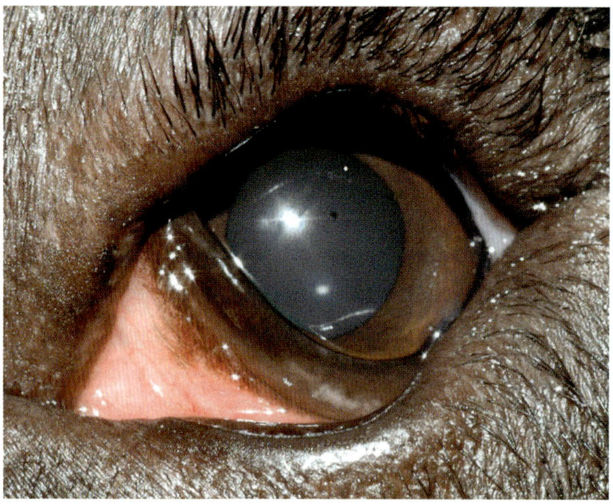

Close-up of the inversion of the palpebral margin of the left eye in the patient shown above.

Breed predisposition

Primary lateral entropion, resulting from a tension disparity between the orbicularis oculi muscle and the lateral canthal ligament, has been described in Rottweilers, Retrievers (Golden and Labrador), Pointers, Dalmatians, and Weimaraners.

Lateral entropion

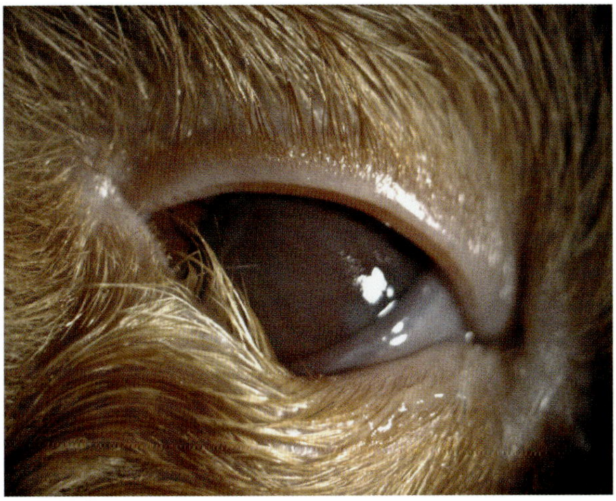

Close-up of the severe inversion of the palpebral margin of the cat pictured below.
Note the amount of hair directed towards the cornea.

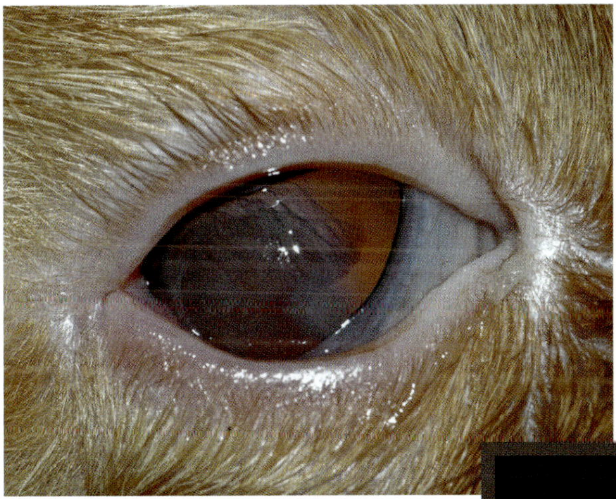

Severe ulcerative keratitis secondary to entropion.

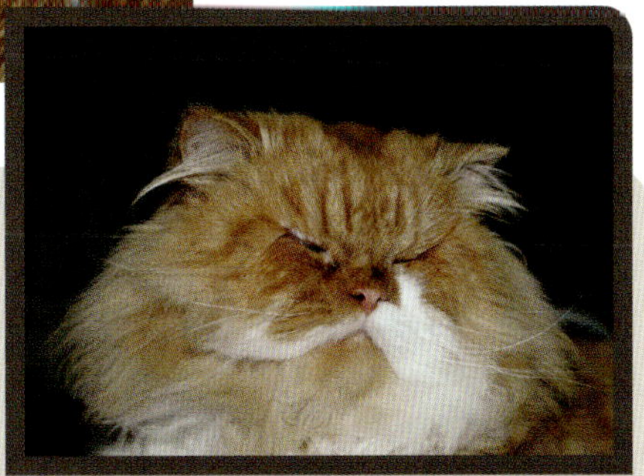

Ten-month-old Persian cat with blepharospasm secondary to lateral entropion.

Important notes

- Entropion is less common in cats than in dogs, but it may cause severe corneal damage in cats.
- Young Persian cats are at the greatest risk, and the lower lid is most commonly affected.

Lateral entropion

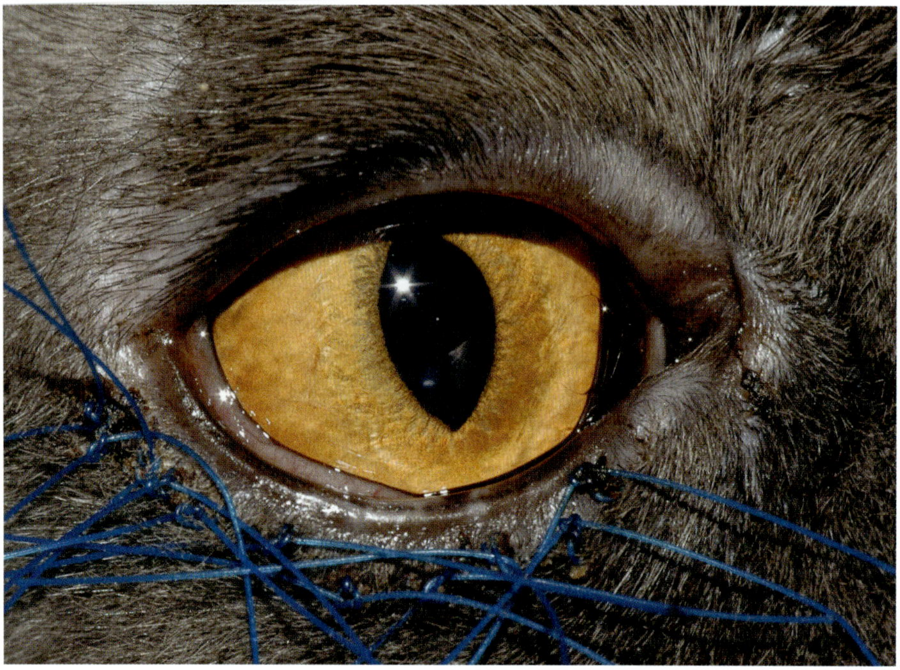

Correction of entropion in the patient pictured below. Ten days postoperatively. Note the correct position of the palpebral margin.

Surgical technique

- The Hotz-Celsus technique is most appropriate for correcting lateral entropion in Persian cats, but recurrence is common.
- The ideal skin suture calibre for cats is 6-0. Nylon or Monosyn (for aggressive patients) can be used.

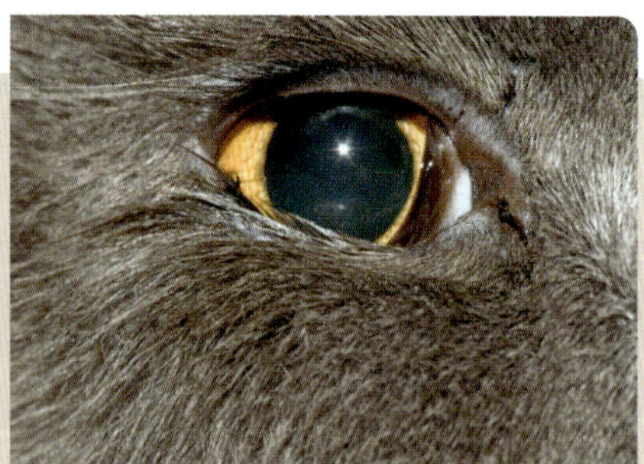

Lateral entropion in an 11-month-old Persian cat.

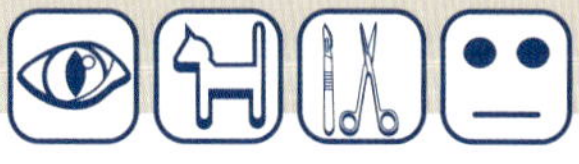

Cicatricial entropion

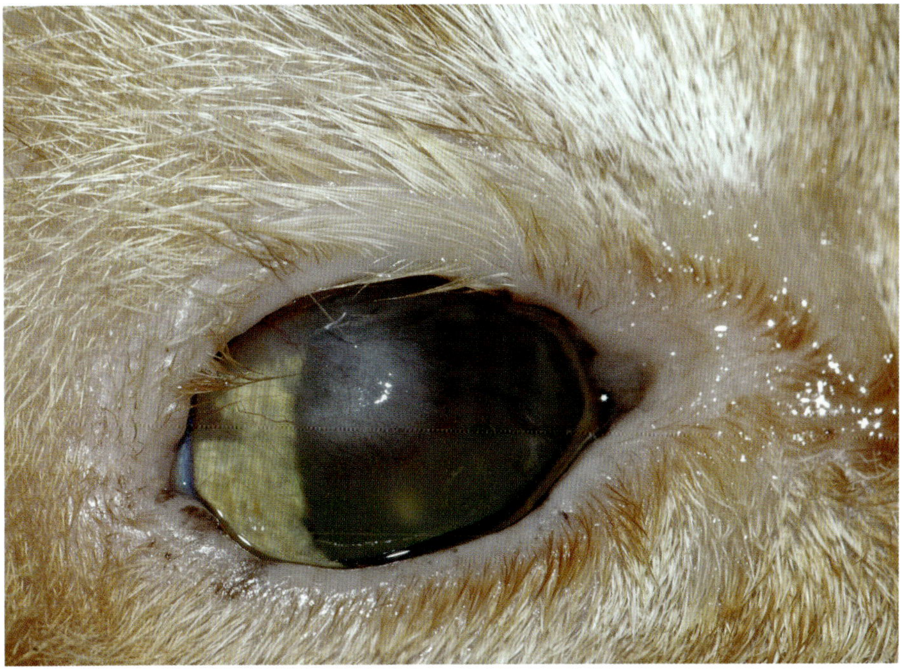

Close-up of the corneal damage from the rubbing of the hairs. Trichiasis of the eyelashes is secondary to cicatricial entropion.

Important notes

- Post-traumatic fibrosis can complicate palpebral surgery in these cases.
- Monitor the direction of hair growth in the palpebral region to ensure hair does not rub against the cornea.

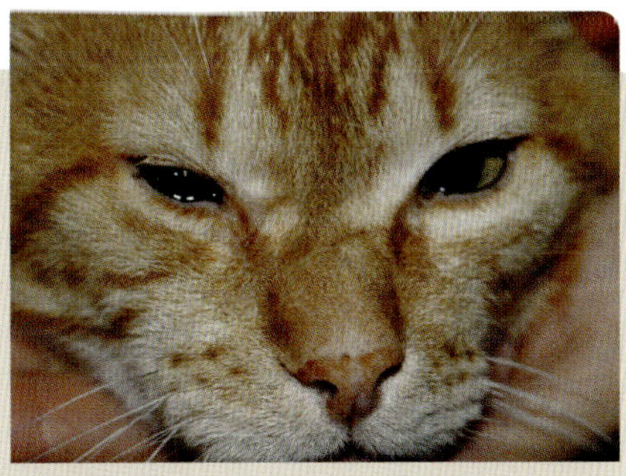

Cicatricial entropion in a four-year-old domestic shorthair cat who was hit by a vehicle.

Cicatricial entropion

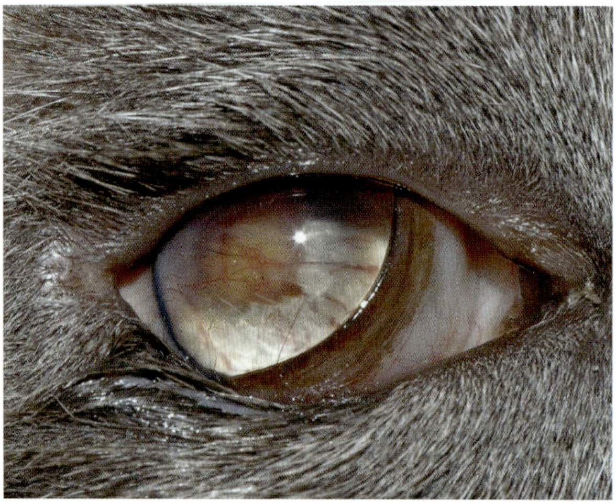

Cicatricial entropion of the central lower eyelid due to a pellet wound in a cat. Note the corneal damage induced by the gunshot.

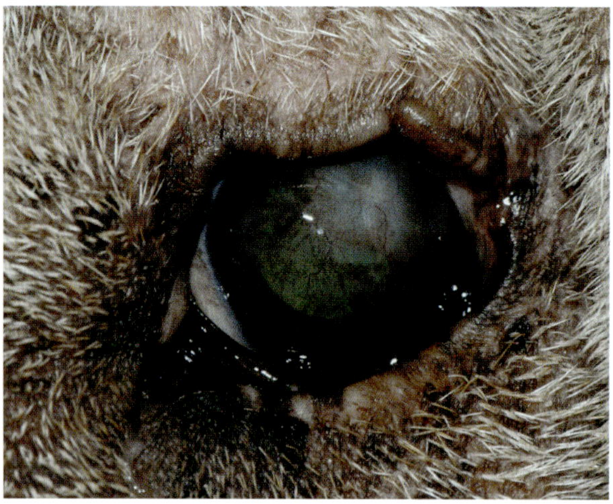

Cicatricial entropion of the upper eyelid of a mixed-breed dog who was hit by a car. Chronic rubbing of the lashes against the cornea caused severe keratitis. Close-up of the corneal opacity (pigment).

i | Skin burns from shotgun pellets can lead to entropion secondary to cicatricial retraction of the palpebral margin.

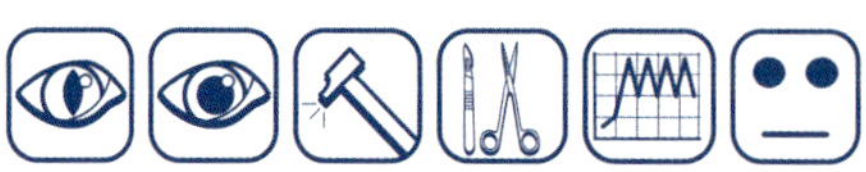

Entropion due to lack of support

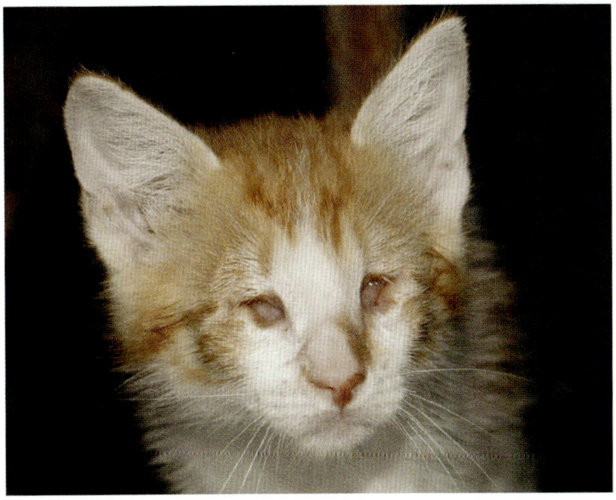

Domestic shorthair cat with bilateral entropion due to lack of support of the palpebral margin.

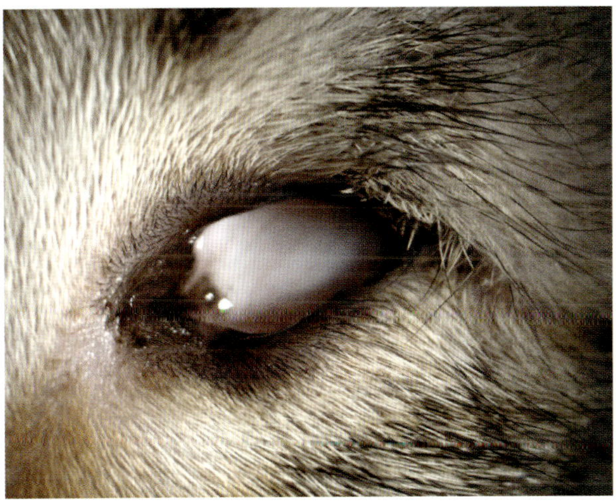

Close-up of the lower lateral entropion due to lack of tension in a two-month-old kitten.

i

Atrophy of the globe (**phthisis bulbi**) favours protrusion of the nictitating membrane and inversion of the palpebral margin.

Most cases in kittens result from viral infection.

Ectropion

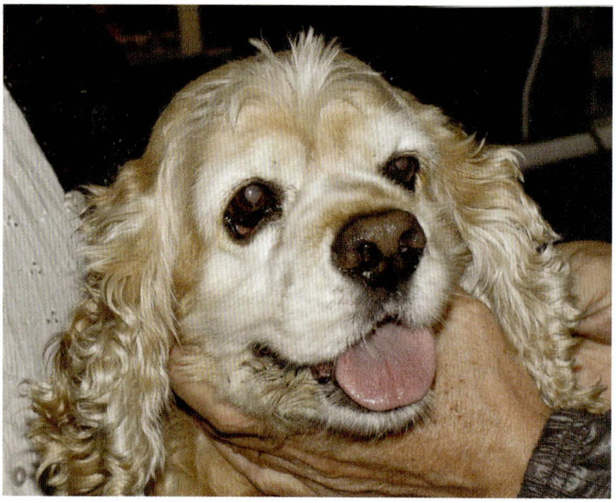

American Cocker Spaniel with bilateral ectropion of the lower eyelids.

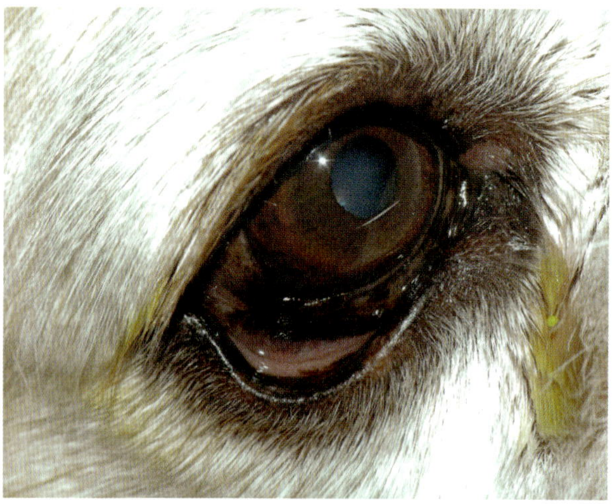

Eversion of the palpebral margin, leaving the conjunctiva exposed. Close-up of the right eye of the patient pictured above.

i | Eversion of the free eyelid margin, leaving the conjunctiva exposed and the cornea unprotected. Generally, it is bilateral and affects the lower eyelid.

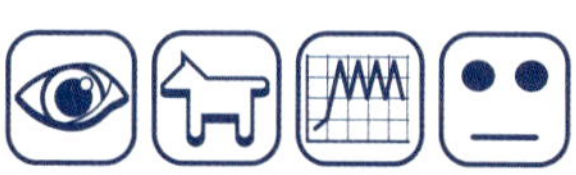

Ectropion

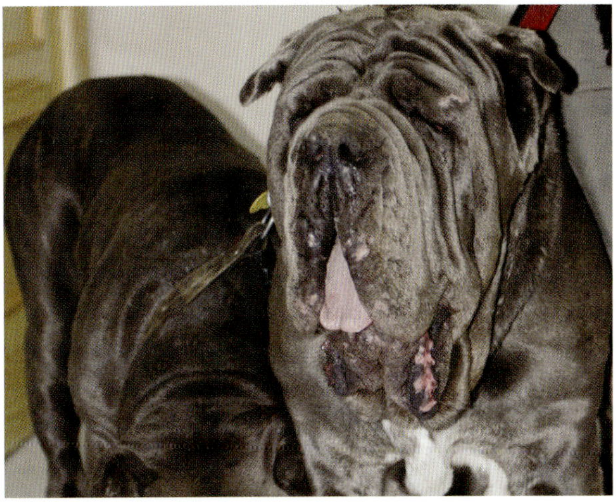

Neapolitan Mastiffs are particularly predisposed to lower lid ectropion.

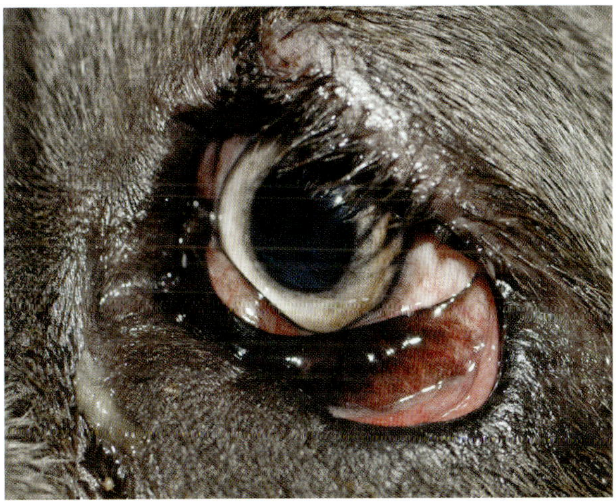

Conjunctival exposure in giant breeds with ectropion is quite significant. Picture of one of the Neapolitan Mastiffs pictured above.

Breed predisposition

Ectropion most commonly affects the Saint Bernard, Neapolitan Mastiff, Boxer, Basset Hound and Cocker Spaniel.

Ectropion

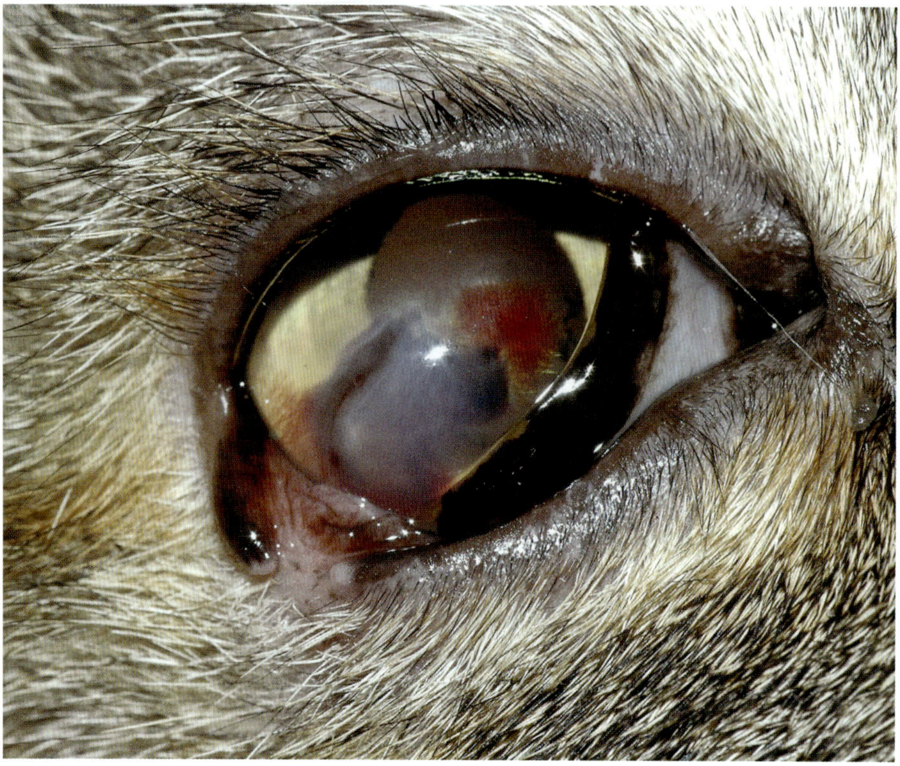

Cicatricial ectropion in a domestic shorthair cat due to palpebral damage caused by a shotgun pellet. The pellet tore through and burned the palpebral margin and then entered the globe, causing severe injury.

Interesting notes

The principal clinical signs of ectropion are conjunctival exposure and epiphora. Chronic exposure keratitis is the major complication of chronic eversion of the palpebral margin.

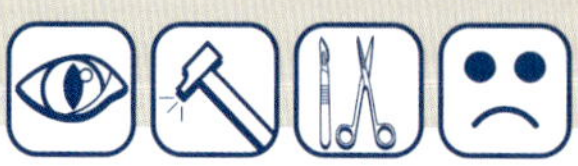

Ectropion

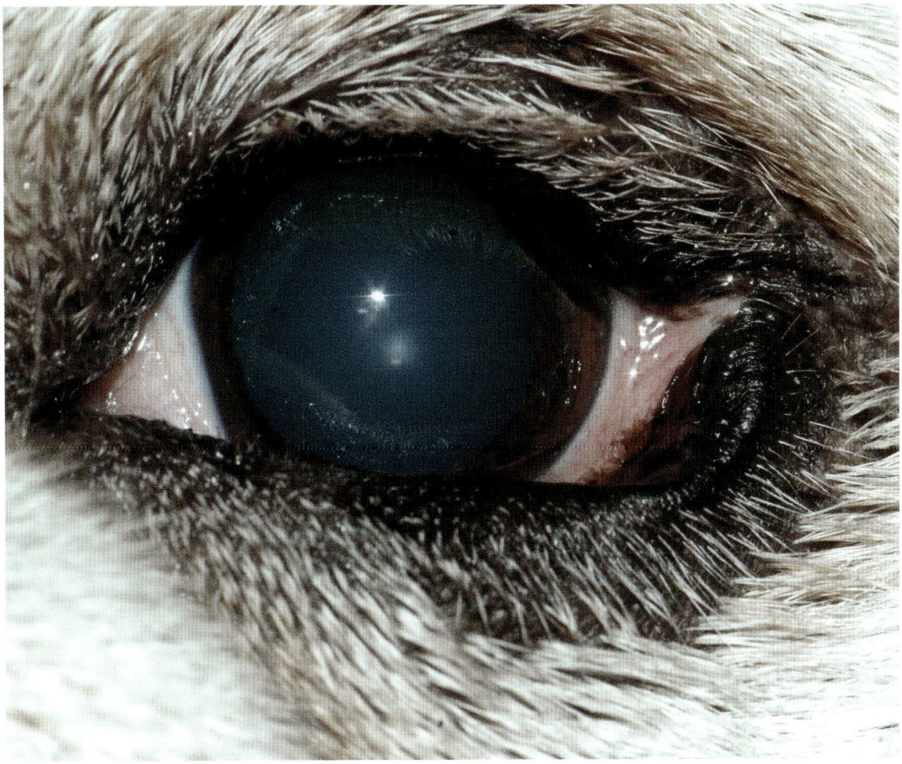

Iatrogenic ectropion in an English Bulldog following surgery for lower lid entropion. Eversion of the palpebral margin in the temporal area reveals the conjunctiva. This abnormal palpebral conformation prevents full coverage of the cornea during blinking.

Important notes

In surgical correction of entropion, it is preferable to remove too little tissue and revise later if needed than to induce iatrogenic ectropion by removing too much.

Ectropion

Surgical techniques

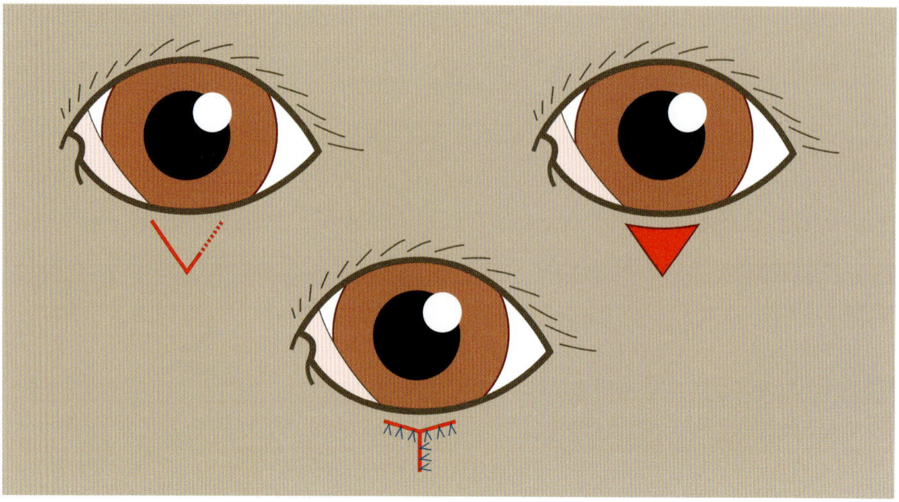

Wharton-Jones technique.

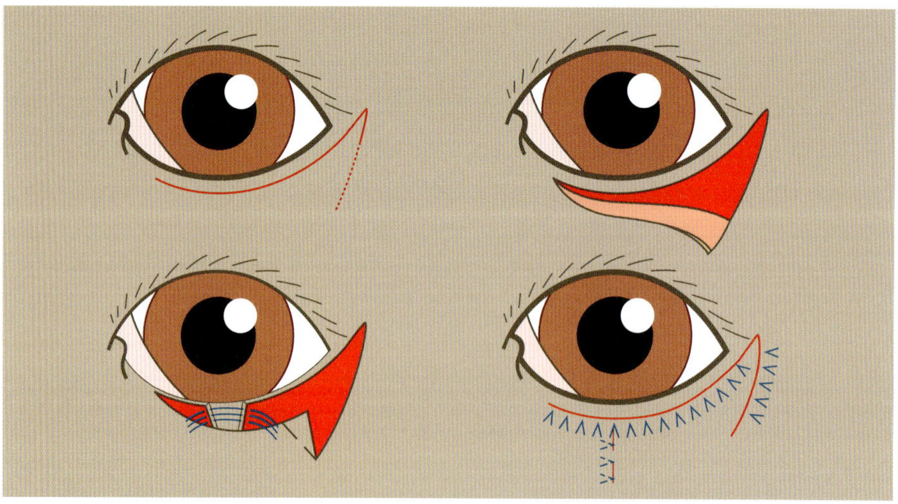

Kuhnt–Szymanowski technique.

- The Wharton-Jones technique is used for cicatricial ectropion and in mild cases.
- The Kuhnt–Szymanowski technique is used in more severe cases or in patients who require shortening of the lower lid.

Entropion/ectropion

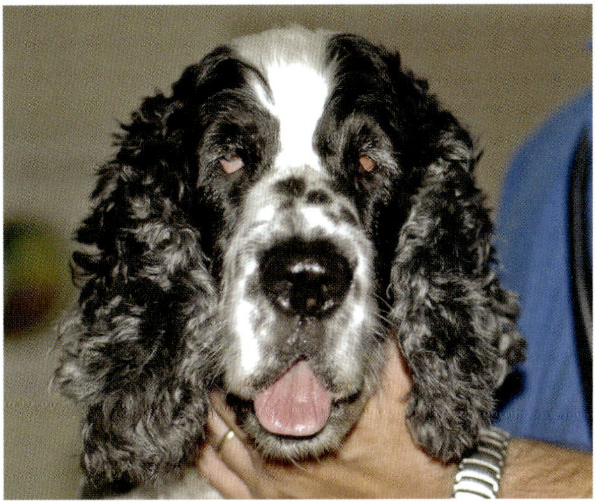

Twelve-year-old English Cocker Spaniel with ectropion of the lower eyelid and entropion of the upper eyelid.
The patient has vision loss due to the abnormal upper eyelid position.

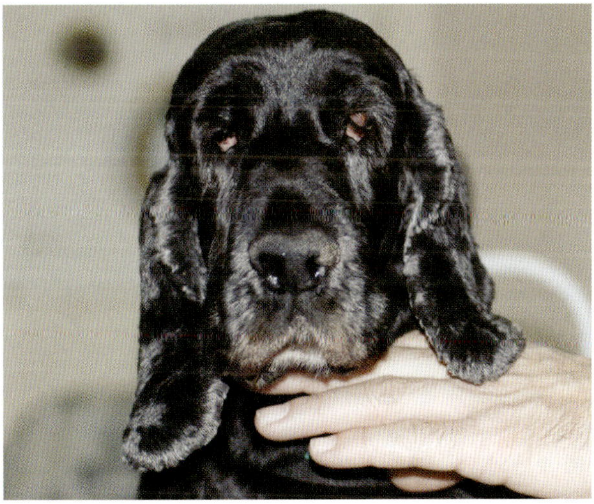

Facial skin laxity and the weight of the ears and lips contribute to entropion/ectropion.

Interesting notes

In older Cocker Spaniels and Basset Hounds, the entropion/ectropion combination often occurs with palpebral ptosis and trichiasis.

Entropion/ectropion

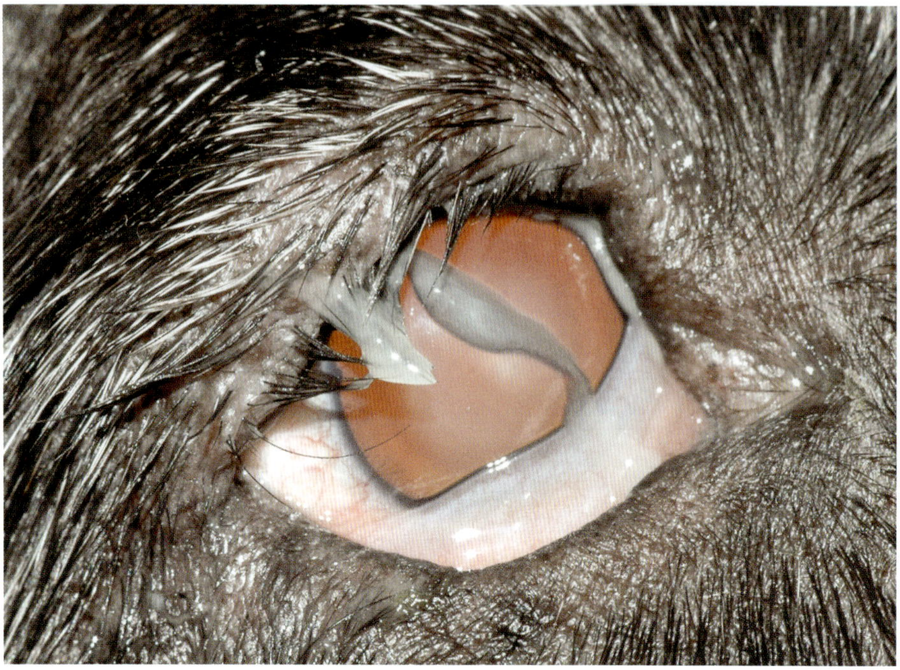

In patients with associated keratoconjunctivitis sicca, corneal and conjunctival damage secondary to entropion/ectropion is much more severe.

Contraindicated

NEVER TRIM THE EYELASHES! The sharp tip of a cut hair can cause even greater corneal damage.

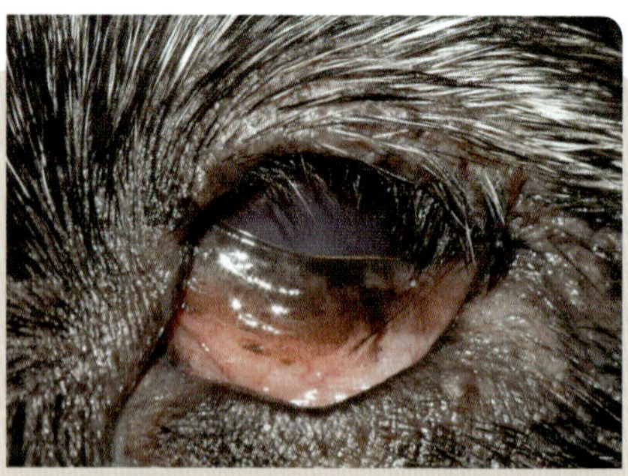

Close-up of upper lid entropion/trichiasis and lower lid ectropion in a nine-year-old English Cocker Spaniel (patient from the previous page). Note the corneal damage from the rubbing of the eyelashes.

Entropion/ectropion

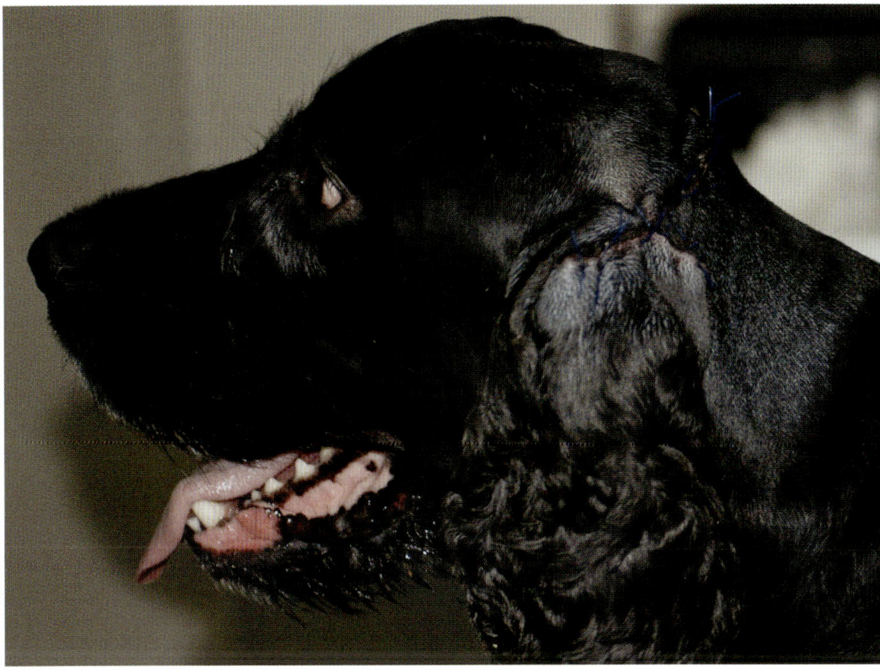

Correction of entropion/ectropion using rhytidectomy. Skin closure with 4-0 nylon. Lateral view.

Surgical technique

- Both problems (entropion and ectropion) can be solved with a single technique: rhytidectomy.
- DO NOT PLACE SKIN SUTURES UNDER TENSION due to the risk of dehiscence.

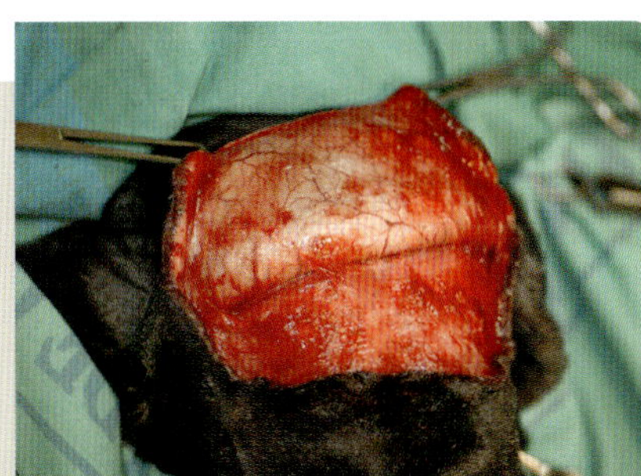

Intraoperative picture of a rhytidectomy in a nine-year-old English Cocker Spaniel (same patient as in the previous pictures). Skin dissection.

Entropion/ectropion

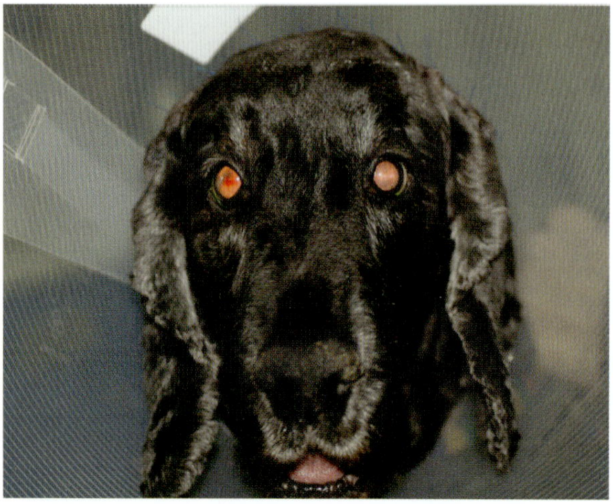

The preceding case four days postoperatively. The corneal damage is still appreciable.

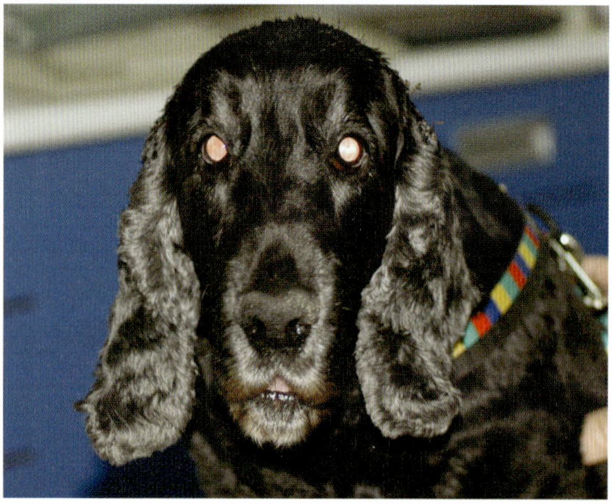

Patient 15 days postoperatively. Note the correct position of the eyelids.

i | After rhytidectomy, owners often comment on the obvious improvement in their pet's vision compared to before surgery.

Entropion/ectropion. Diamond eye

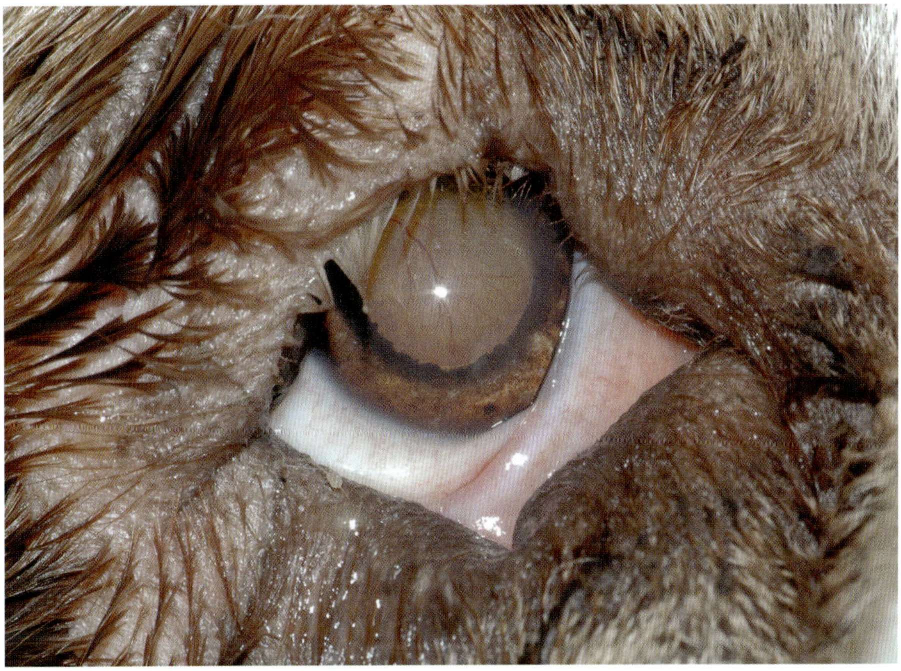

One-year-old Saint Bernard with lateral entropion and central ectropion.
Close-up of the corneal damage caused by the rubbing of the eyelashes against the cornea.
Corneal oedema and neovascularisation (keratitis) are present.

Breed predisposition

In giant breeds like Saint Bernards, Great Danes, and Neapolitan Mastiffs, the upper and lower lids may form a triangle that creates an abnormal palpebral fissure known as "diamond eye".

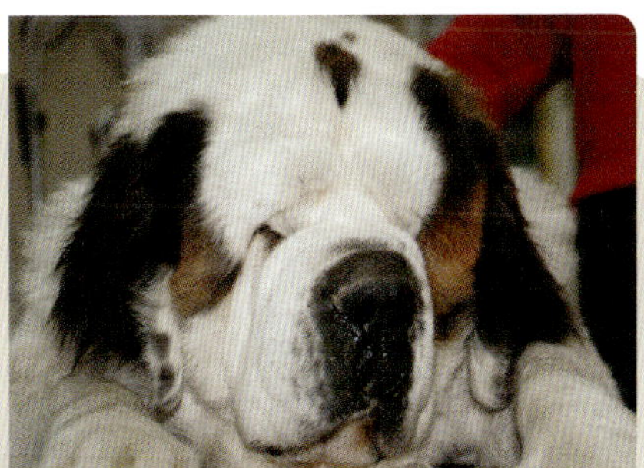

Saint Bernards are one of the breeds most highly predisposed to diamond eye.

Entropion/ectropion. Diamond eye

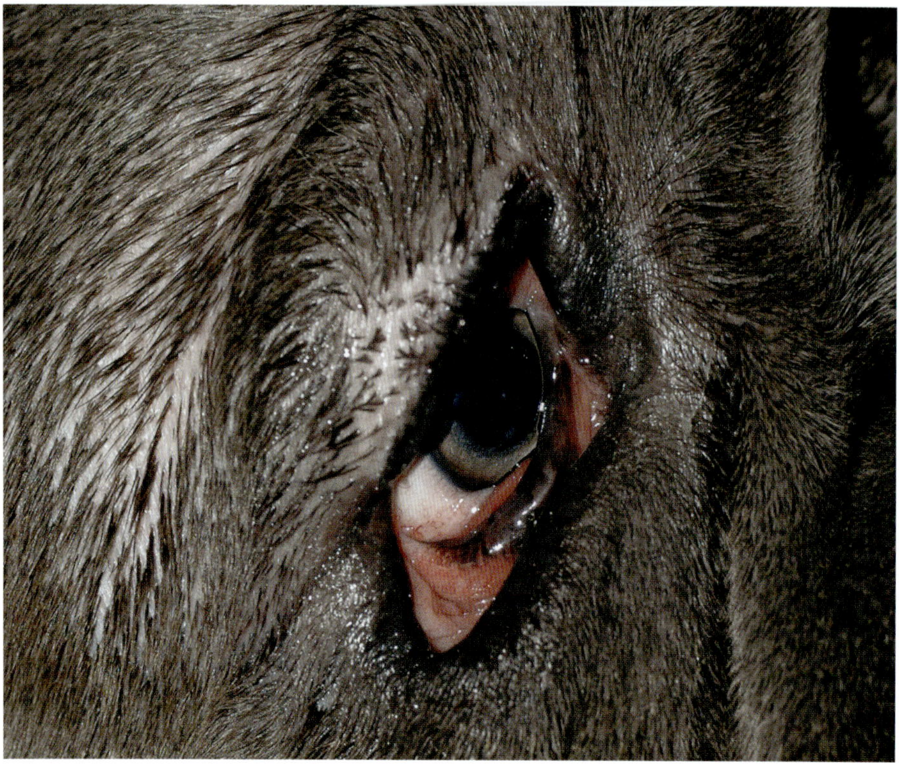

Diamond eye in a 13-month-old Neapolitan Mastiff. Note the triangular eyelid conformation and abnormal corneal and conjunctival exposure.

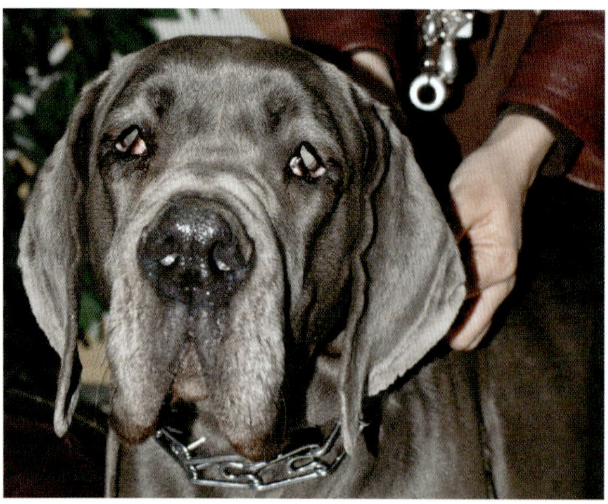

One-year-old Great Dane with bilateral entropion/ectropion. Abnormal eyelid conformation, protrusion of the nictitating membrane, and enophthalmos (secondary to ocular irritation) cause vision loss in these patients.

Entropion/ectropion. Diamond eye

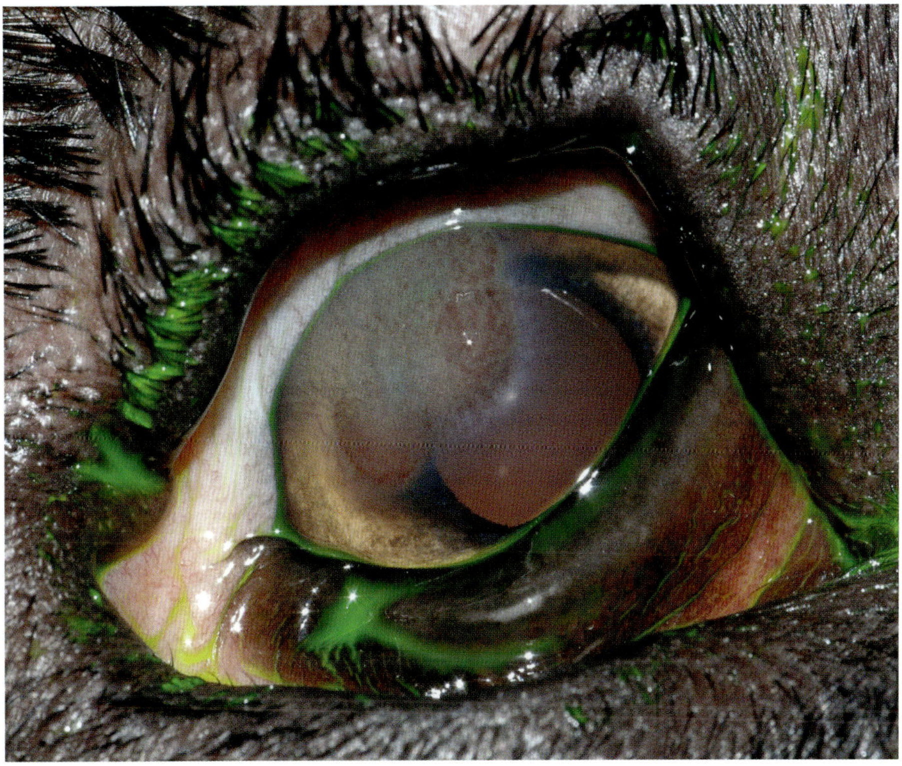

Close-up of the severe corneal damage caused by the rubbing of the lashes in a 10-month-old Saint Bernard with diamond eye.

Important notes

- In most cases, the central peak of the ectropion must be eliminated to align the eyelids.
- The skull conformation in these giant breeds and their enlarged palpebral fissures (euryblepharon) predispose them to diamond eye.

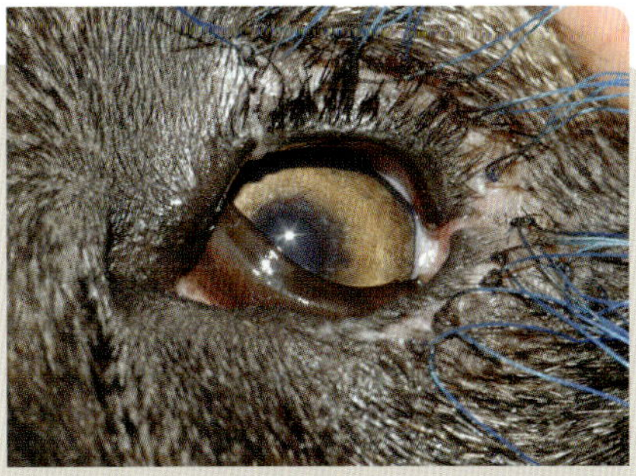

Patient treated surgically.
The correction of the palpebral margins creates a normal palpebral fissure.

Euryblepharon

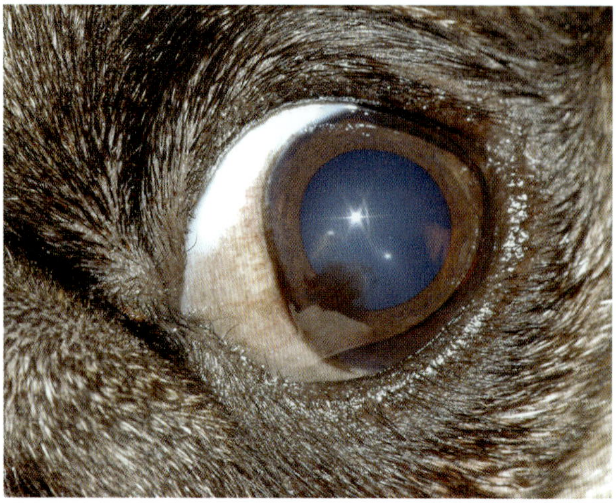

Ten-month-old Pug with euryblepharon, or macropalpebral fissure.

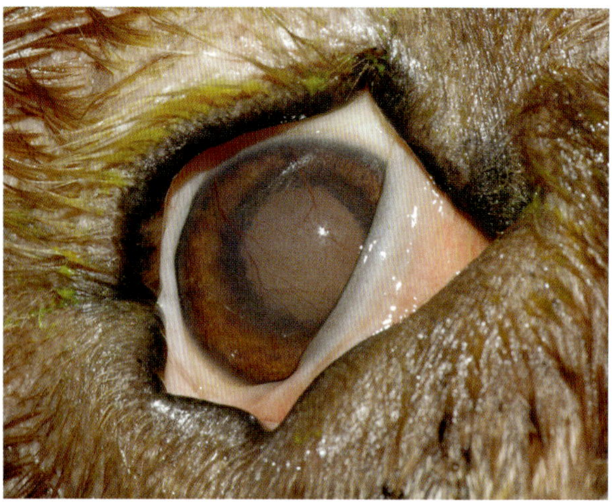

Euryblepharon is often accompanied by diamond eye. Thirteen-month-old Saint Bernard.

i | The enlarged palpebral fissure exposes an abnormally large portion of the sclera and conjunctiva.

Important notes

- Increased corneal exposure.
- Predisposes to entropion.

Euryblepharon

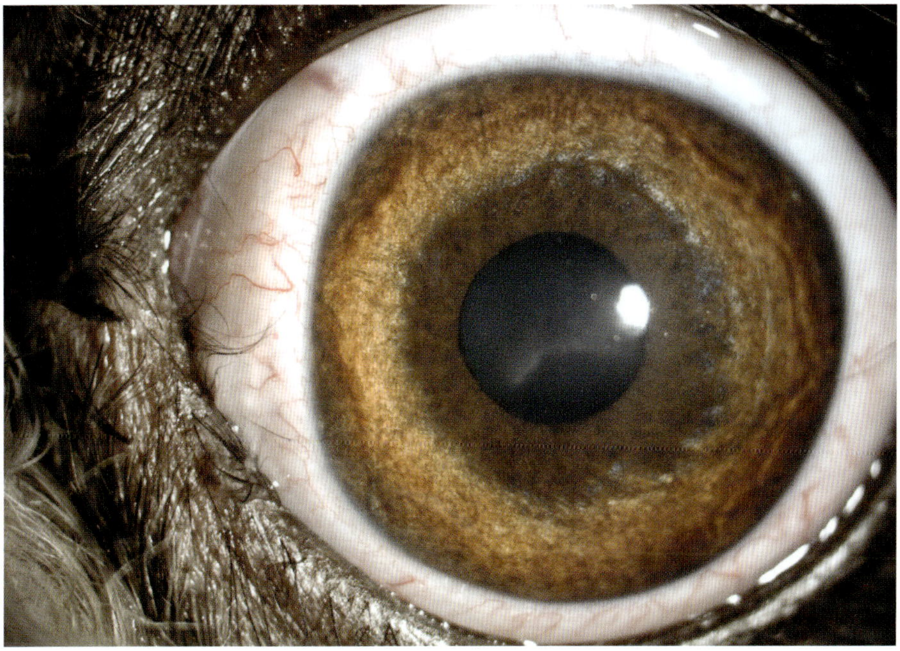

Shih-Tzu with euryblepharon. Note the increased exposure of the globe.

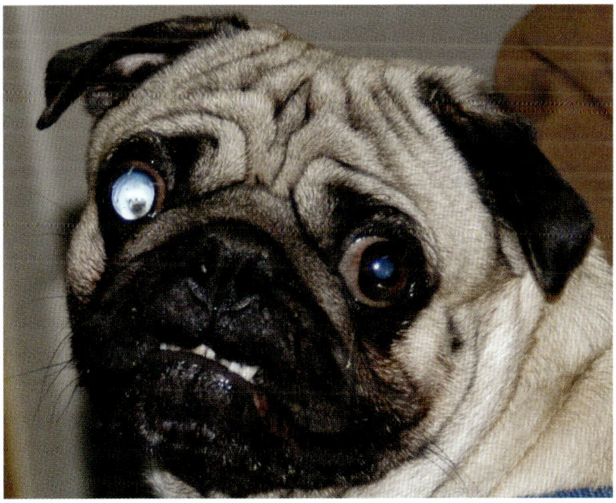

Pug with euryblepharon. The presentation is always bilateral.

Breed predisposition

The most commonly affected breeds are the Shih-Tzu, Pug, Lhasa Apso, and Pekingese.

Euryblepharon

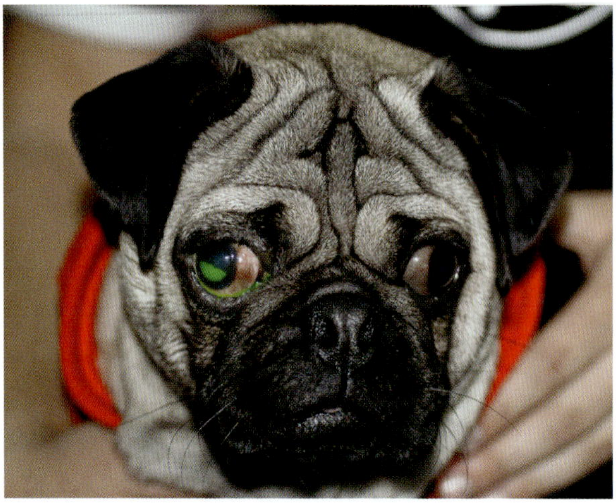

Corneal ulcer due to exposure in a one-year-old Pug with macropalpebral fissure.

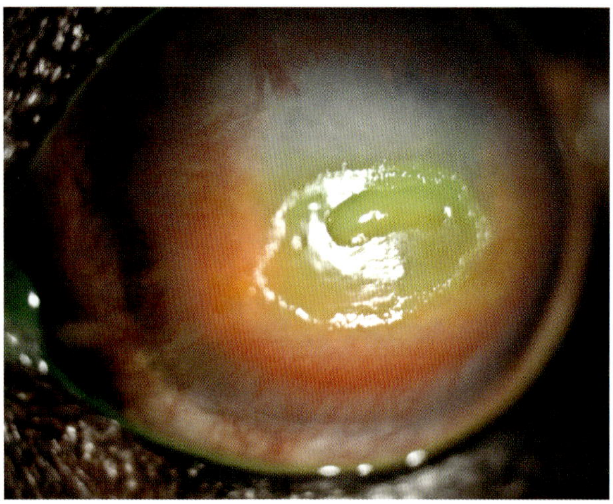

Corneal lesion in a Pug. Note the fluorescein uptake at the centre of the cornea.

Important notes

- Brachycephalic patients with euryblepharon are more prone to corneal ulcers and proptosis.

Euryblepharon

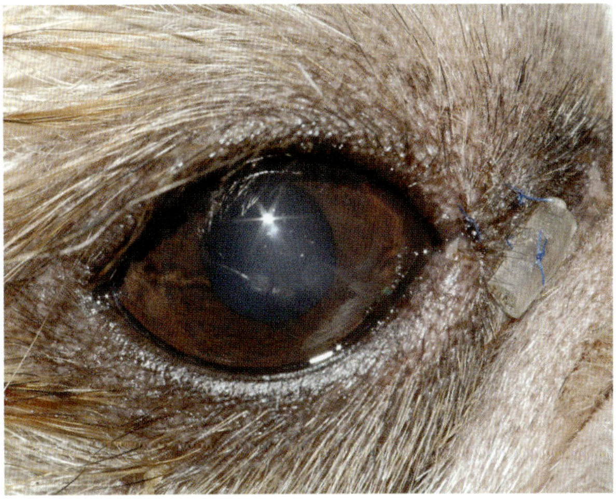

Roberts–Jensen technique for correcting euryblepharon.

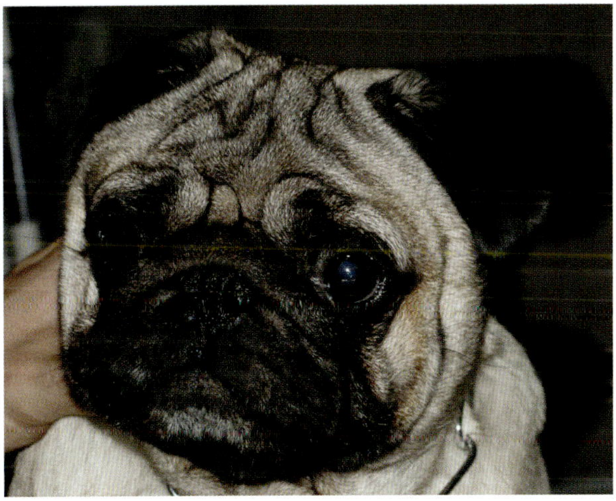

Patient treated surgically for euryblepharon. Note the correct size of the palpebral fissure.

Surgical technique

Medial canthoplasty is indicated for correcting euryblepharon.

Contraindicated

Do not damage the lower lacrimal punctum or canaliculus.

Palpebral laceration

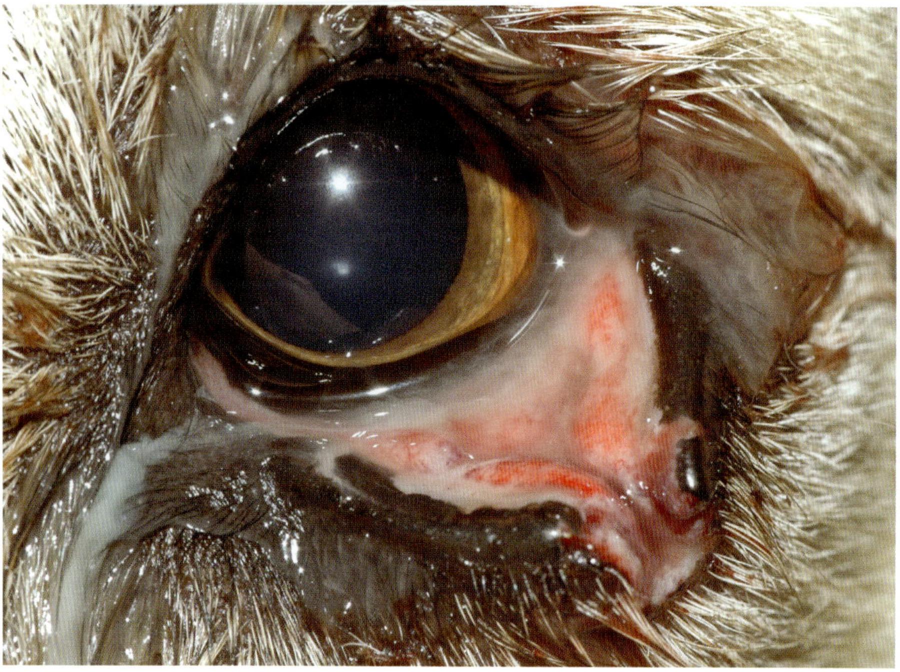

Four-year-old mixed-breed dog. Aspect of the wound five hours after it happened. Note the extensive damage to the palpebral margin caused by a wire.

Surgical technique

- Emergency surgical reconstruction is performed to avoid cicatricial retraction.
- Align the wound edges (figure-of-8 suture pattern).

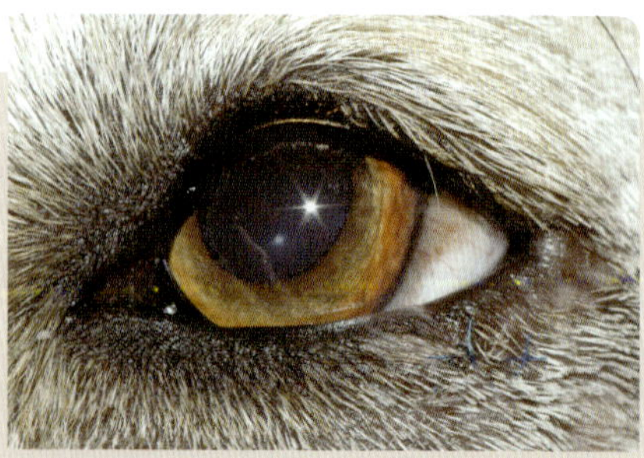

Eye 72 hours after the wounding event.

Palpebral laceration

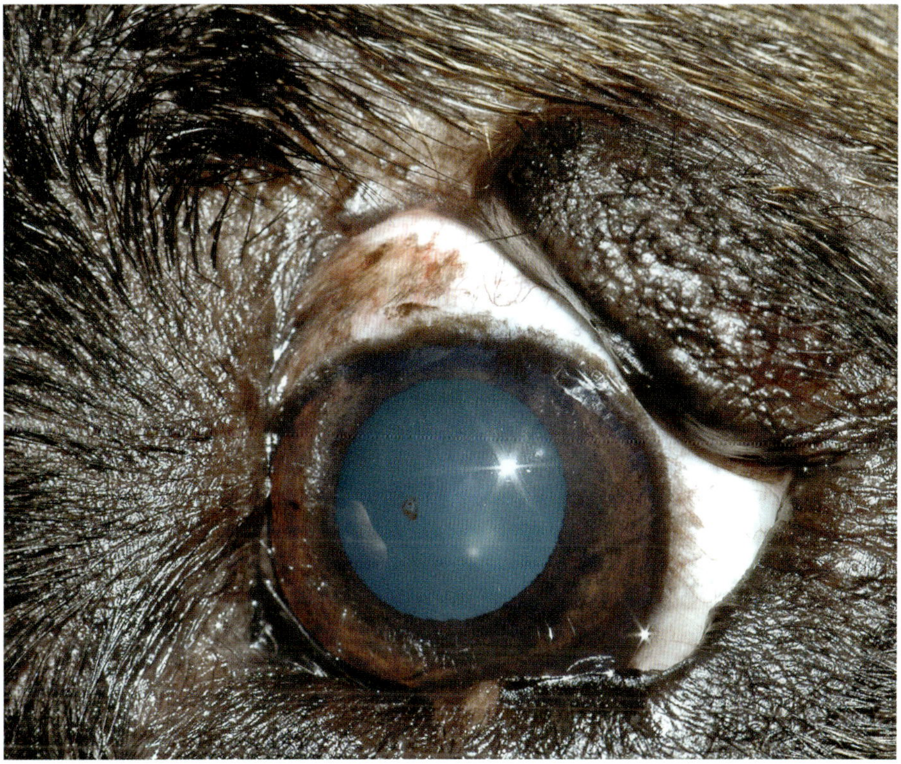

Eight-year-old Boxer whose upper left eyelid was torn in a fight seven months prior to this picture. Note the cicatricial retraction of the eyelid and exposure damage to the cornea.

Important notes

- Palpebral lacerations should be repaired within the first 24 hours. If not, the risk of cicatricial retraction increases markedly.

Contraindicated

- NEVER allow healing by second intention, as it may lead to keratitis and corneal ulcers resulting from lagophthalmos.

Fungal blepharitis

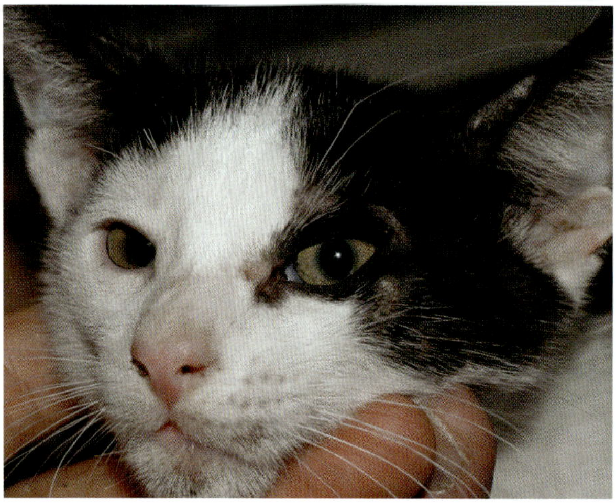

Three-month-old cat with fungal blepharitis. Note the hyperkeratotic plaques and alopecic, crusted lesions, as well as localised desquamation of the eyelids and ears.

Inflammatory disease of the eyelid or eyelids.
It may be unilateral or bilateral, focal or diffuse.

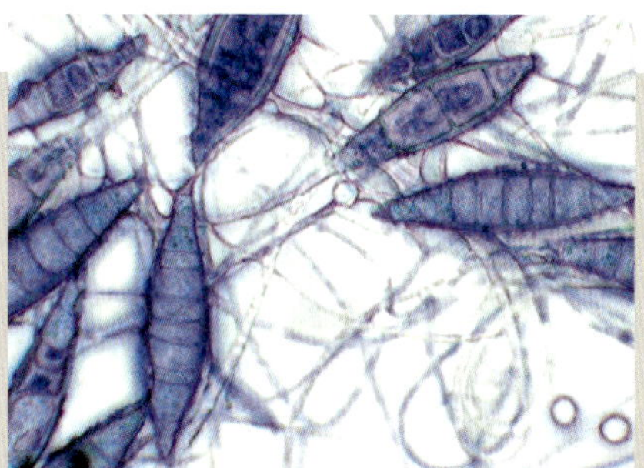

Microsporum canis (macroconidia, 40×)
Image courtesy of Cristina Fernández Algarra.

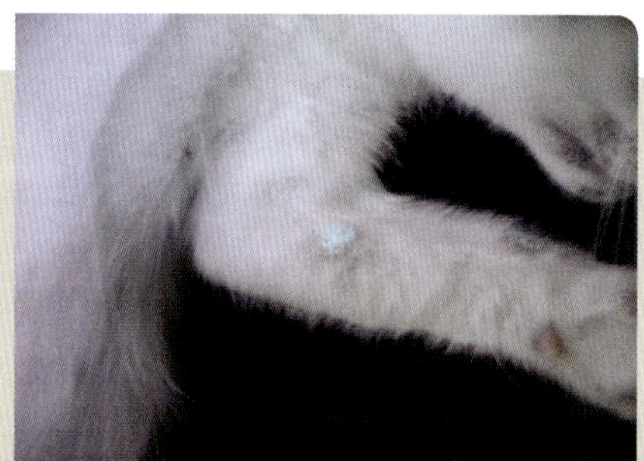

Use of a Wood's lamp to assist in diagnosis of dermatophytosis.

Important notes

- The most affected patients are the young or immunosuppressed (rule out FIV).
- IT IS A CUTANEOUS ZOONOSIS.
- The lesions tend to be non-pruritic.

Fungal blepharitis

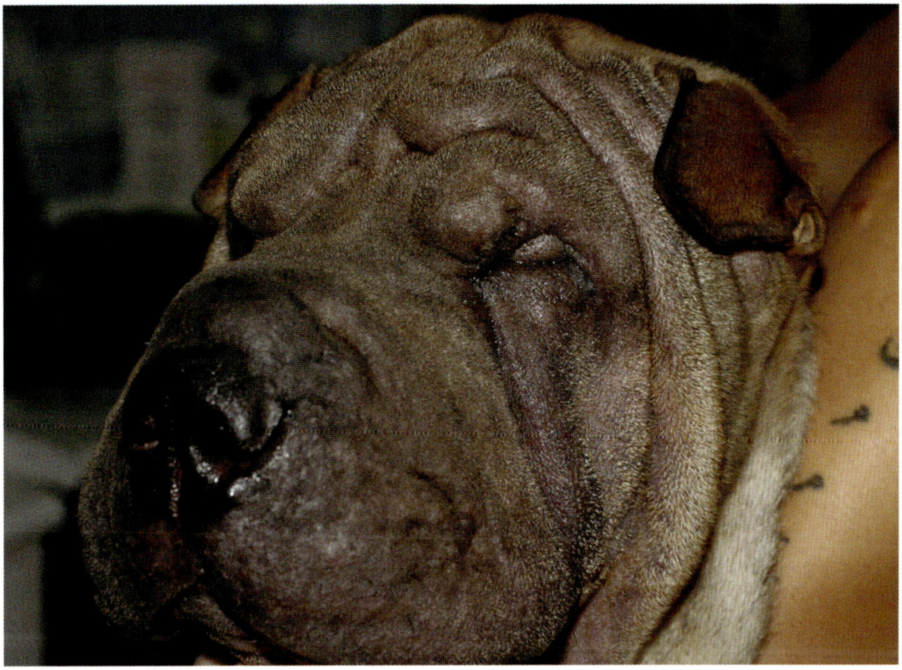

Shar Pei with blepharitis and generalised *Malassezia* dermatitis complicated by bacterial infection. Note the skin erythema, alopecia, and hyperpigmentation.

Important notes

- PRURITIC
  (place Elizabethan collar).
- Medical treatment (oral antifungals and therapeutic baths) should continue at least 15 days after resolution of the clinical signs.

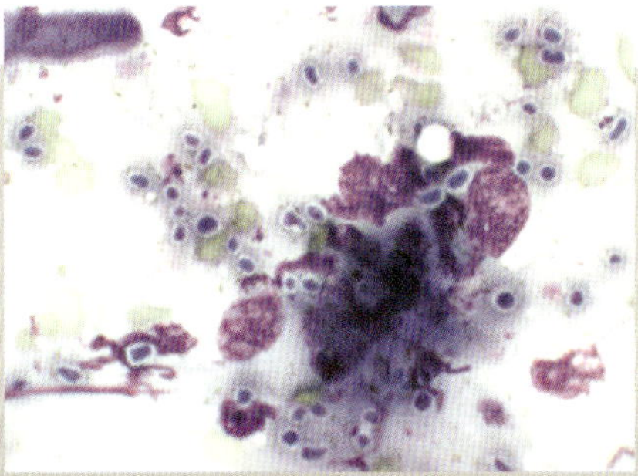

Malassezia pachydermatis (100×).
Image courtesy of Cristina Fernández Algarra.

Bacterial blepharitis

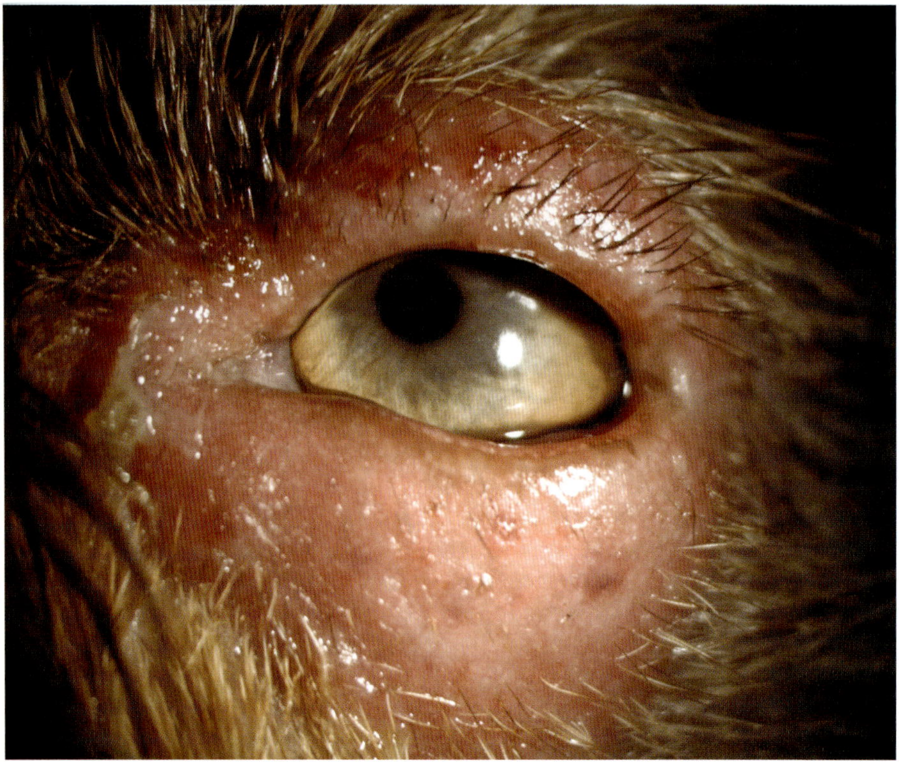

Severe bacterial blepharitis due to *Staphylococcus* (juvenile pyoderma). Eight-month-old patient with hyperaemic, alopecic, ulcerative, oedematous lesion.

Interesting notes

- Pruritus in these patients is the result of an allergenic cascade triggered by toxins released by *Staphylococcus* (treat with corticosteroids).
- Use broad-spectrum systemic antibiotics (cephalosporins or macrolides).

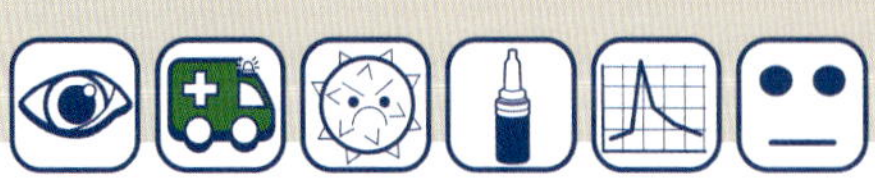

Bacterial blepharitis

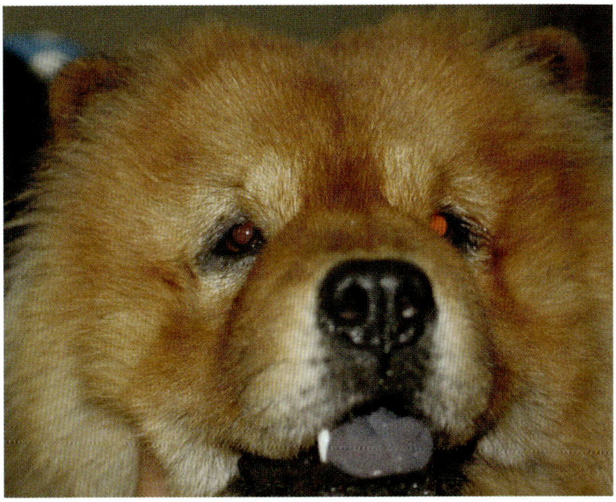

Thirteen-month-old Chow Chow with chronic bilateral blepharitis.

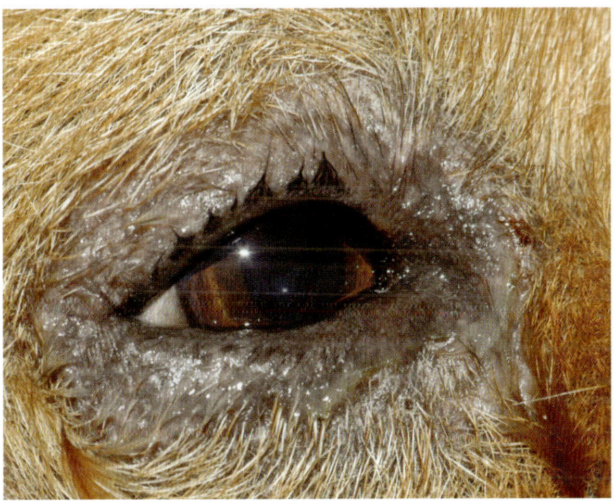

Close-up of blepharitis in the patient pictured above. Note the alopecia and hyperpigmentaton, signs of chronicity.

Interesting notes

- Bacterial blepharitis with a chronic presentation may be linked to systemic processes (endocrine, immune-mediated, seborrhoeic).

Parasitic blepharitis

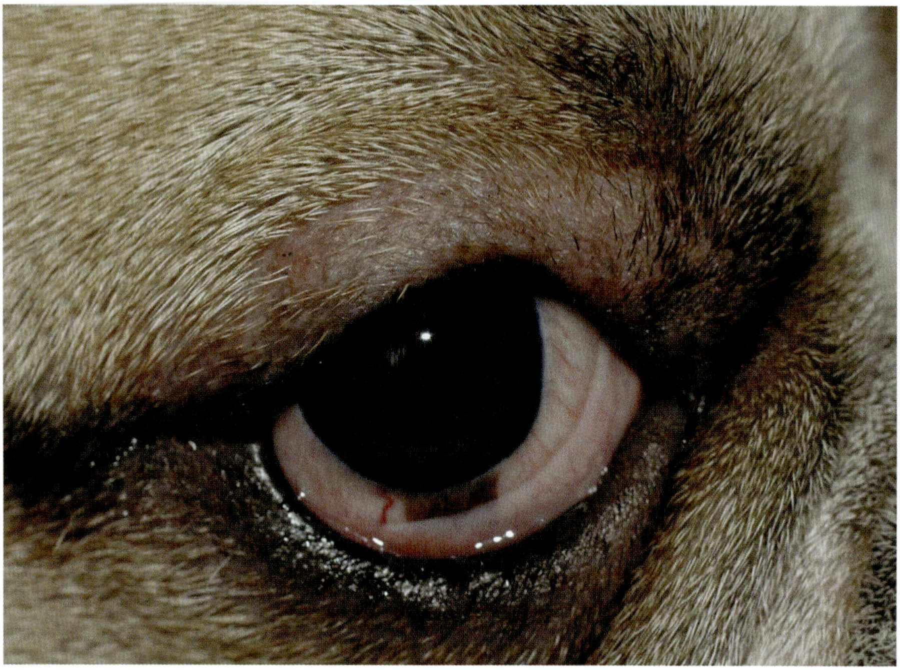

Blepharitis caused by *Demodex* in the upper eyelid of a six-month-old English bulldog puppy.

Parasitic blepharitis from *Demodex* is more common in short-haired breeds (Bulldog, Boxer, Pug, Pit Bull).

It most commonly occurs in young animals or immunosuppressed adults with comorbidities.

Hyperaemia, alopecia and pruritus are commonly observed.

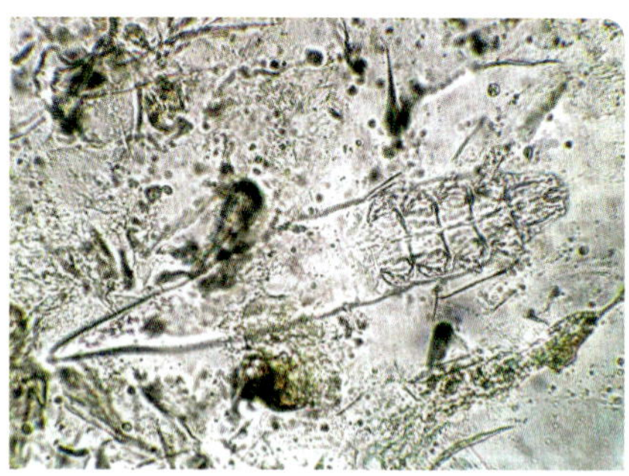

Demodex canis (40×). Image courtesy of Cristina Fernández Algarra.

Parasitic blepharitis

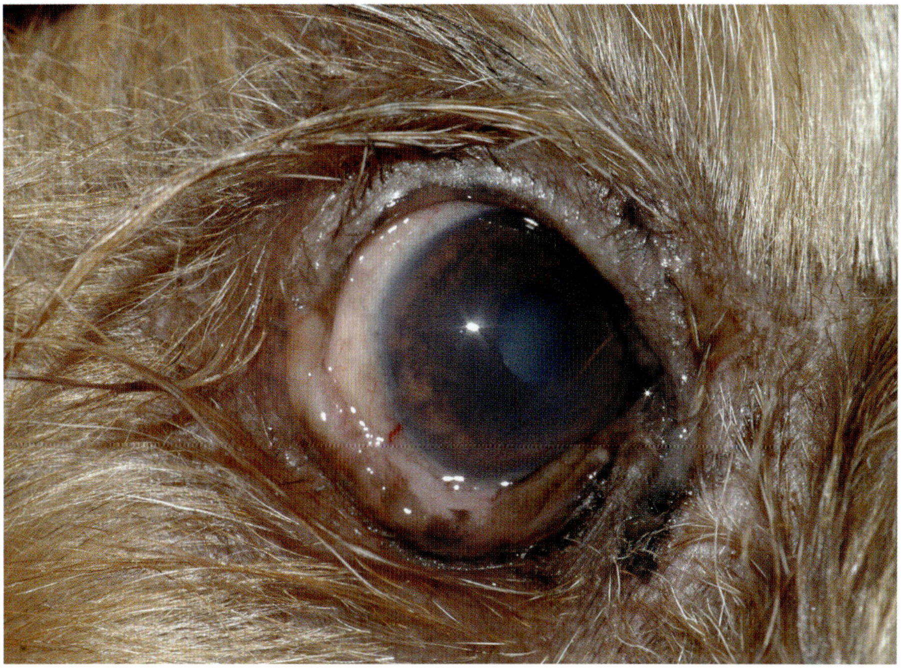

Patient with chronic blepharitis due to *Leishmania*.
Note the associated keratouveitis.

Interesting notes

- Palpebral lesions associated with *Leishmania* are generally granulomatous, alopecic, and/or ulcerative.
- They may appear in isolation or with other ophthalmological disorders (uveitis or keratouveitis) or systemic processes (see picture below).

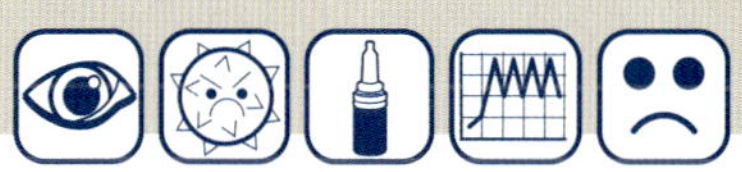

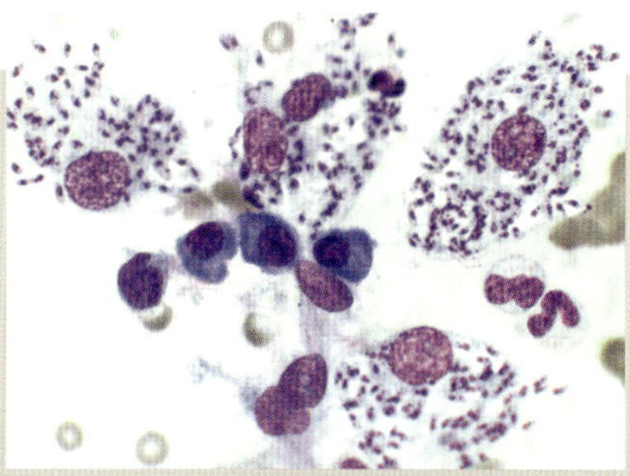

Leishmania infantum and humoral response with plasma cells (100×).
Image courtesy of Cristina Fernández Algarra.

Parasitic blepharitis

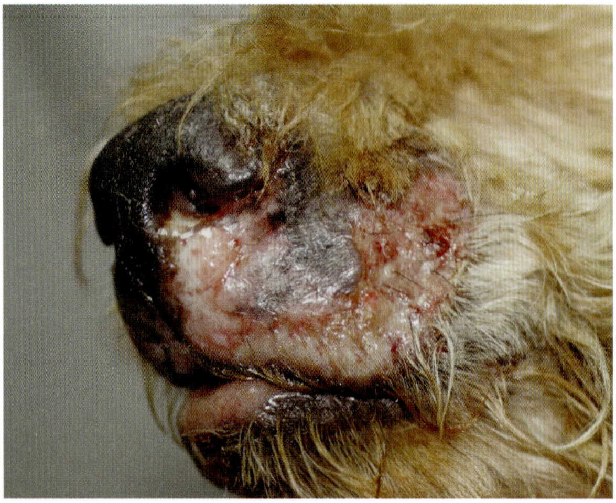

Four-year-old Airedale Terrier with cutaneous leishmaniasis.

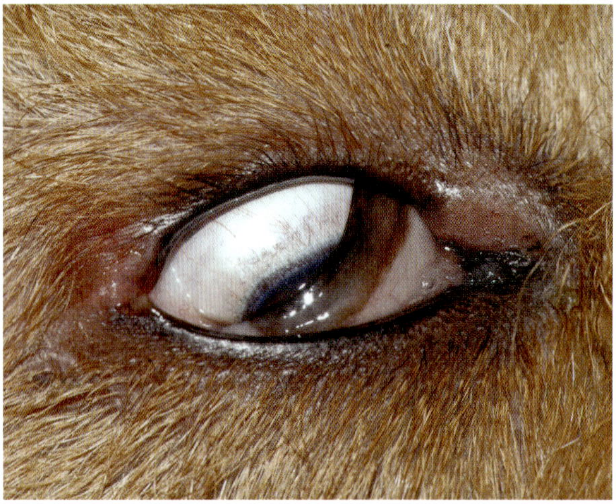

Alopecic ulcerative blepharitis of the right eye.

Recommendations

- Systemic treatment: antimonials, miltefosine, or marbofloxacin, along with allopurinol (per clinician's discretion).
- Treatment with intralesional corticosteroids in the palpebral area can help improve the clinical condition.

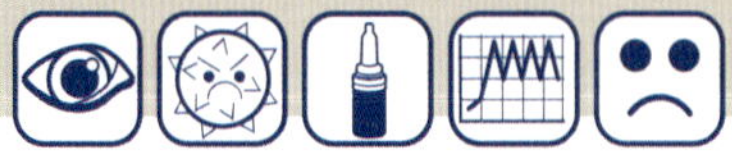

Blepharitis

Hypersensitivity

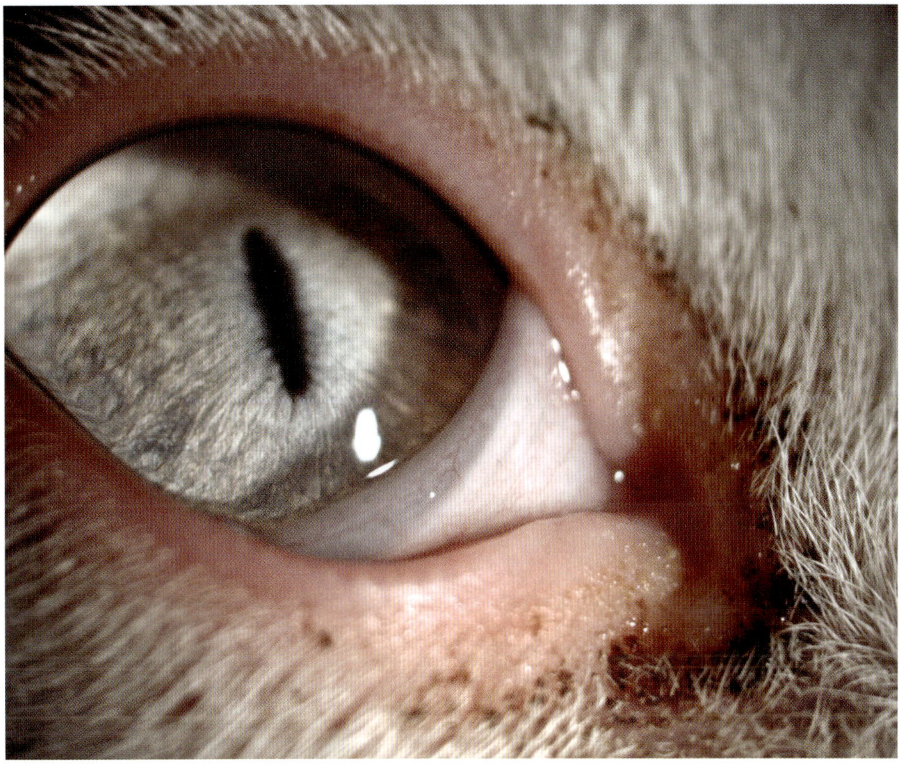

Allergic blepharitis from topical neomycin in a four-year-old cat. The patient improved when the topical medication was discontinued.

Contraindicated

- If ophthalmological signs appear after administration of a drug, consider this in the differential diagnosis.

Important notes

- Any adverse reaction must be reported.

Blepharitis

Hypersensitivity

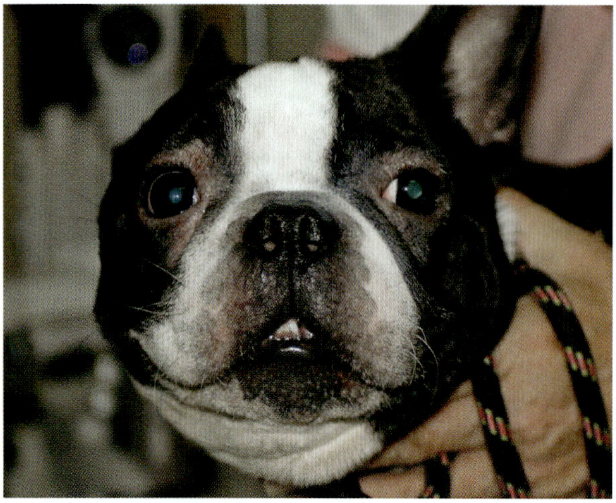

Atopic blepharitis in a two-year-old French bulldog.

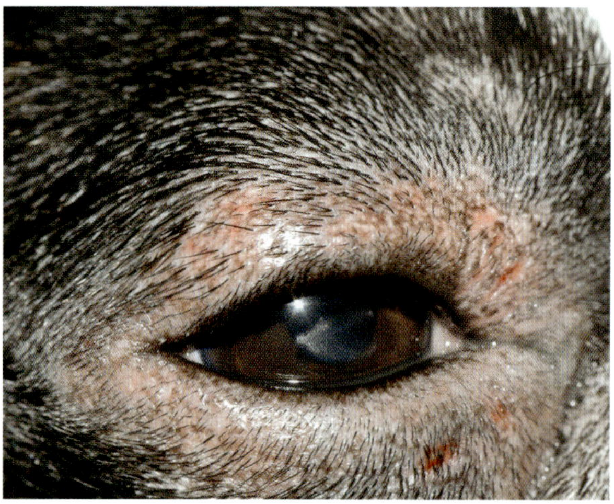

Close-up of the patient's right eyelids. Note the blepharitis and erythema.

Important notes

- Initial signs of atopic dermatitis are pruritus and erythema.
- The most common areas affected on the head are the periocular region, the nose, and the pinnae.

Blepharitis

Hypersensitivity

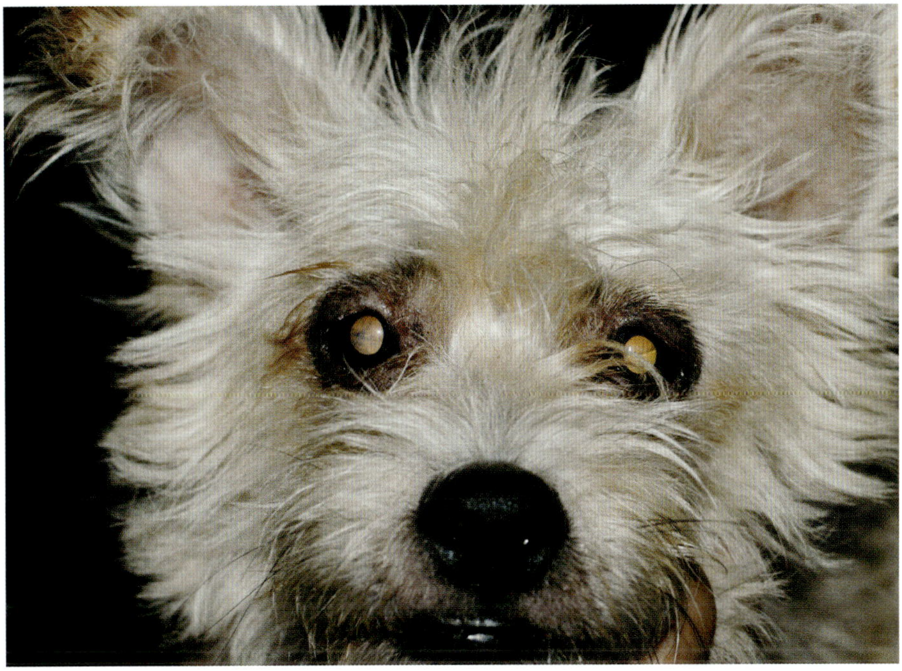

West Highland White Terrier with atopic blepharitis. Alopecia, skin thickening, erythema, and skin hyperpigmentation are evident.

Breed predisposition

- The breeds most predisposed to atopic blepharitis are as follows: English bulldog, French bulldog, Bull Terrier, West Highland White Terrier, Boxer, Labrador and Golden Retriever.
- Hyperpigmentation, hyperkeratosis, and lichenification are common in chronic cases of atopic dermatitis.

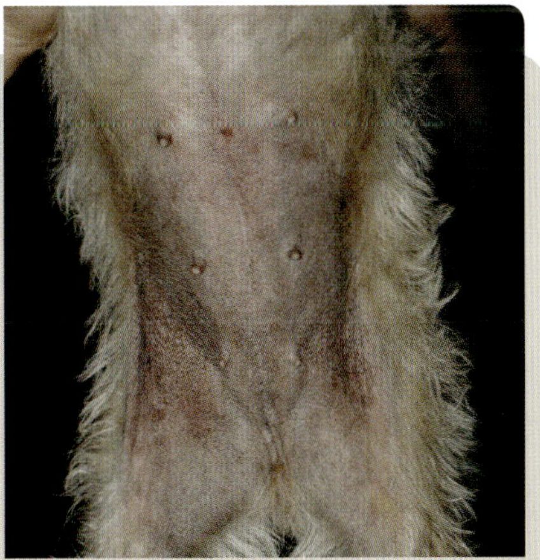

Ventral abdominal area of patient.

Blepharitis

Hypersensitivity

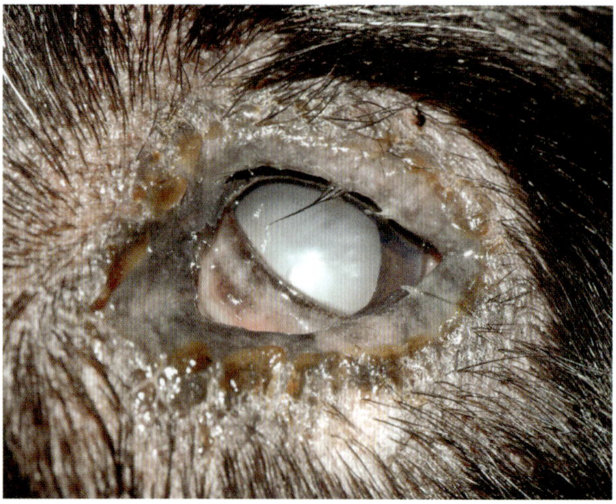

Cocker Spaniel with chronic atopic blepharitis. Note the hyperpigmentation and secondary bacterial infection.

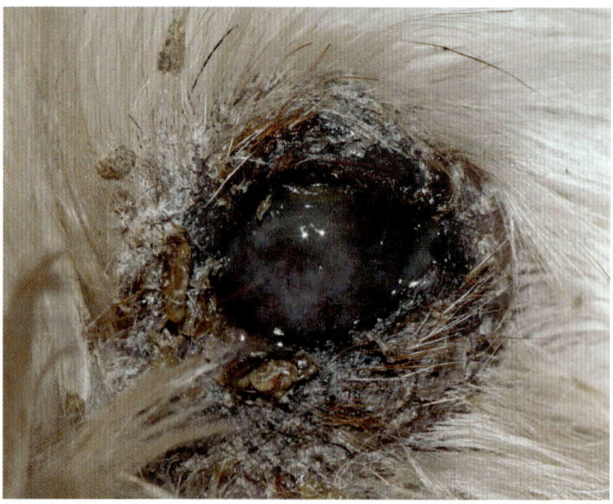

West Highland White Terrier with chronic blepharitis. Close-up of periocular crusting.

Interesting notes

Secondary pyodermas and seborrhoeic disorders may occur with the chronic phase of atopic blepharitis.

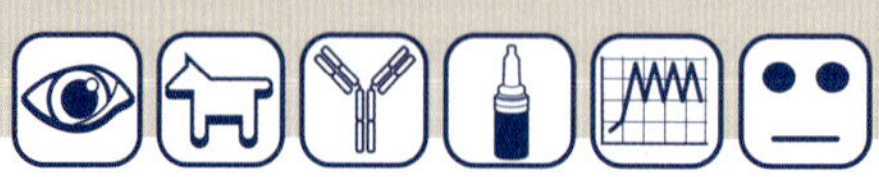

Immune blepharitis

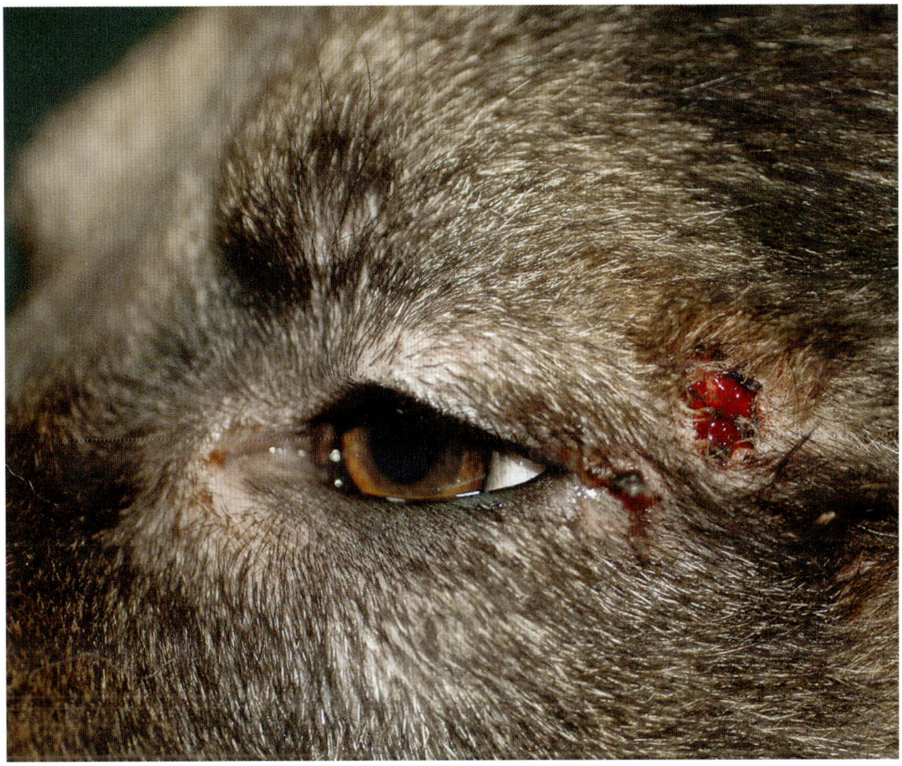

Three-year-old female German Shepherd with discoid lupus erythematosus. Close-up of the erythematous, ulcerative lesions and depigmentation.

In patients with discoid lupus erythematosus (DLE), lesions are localised to mucocutaneous junctions and the face.

Breed predisposition

German Shepherds and Belgian Shepherds are predisposed breeds.

Treatment

Use of topical corticosteroids, cyclosporine or tacrolimus (lotion) may be sufficient to control the palpebral disease. Systemic corticosteroids (prednisone) and fatty acids should be added in severe cases.

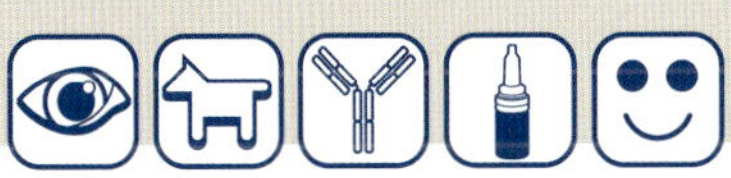

Immune blepharitis

Idiopathic facial dermatitis in Persian cats

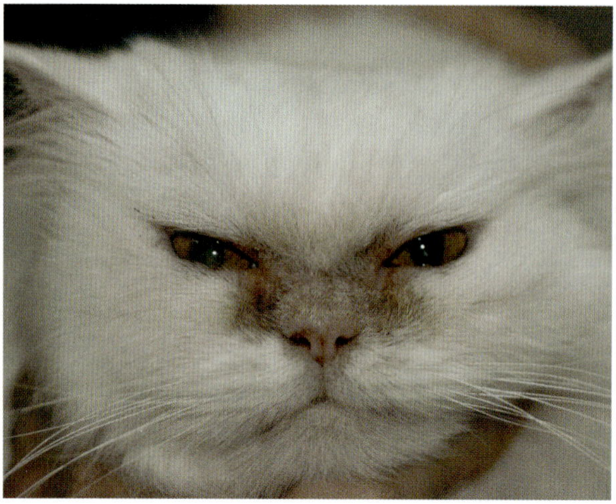

Four-year-old Persian cat with idiopathic facial dermatitis.

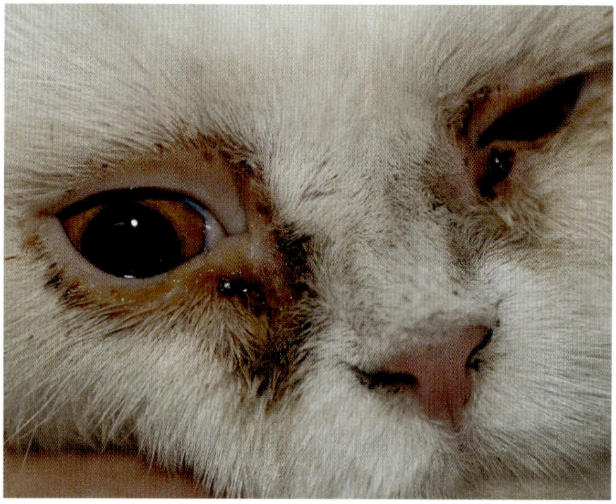

Erythematous and ulcerative lesions in a five-year-old Persian cat with idiopathic facial dermatitis. Close-up of serous blackish exudate.

Interesting notes

The exact aetiology of idiopathic facial dermatitis in Persian cats is unknown. Also called "dirty face syndrome", its response to cyclosporine suggests a possible immune-mediated disorder.

Palpebral neoplasms

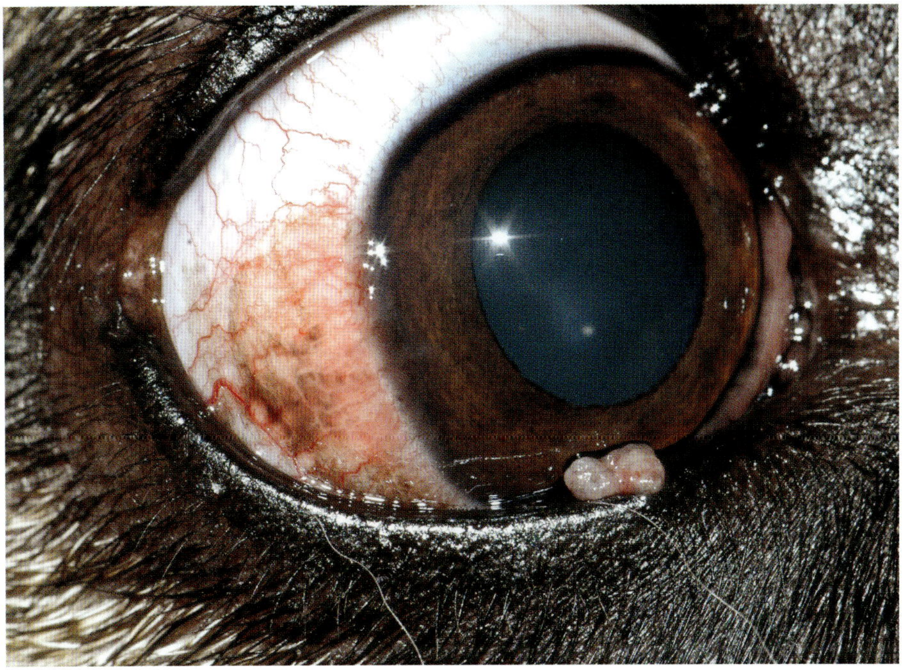

Meibomian gland adenoma in an 11-year-old German Shepherd.

Important notes

- Sebaceous adenoma of the Meibomian gland is the most common palpebral neoplasm in older dogs, and it is benign.
- It starts at the base of the gland and emerges through the secretory duct.

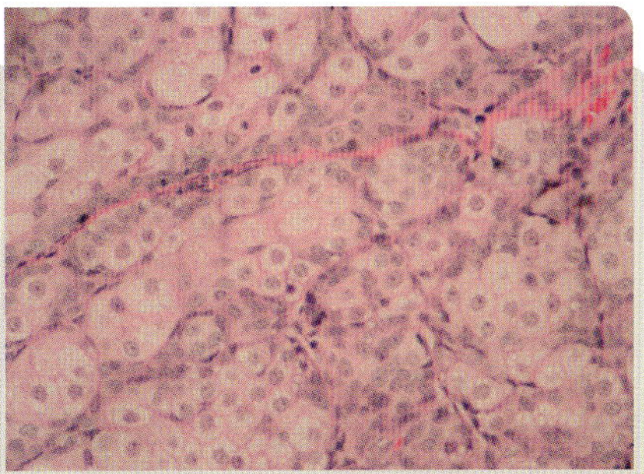

Histopathological image of a Meibomian gland adenoma courtesy of Dr Elena Alonso Fernández-Aceytuno.

Palpebral neoplasms

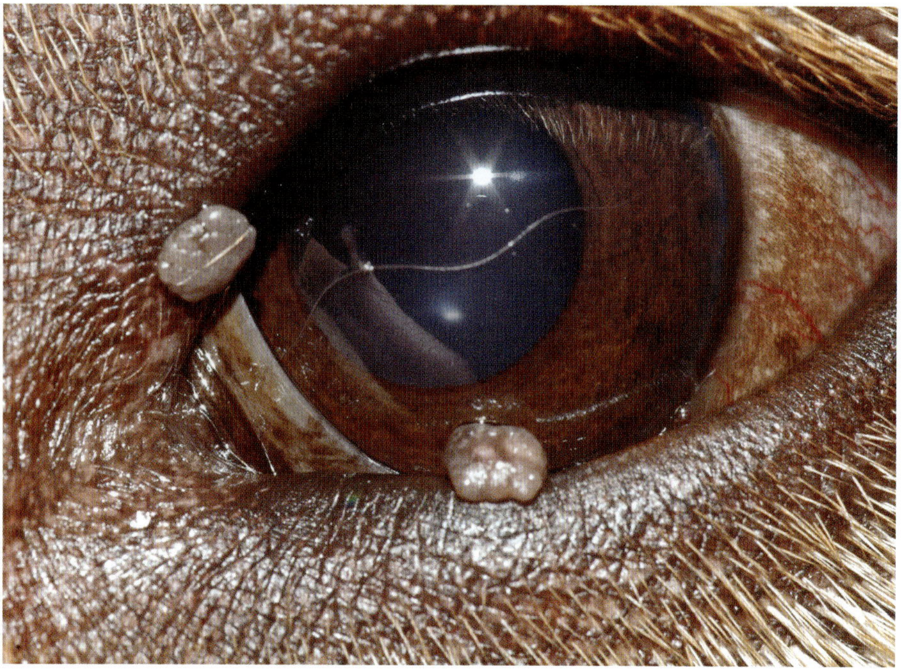

Meibomian gland adenomas in a 13-year-old mixed breed dog.

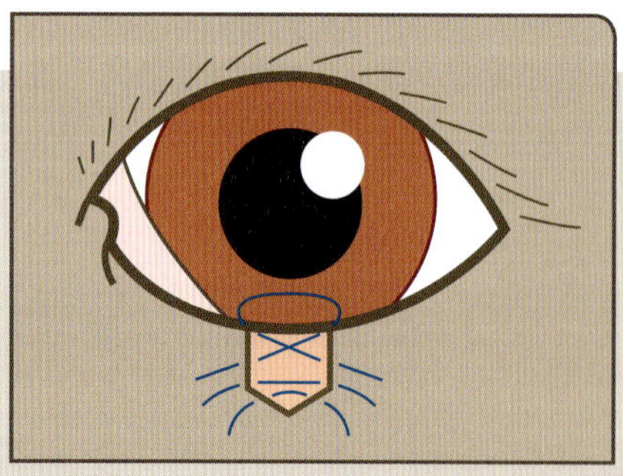

Diagram of closure following tumour resection.

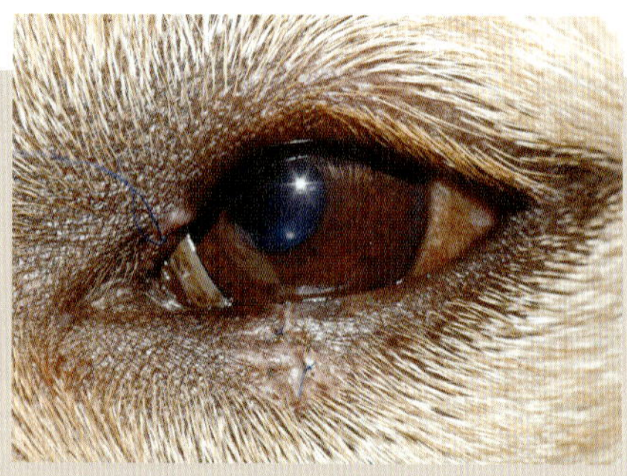

Patient 10 days postoperatively.

Surgical techniques

- If the surgical defect covers less than ¼ of the length of the eyelid, a V-shaped excision or inverted house-shaped excision may be used.
- A figure-of-8 suture is essential to align the palpebral margin.

Palpebral neoplasms

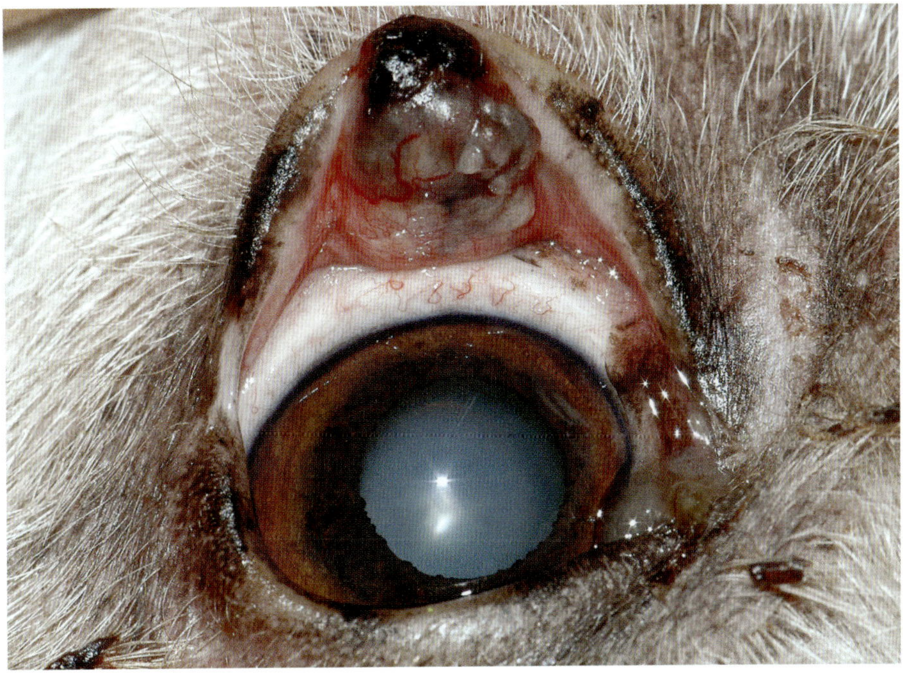

Thirteen-year-old mixed-breed dog with Meibomian gland epithelioma.
Note the size of the neoplasm.

Interesting notes

Sebaceous epithelioma of the eyelid is considered low-grade malignant, and complete excision is considered curative.

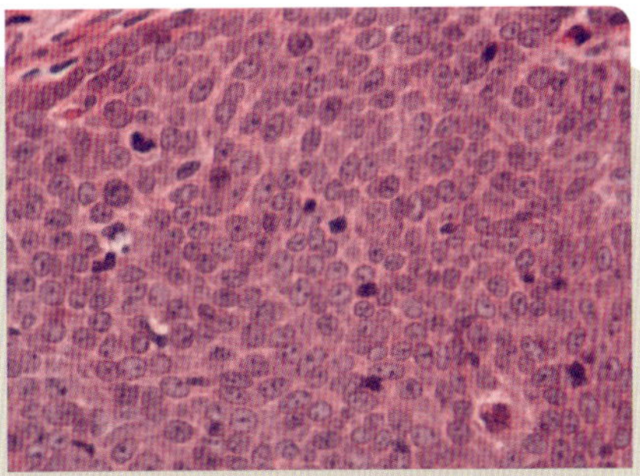

Histopathological image of the sebaceous epithelioma courtesy of Dr Elena Alonso Fernández-Aceytuno.

Palpebral neoplasms

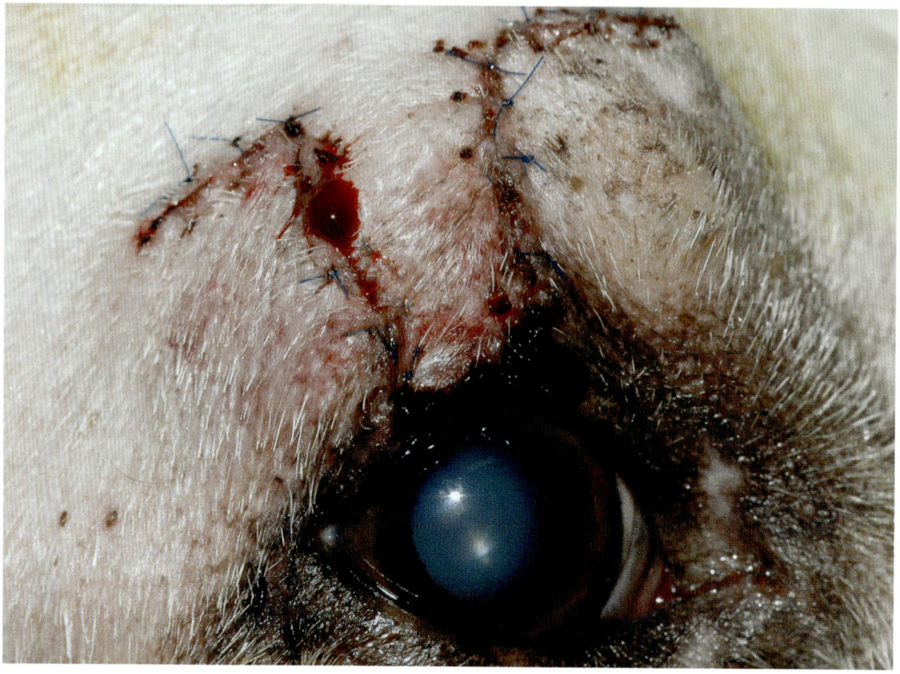

H-blepharoplasty used for surgical excision of the epithelioma pictured previously.

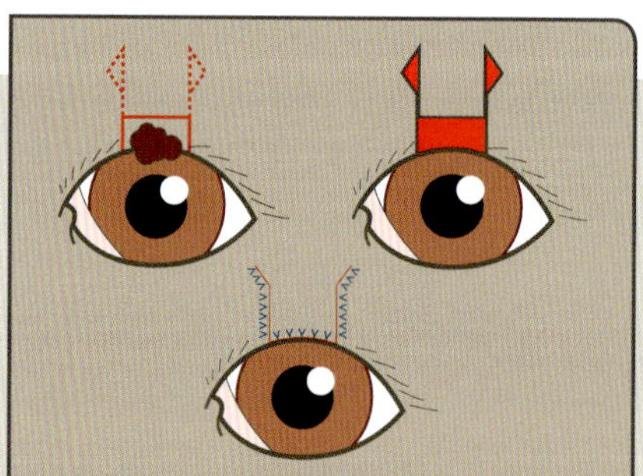

Tumour resection with H-blepharoplasty.

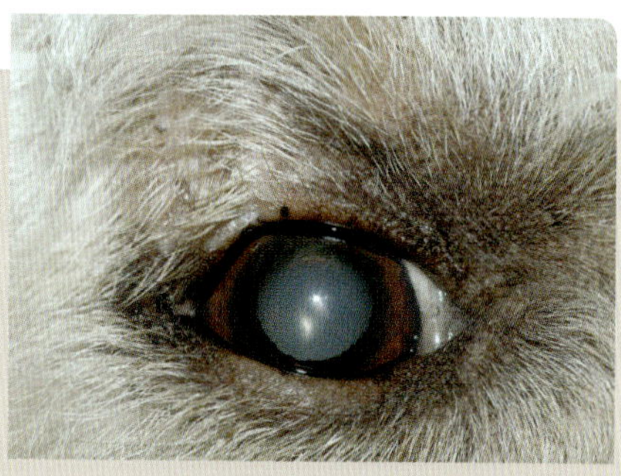

Results of the H-blepharoplasty two months after surgery.

Surgical techniques

- If the surgical defect created by tumour excision exceeds ¼ of the length of the eyelid, perform blepharoplasty.
- For large, centrally located eyelid tumours, H-blepharoplasty is most often used.

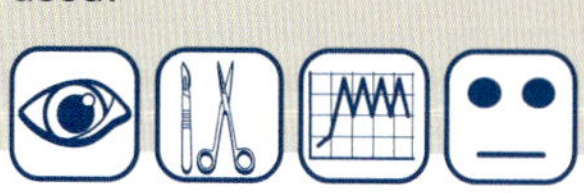

Palpebral neoplasms

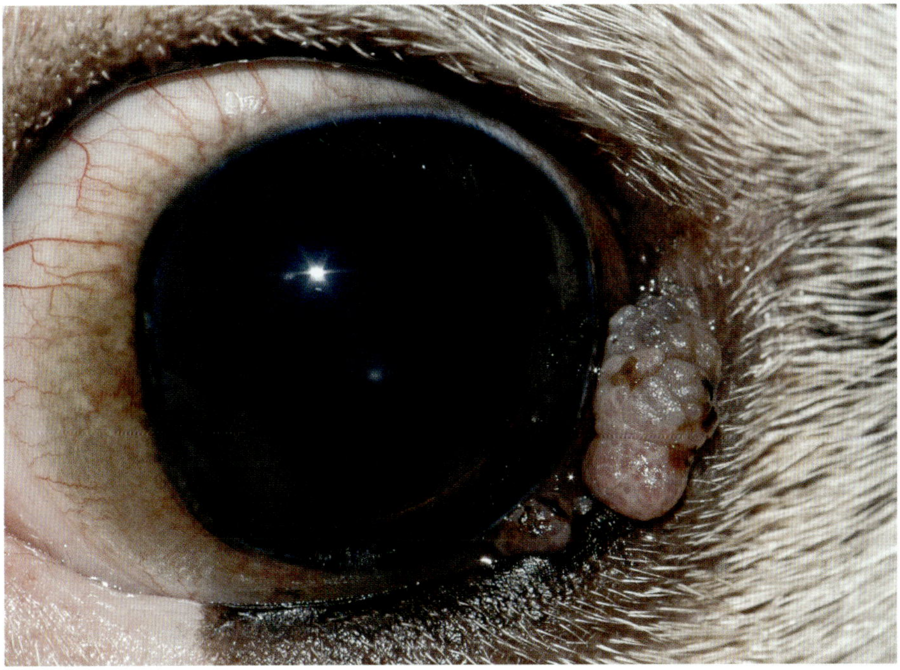

Close-up of palpebral papillomatosis of the left eye in the patient pictured below.

Interesting notes

- Palpebral papillomas appear in young animals, are often viral in origin, and may be associated with oral papillomatosis.
- These may be self-limiting but usually require surgery.

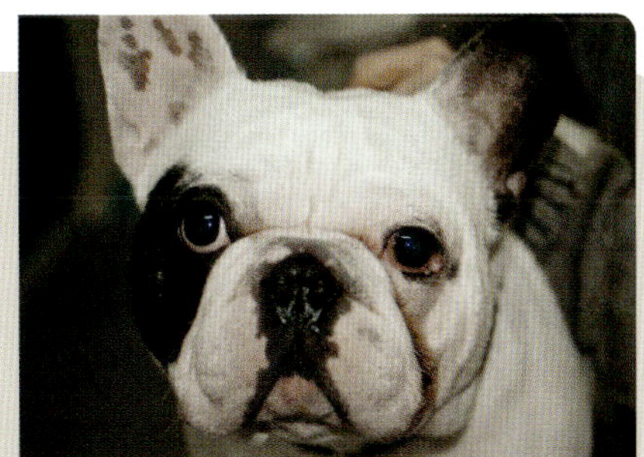

Eight-month-old French Bulldog with palpebral papilloma.

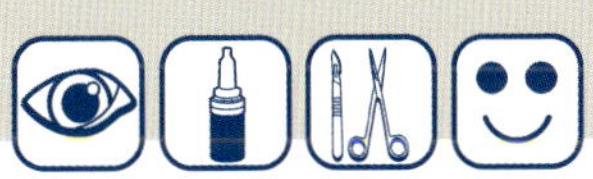

Palpebral neoplasms

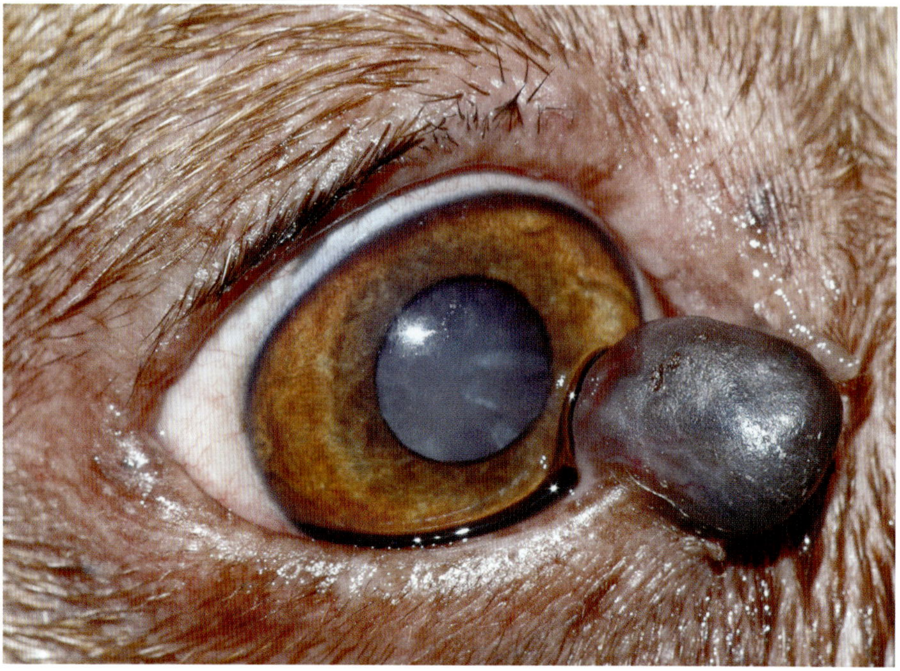

Palpebral melanoma of the lower eyelid in an eight-year-old Pit Bull.

Important notes

- Melanomas in dogs often show histological characteristics of malignancy (mitotic index and atypical cells). In spite of this, melanocytic tumours of the eyelids (in dogs) are generally benign in behaviour.

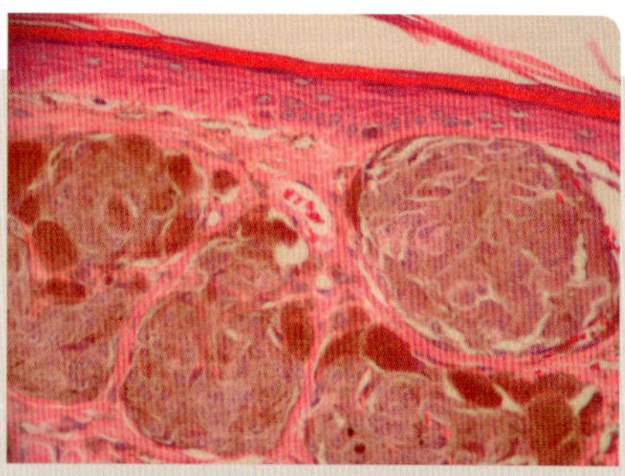

Histopathological image of melanoma. Courtesy of Dr Elena Alonso Fernández-Aceytuno.

Palpebral neoplasms

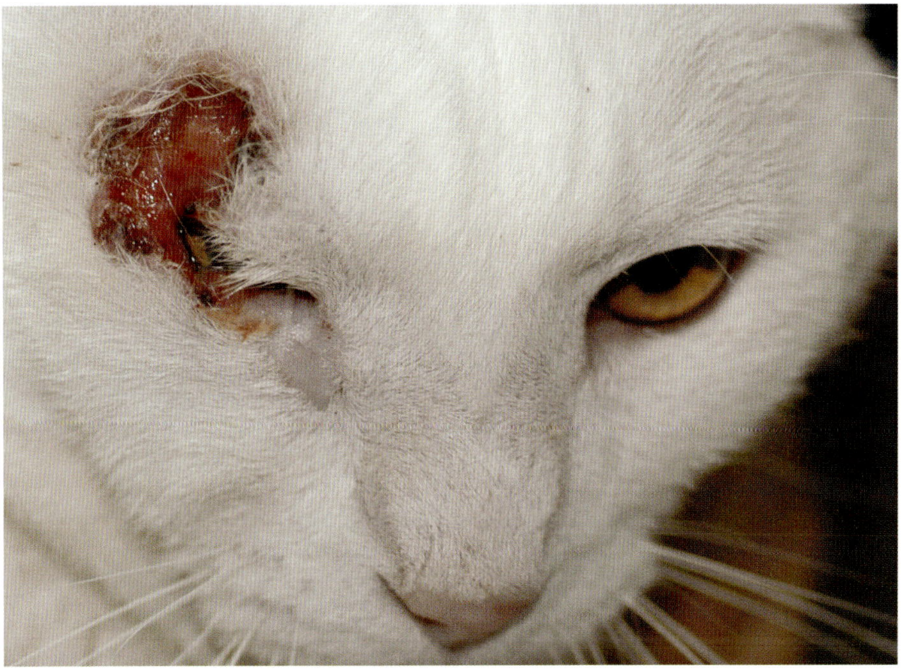

Close-up of the SCC in the cat pictured below. Note the erosive lesion of the upper eyelid.

Important notes

- Squamous cell carcinoma (SCC) in cats is malignant and highly invasive.
- These generally appear in cats with white fur.

Contraindicated

DO NOT CONFUSE WITH A PALPEBRAL WOUND.

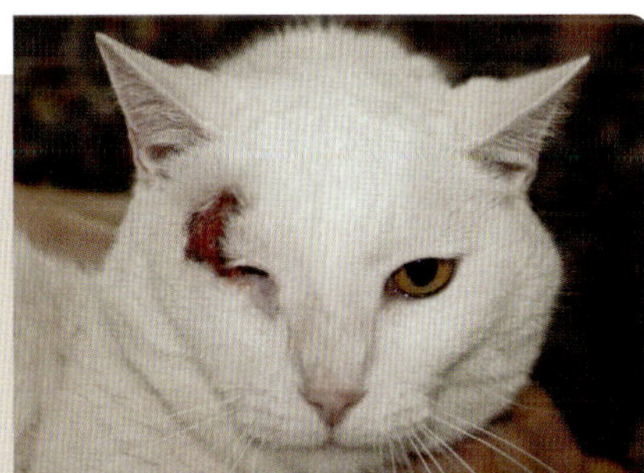

Feline patient with a squamous cell carcinoma (SCC) affecting the right upper eyelid.

Palpebral neoplasms

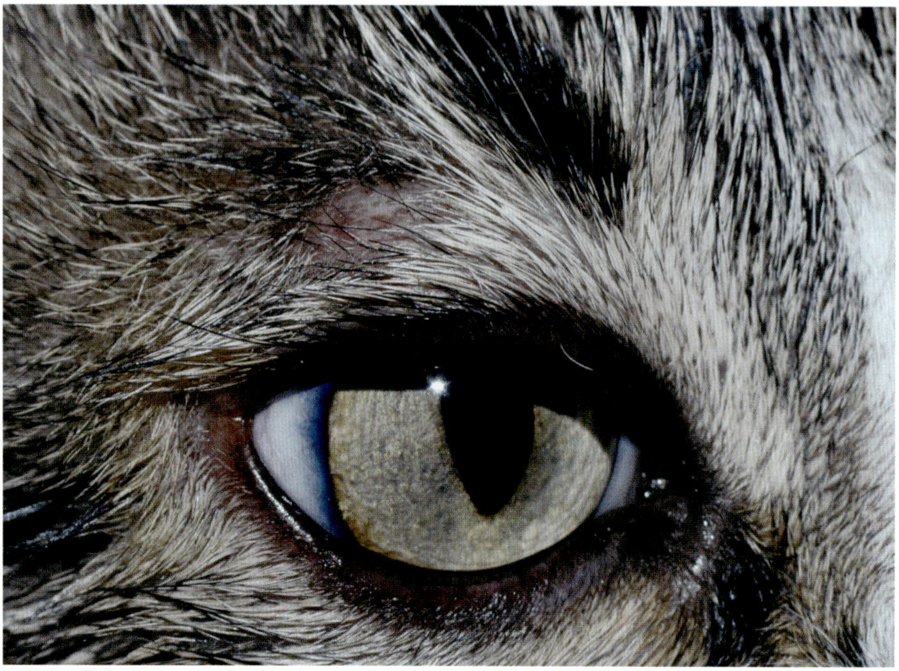

Mast cell tumour on the upper eyelid of a nine-year-old domestic shorthair cat.

Cutaneous mast cell tumours are less common in cats than in dogs.

These should be considered malignant in general, though their behaviour varies by grade of differentiation.

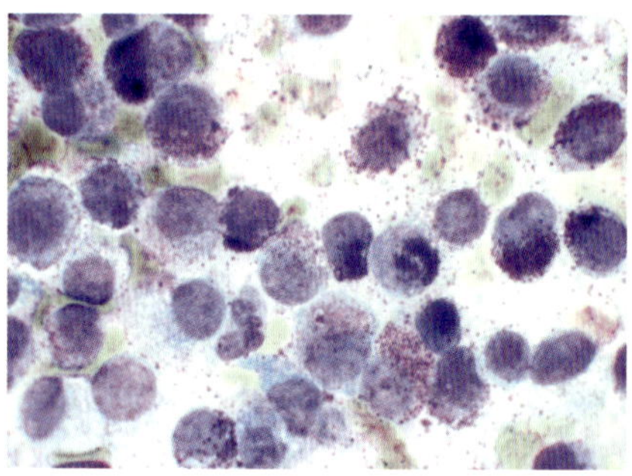

Cytology of the eyelid allows an approximate diagnosis (100×). Image courtesy of Cristina Fernández Algarra.

Distichiasis

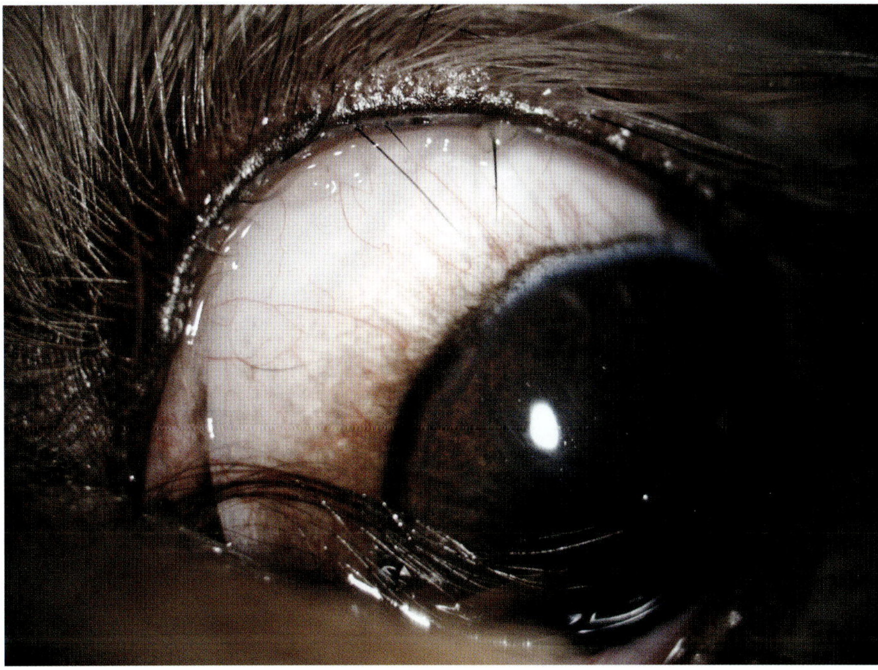

Distichiasis in a two-year-old Shih-Tzu. Close-up of the abnormal position of the hairs emerging from the excretory duct of the Meibomian glands.

i Presence of additional eyelashes in abnormally located follicles, growing towards or away from the cornea.

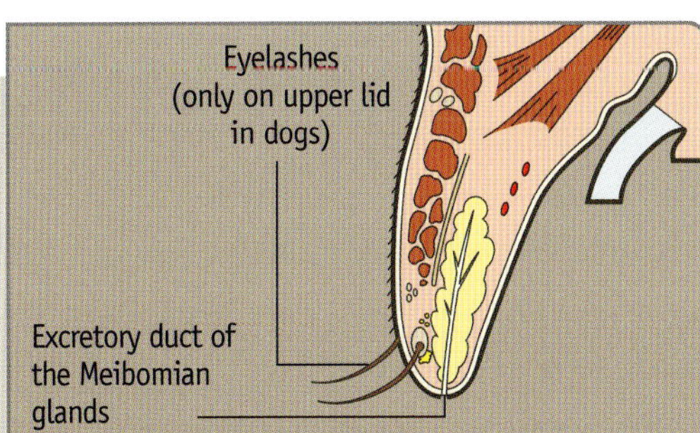

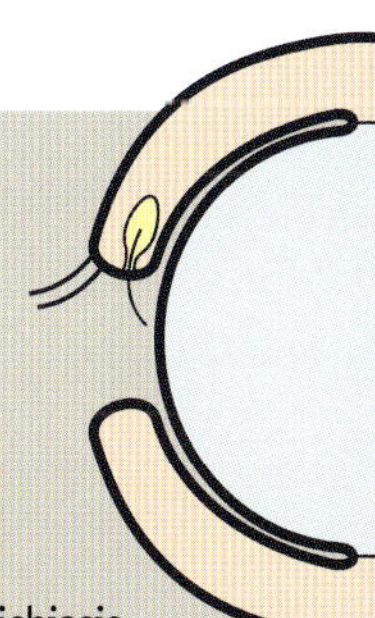

Distichiasis.

Interesting notes

These eyelashes generally emerge from the excretory ducts of the Meibomian glands.

Distichiasis

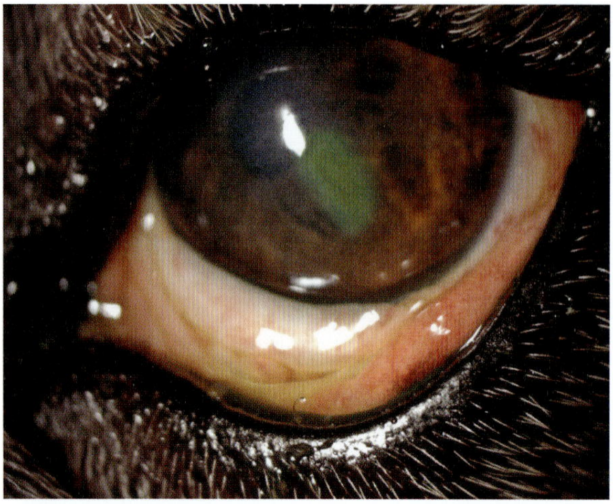

Two-year-old English Bulldog with distichiasis of the lower eyelid. The presence of a teardrop on the hair helps in its localisation. Corneal ulcers often occur along with distichiasis.

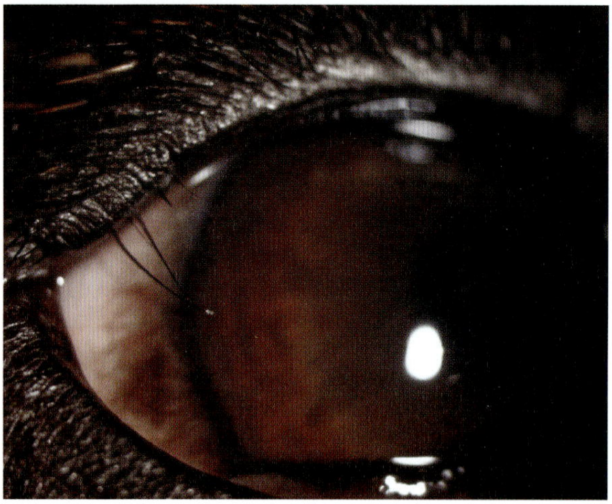

Four-year-old English Bulldog with distichiasis of the upper eyelid.

Breed predisposition

- The breeds most predisposed to distichiasis are the English Bulldog, Pug, Poodle, Shih-Tzu and Pekingese.
- The upper eyelid is more commonly affected.

Districhiasis

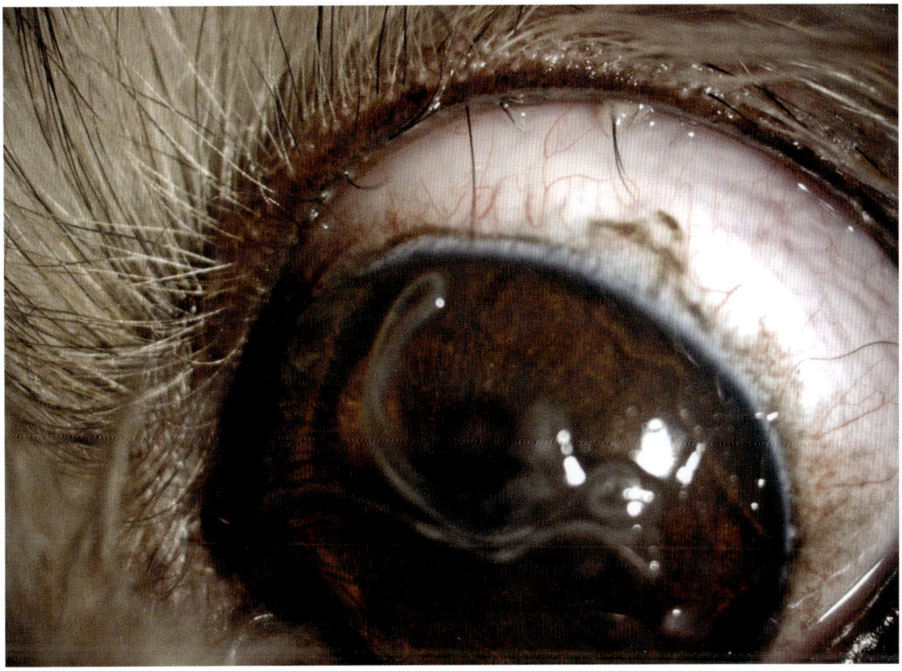

Shih-Tzu with districhiasis of the upper eyelid.

i This is essentially the same disorder as distichiasis, but in districhiasis, more than one hair grows out of the Meibomian gland duct.

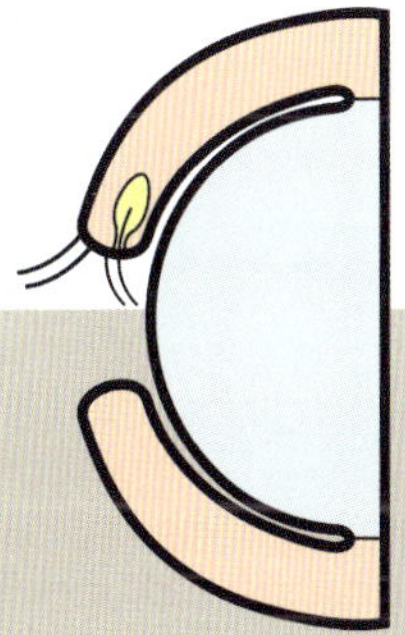

Districhiasis.

Treatment consists of manual depilation, electrodepilation, or surgery. It depends on the number of hairs and patient cooperation.

Ectopic cilia

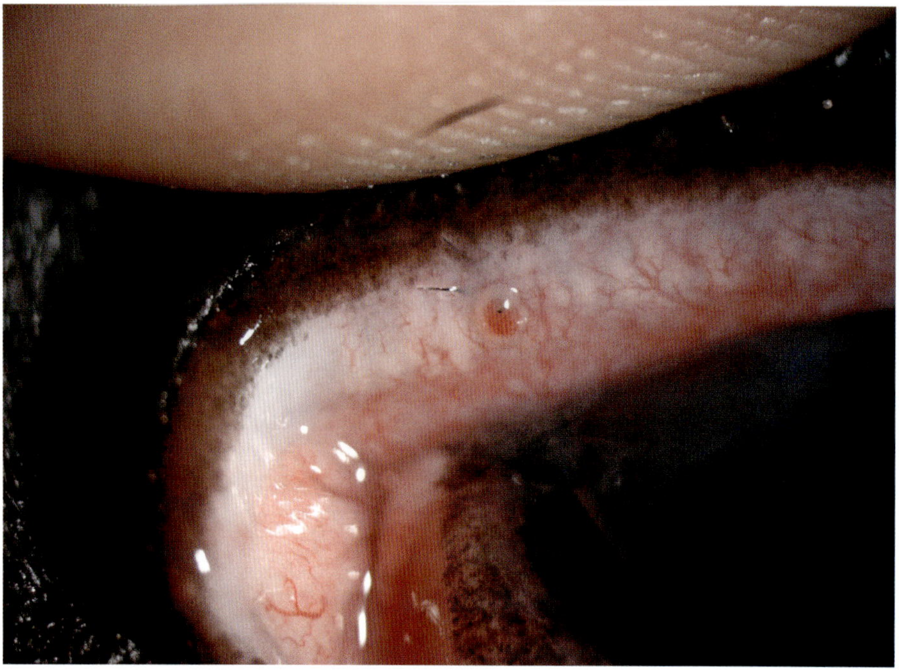

French Bulldog with ectopic cilia of the upper lid.

It involves hairs emerging from hair follicles located inside the Meibomian glands or within the palpebral conjunctiva. Instead of growing from the glandular excretory duct, they grow through the conjunctiva and towards the cornea.

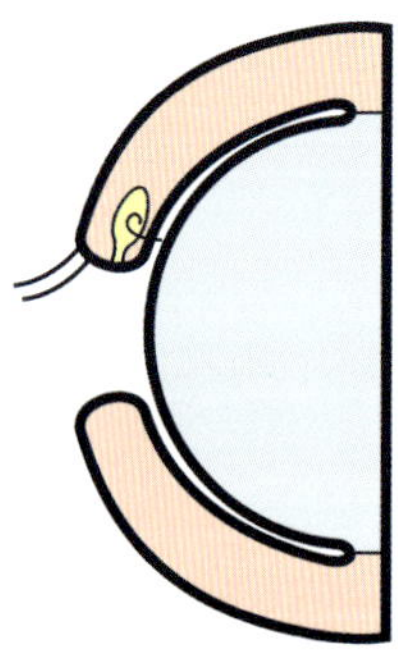

Ectopic cilium.

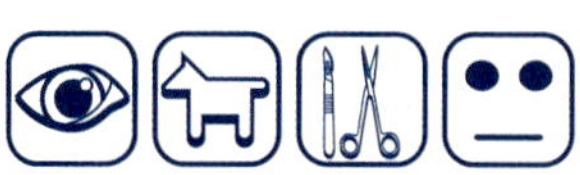

Ectopic cilia

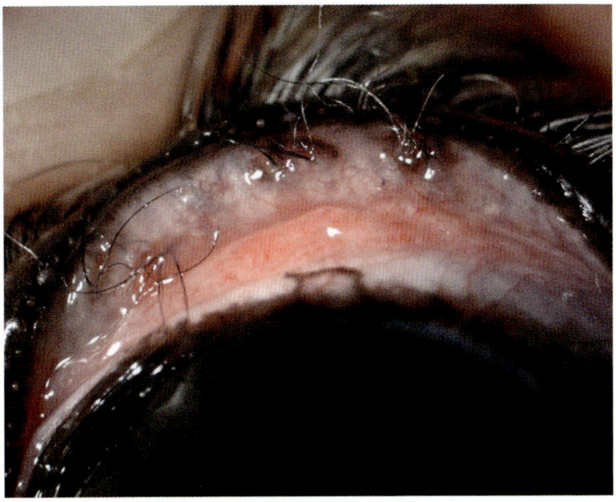

One-year-old Shih-Tzu with several ectopic cilia coming through the upper palpebral conjunctiva.

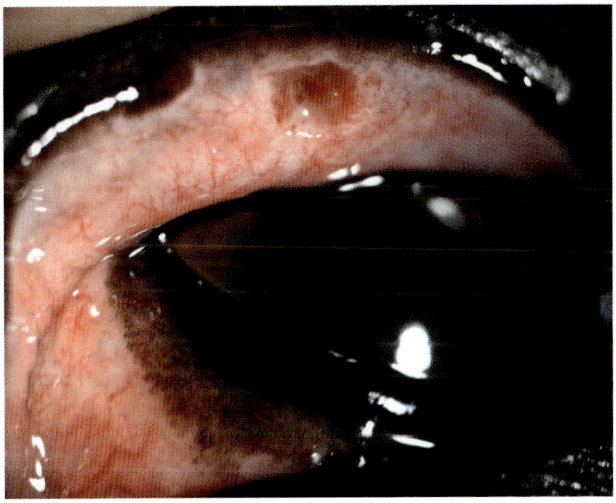

Patient from the previous page after removal of the Meibomian gland from which the hair was growing.

Important notes

- Evert the eyelid well and scan within 4 mm of the palpebral margin.
- It occurs more frequently in the upper eyelid.
- Different Meibomian glands may be affected at various times in the patient's life.

Trichiasis

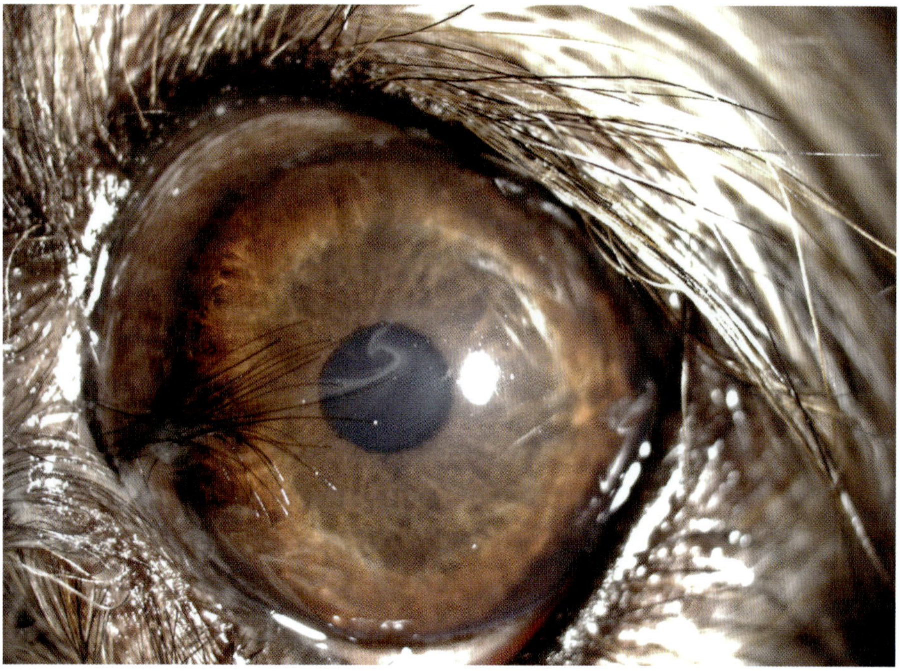

Trichiasis in a 10-month-old Lhasa Apso, with hairs growing towards the cornea from the lacrimal caruncle.

Hairs that grow from a normal location but are directed towards the cornea or conjunctiva, causing lesions of variable severity.

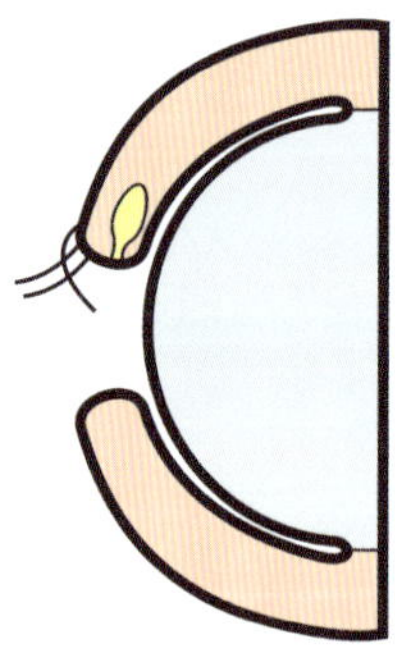

Trichiasis.

Trichiasis

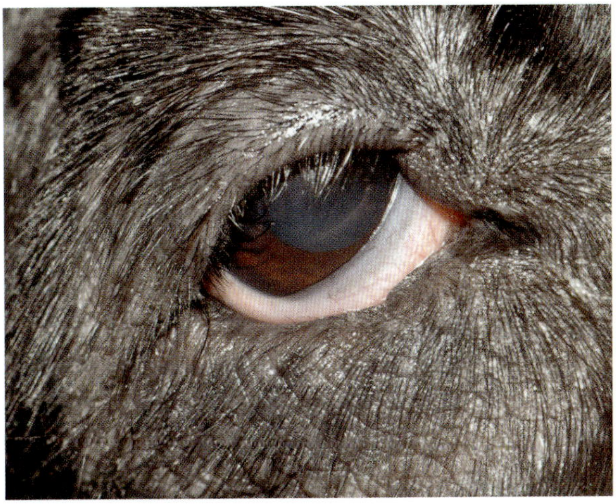

Trichiasis in an 11-year-old English Cocker Spaniel. In this case, the eyelashes, which emerge from their normal location, grow towards the cornea. Blepharitis also occurs due to the excess humidity.

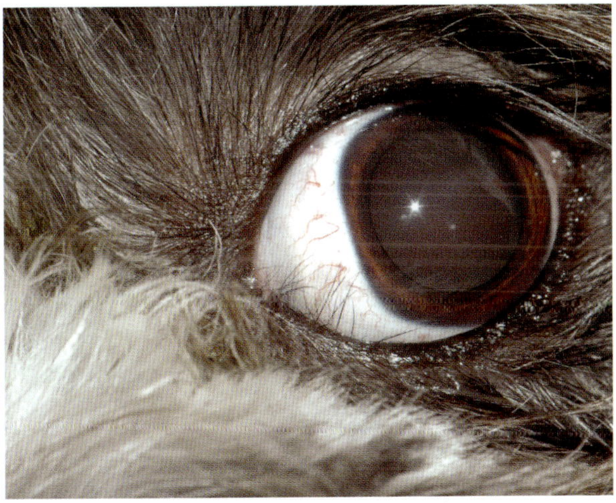

Trichiasis of hairs growing from the face towards the cornea in a two-year-old Lhasa Apso.

Considerations

- Hairs growing towards the cornea must be redirected to avoid keratitis; this can be done manually or by surgical correction (nasal fold resection, entropion surgery, or lacrimal caruncle excision).

Trichomegaly

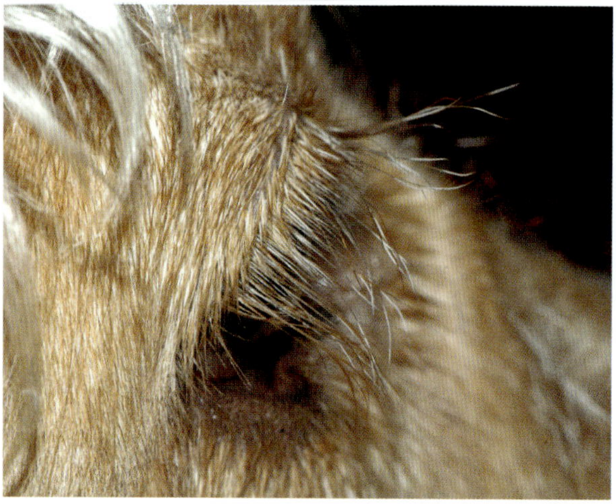

Seven-year-old Cocker Spaniel with trichomegaly.

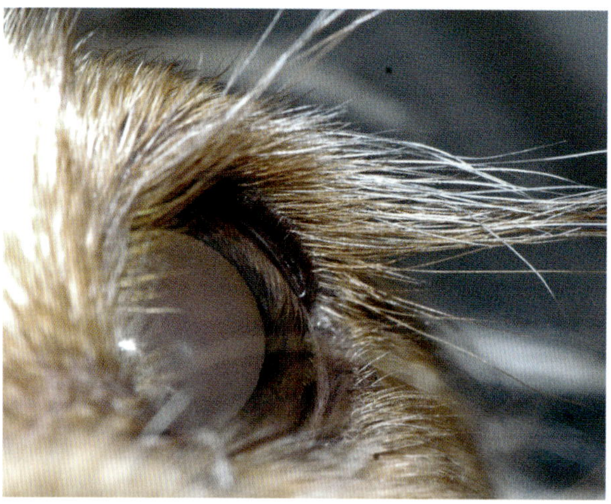

Close-up of the eyelash length in an English Cocker Spaniel.

i

Extremely long eyelashes growing from their normal position.

Physiological condition limited almost entirely to the Cocker Spaniel.

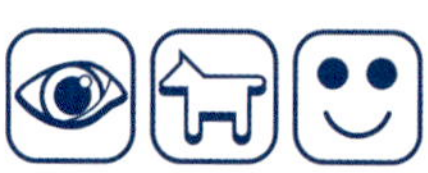

Palpebral ptosis

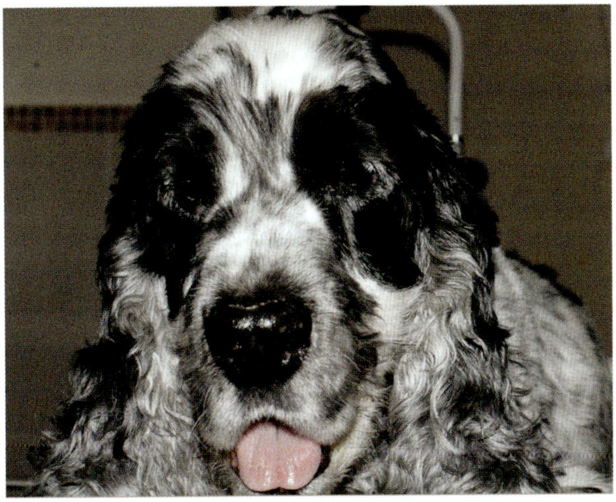

Bilateral palpebral ptosis in a 13 year-old English Cocker Spaniel.

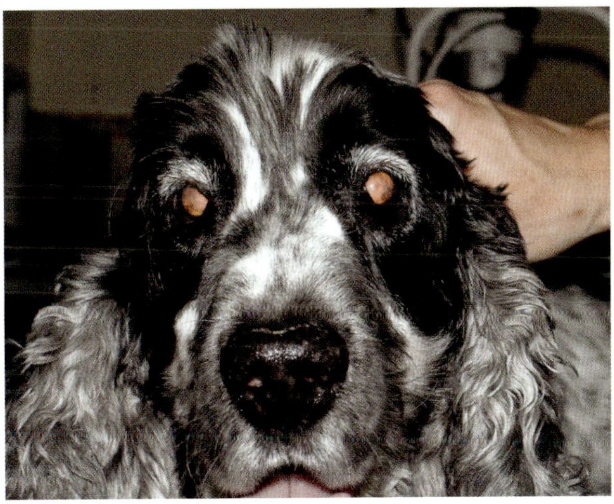

Facial positioning that reveals the physiological position of the patient's eyelids.

i | Droop of the upper eyelid onto the globe. It may be associated with a loss of skin elasticity (pictures above) or neurological problems (Horner's syndrome).

Palpebral ptosis

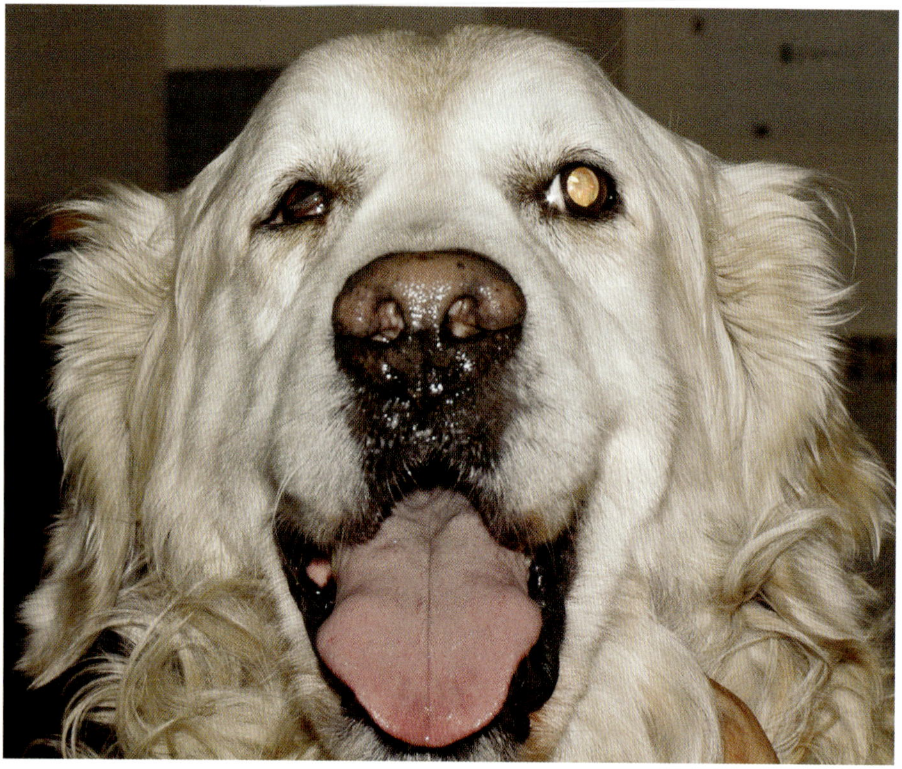

Palpebral ptosis in a Golden Retriever with Horner's syndrome. The drooping upper eyelid and protruding nictitating membrane limit the patient's vision.

Important notes

- In Horner's syndrome, palpebral ptosis is due to a sympathetic nervous system dysfunction and is accompanied by miosis (main sign), protrusion of the nictitating membrane, and enophthalmos.
- Any disorder or disturbance to the central, pre-, or postganglionic neurons may induce this syndrome. These lead to primary, secondary, and tertiary Horner's syndrome, respectively.

Lagophthalmos

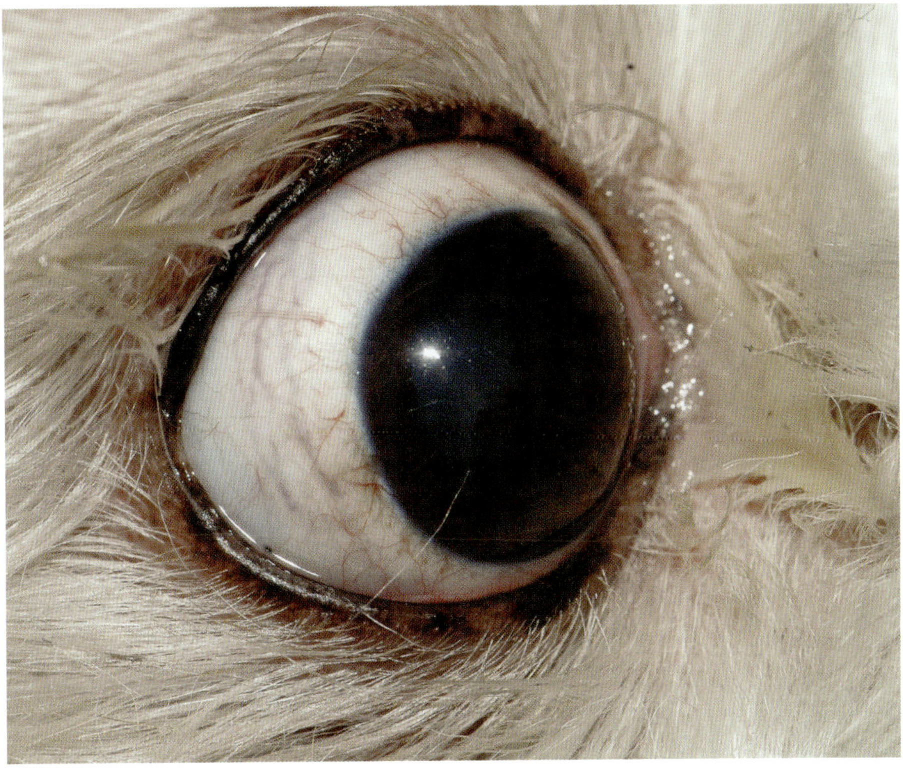

Two-year-old Shih-Tzu with lagophthalmos. Close-up of excessive ocular exposure and chronic corneal damage.

Impossible to close eyelids physiologically.
This carries a risk of increased exposure of the eye surface and thus a predisposition to keratitis and conjunctivitis.

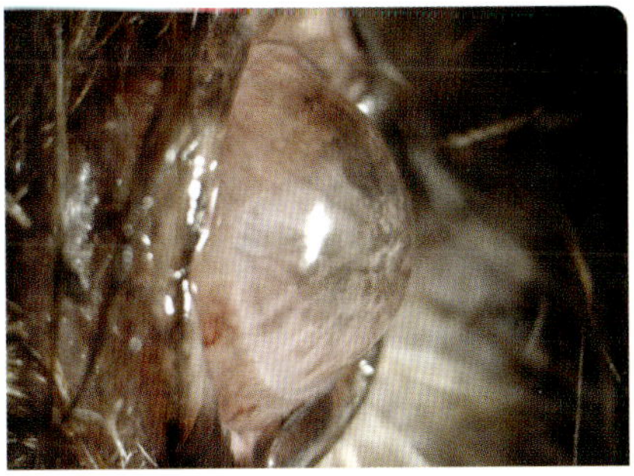

Changes in the shape of the eyeball can also cause lagophthalmos.
Patient with keratoconus.

Chalazion

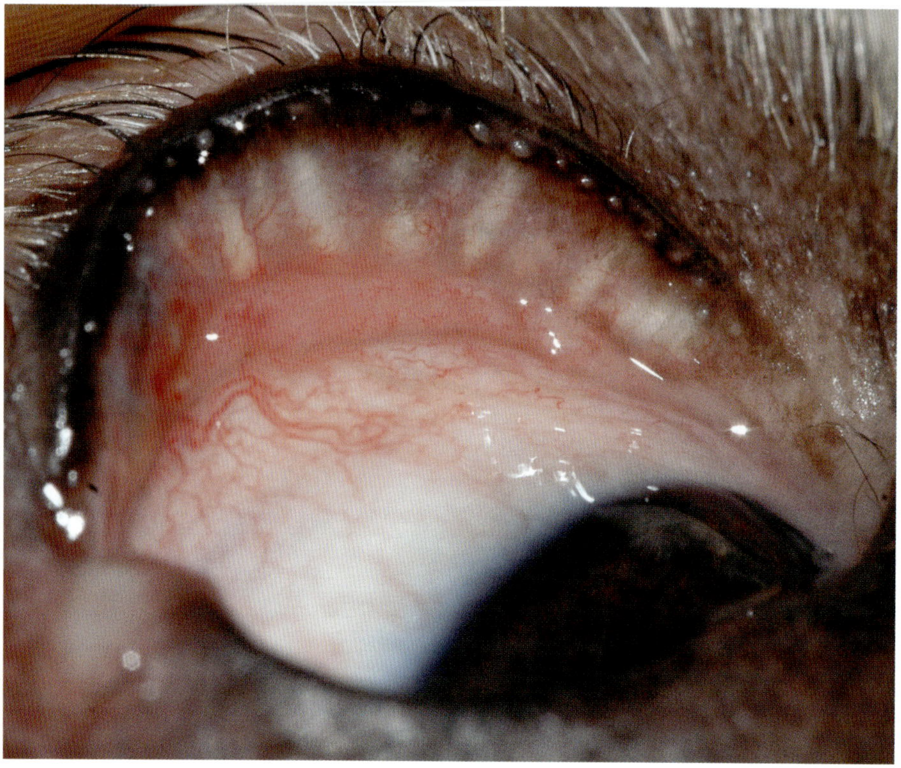

Three-year-old Bichon Maltese with chalazion.

i

Chronic inflammation of one or more Meibomian glands. This is a lipogranuloma.

It often presents as a whitish lesion corresponding to the affected gland.

Interesting notes

- Acute inflammation is known as meibomitis.
- It often recedes with antibiotic and anti-inflammatory treatment.

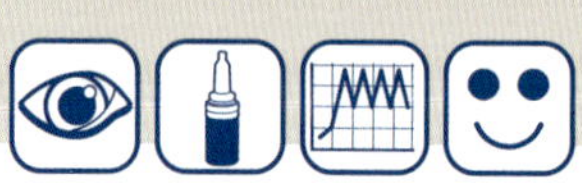

Hordeolum

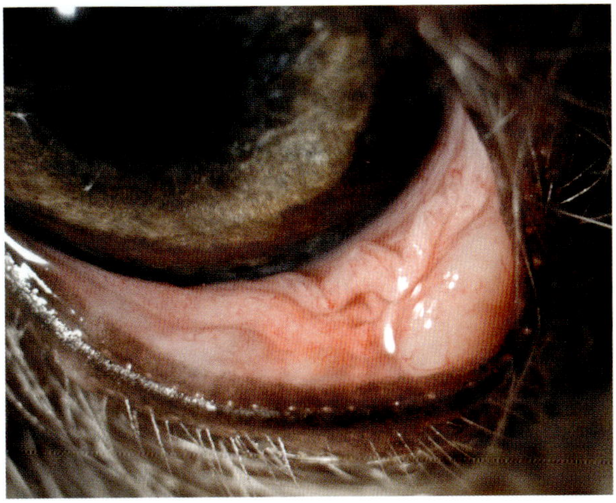

Three-year-old Shih-Tzu with internal hordeolum.

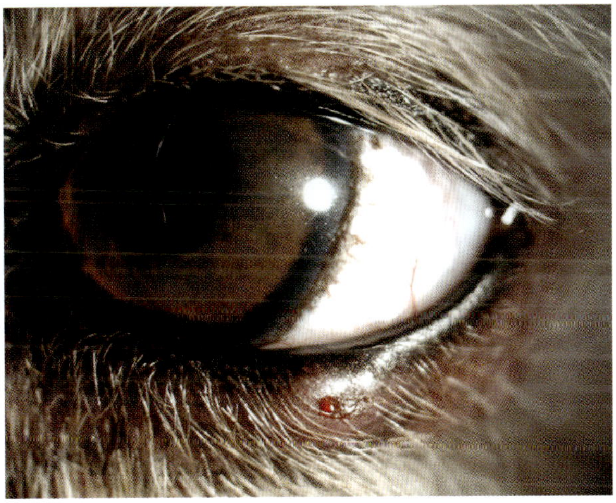

External hordeolum in a nine-year-old Poodle.

i | Internal hordeolum is considered a Meibomian gland infection, while external hordeolum tends to affect the glands of Zeis or Moll.

Lentigo

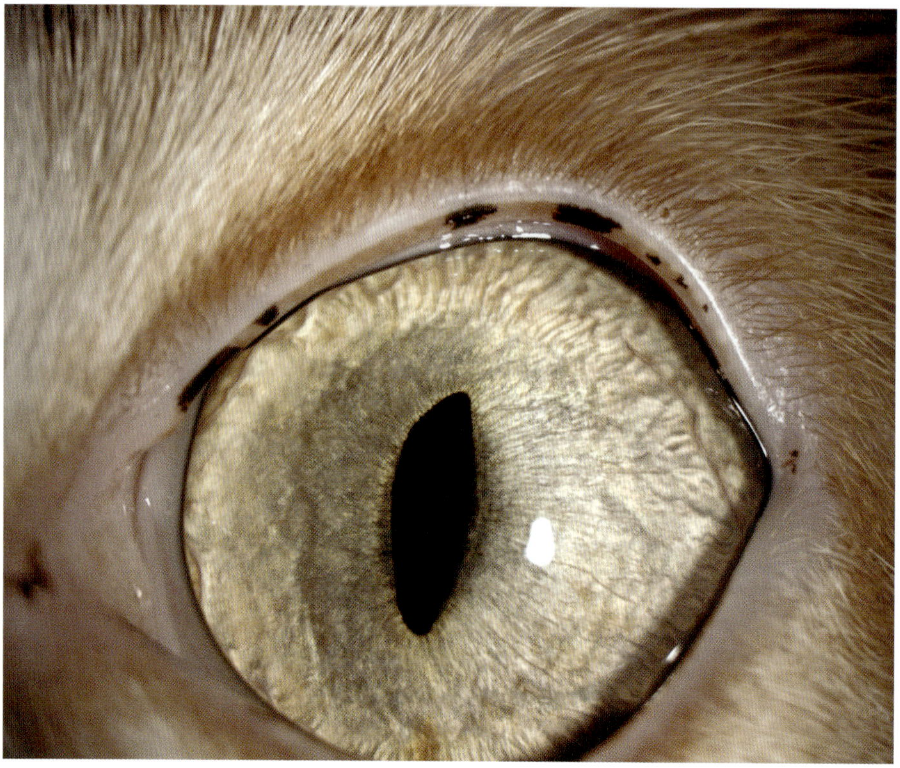

Sixteen-year-old domestic cat with lentigo of the palpebral margin.

This is an asymptomatic disease characterised by pigmented areas or spots 1–10 mm long. In cats, they may appear on the palpebral margin or the lips.

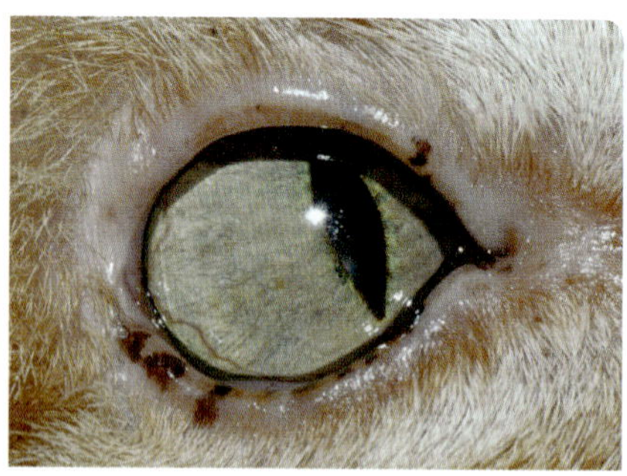

Right eye of a domestic cat with an orange coat and lentigo in both eyelids.

Foreign bodies

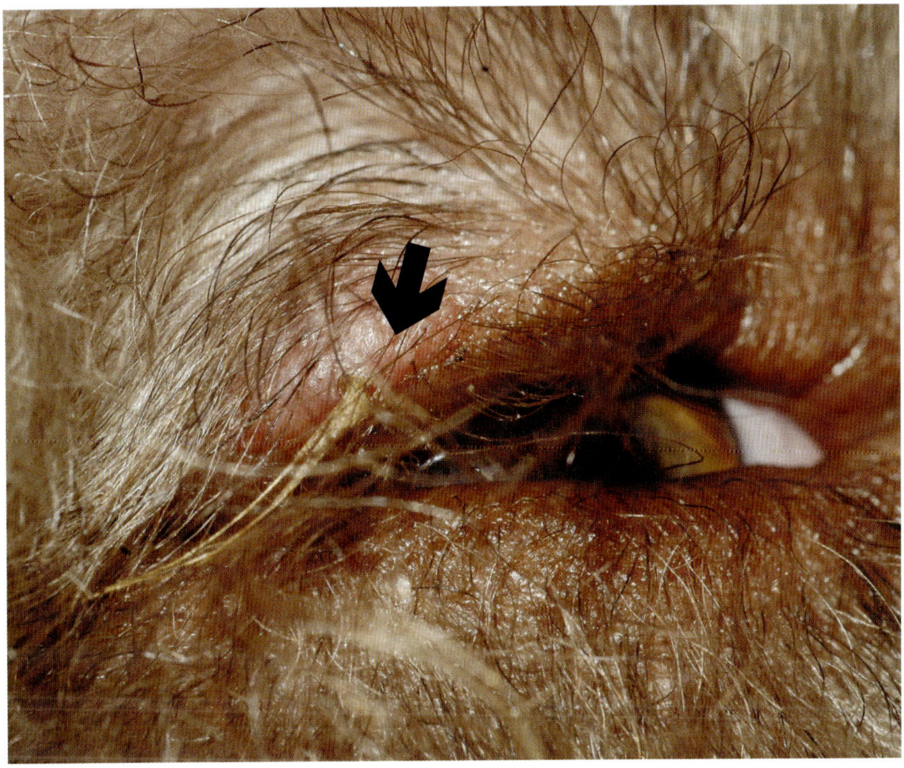

Four-year-old hound with a grass awn embedded in the upper lid after a day of hunting. Close-up of the palpebral inflammation.
Time since injury: three days.

Treatment

Manual removal with tweezers and antibiotics.

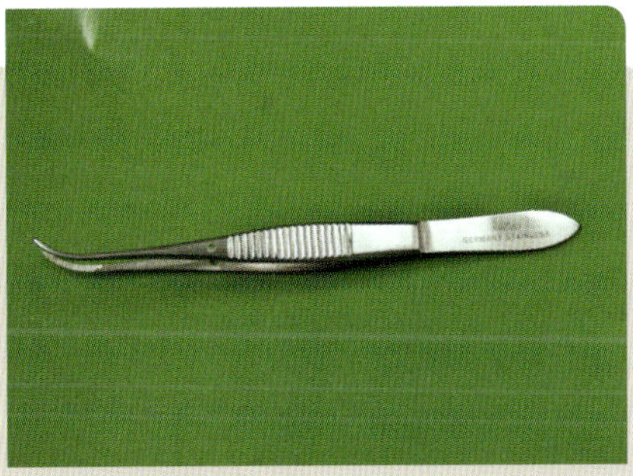

Nictitating membrane

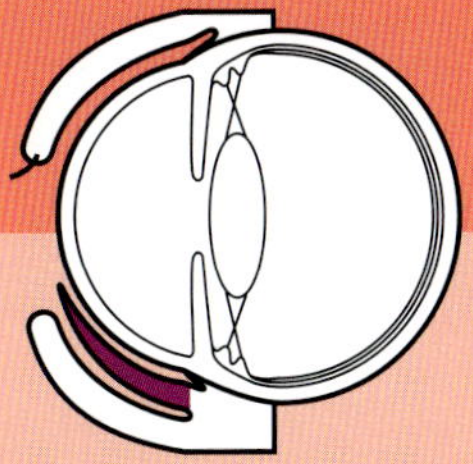

Prolapse of the nictitating membrane gland

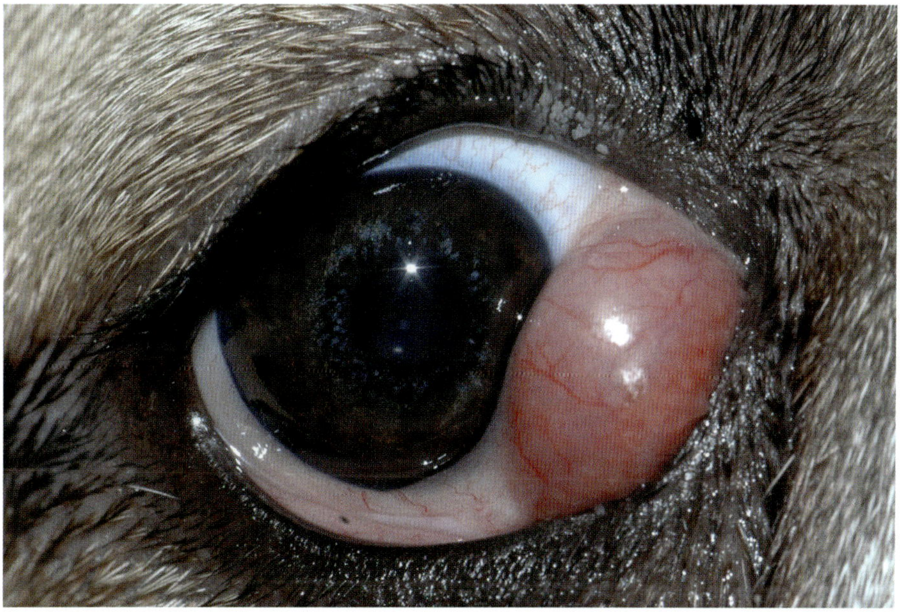

Prolapse of the nictitating membrane gland (NMG).

This is a luxation of the NMG (also called "cherry eye").

It appears to be due to laxity of the connective tissue that anchors the gland inside the orbit.

Glandular hyperplasia can contribute to the condition.

Breed predisposition

The most predisposed breeds are the English Bulldog, Shar Pei, Shih-Tzu, Beagle, Pekingese, Neapolitan Mastiff, and Boxer (among others).

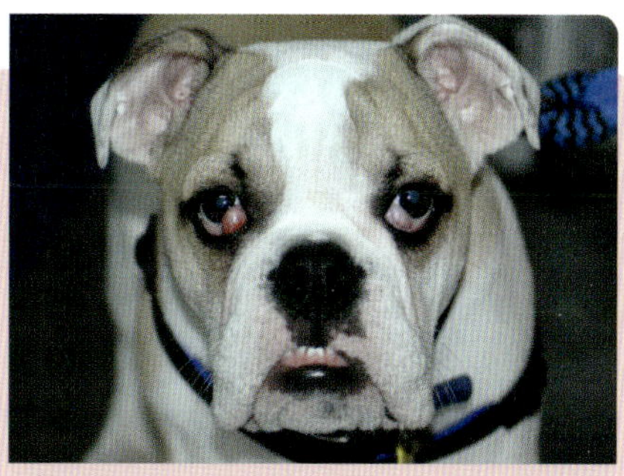

Three-month-old English Bulldog with bilateral prolapse of the NMG.

Prolapse of the nictitating membrane gland

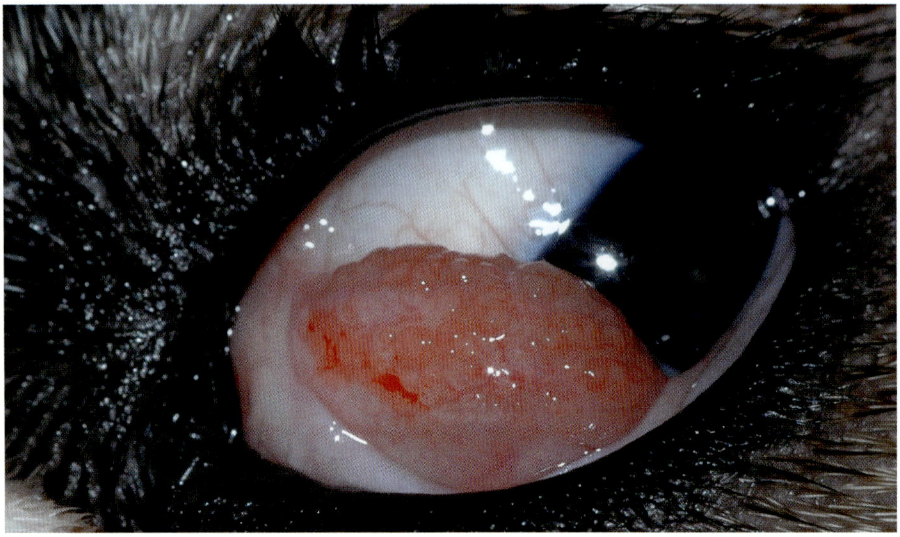

Follicular hyperplasia and conjunctival hyperaemia in a prolapsed NMG after two months.

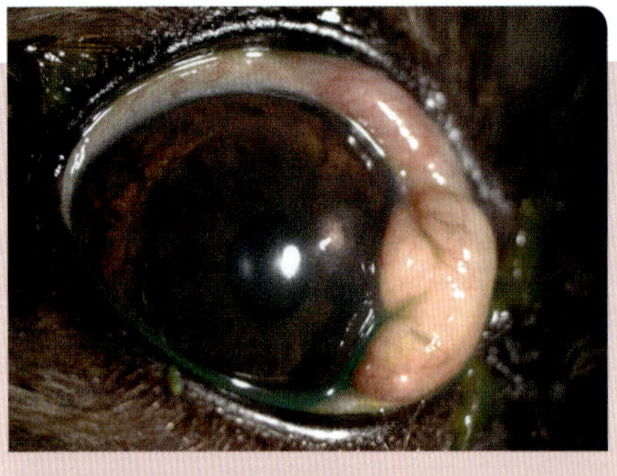

Partial excision of the NMG.

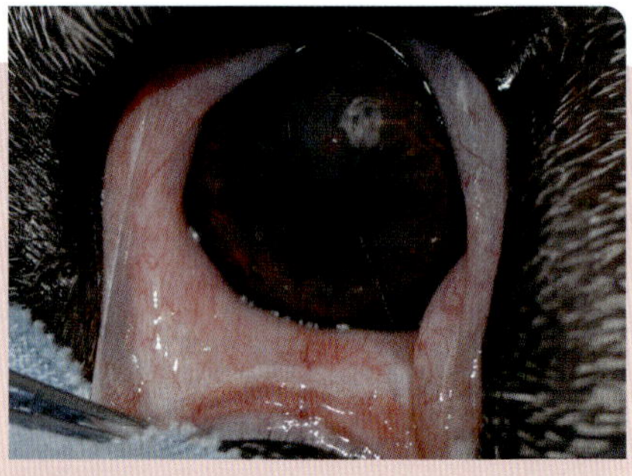

Scar characteristic of complete excision of the NMG in an English Bulldog.

Surgical treatment

Surgical repositioning of the NMG should be performed promptly to avoid glandular damage.
The Morgan pocket technique is recommended.

Contraindicated

Never fully excise the NMG (except in cases of neoplasm) due to the risk of inducing an iatrogenic keratoconjunctivitis sicca.

Prolapse of the nictitating membrane gland

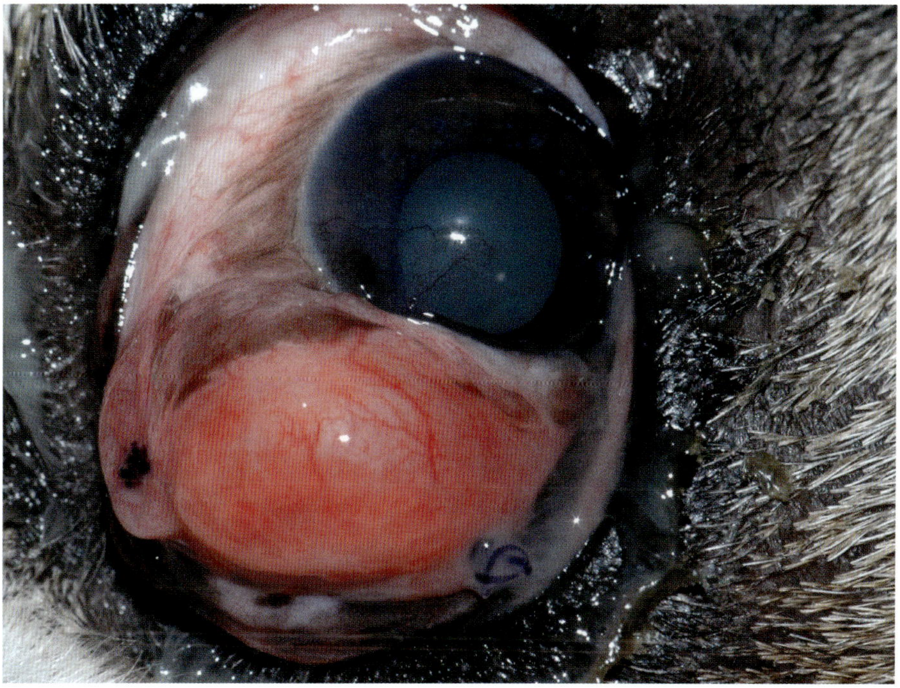

Recurrence. NMG luxation, seven days postoperatively. Note the suture knots.

Complications

The risk of recurrence is minimised by creating a deep pocket with small suture in a simple continuous pattern.

Contraindicated

The ends MUST NOT rub on the cornea due to RISK OF PERFORATION! (They must be buried or transfixion sutures.)

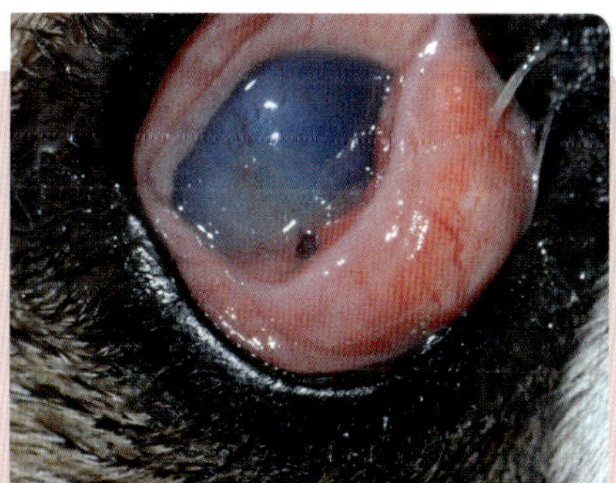

Severe corneal damage caused by sutures rubbing on the cornea.

Prolapse of the nictitating membrane gland

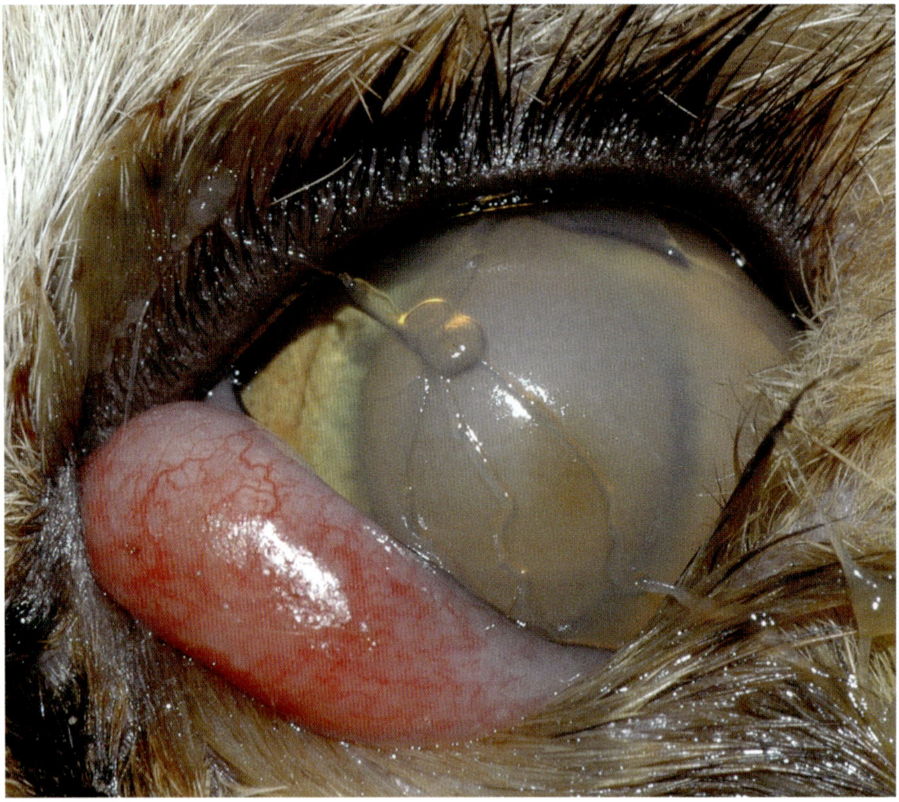

Prolapsed NMG in a six-month-old Persian cat. Note the associated entropion and extensive corneal ulcer.

i

NMG luxation is less common in cats than in dogs.

It has been described in Persian, Siamese, and Burmese cats.

It may be associated with viral conjunctivitis.

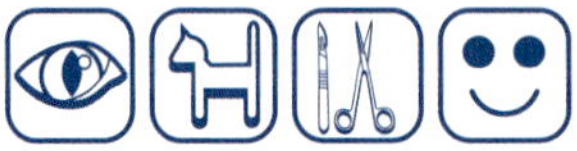

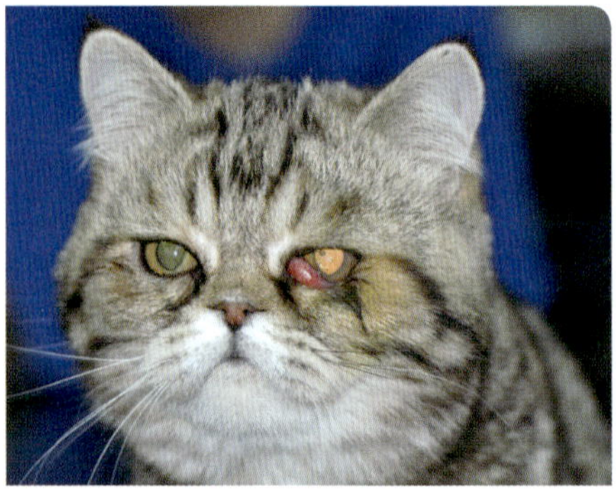

Patient pictured above.

Cartilage eversion

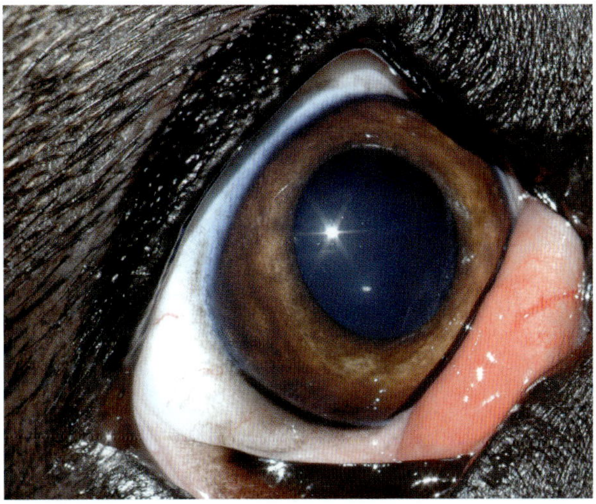

Cartilage eversion of the nictitating membrane in a six-month-old Great Dane.

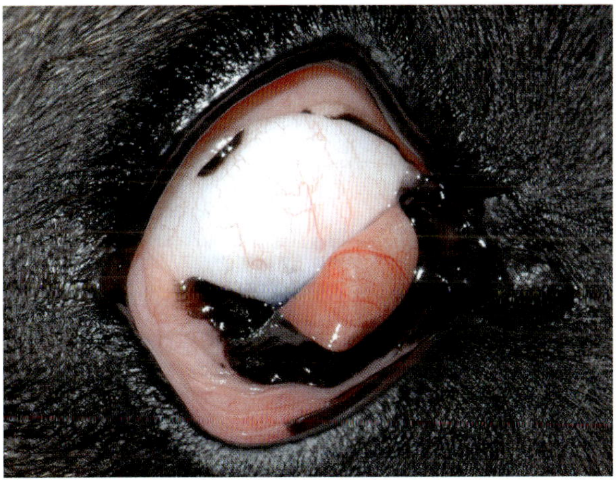

Close-up of cartilage eversion preoperatively.

This is an outward rolling of the vertical part of the cartilage. It alters the physiological position of the free edge of the nictitating membrane. In certain cases, it may roll inwards (inversion).

Important notes

- Do not confuse with a prolapsed nictitating membrane gland.
- More common in young animals.

Cartilage eversion

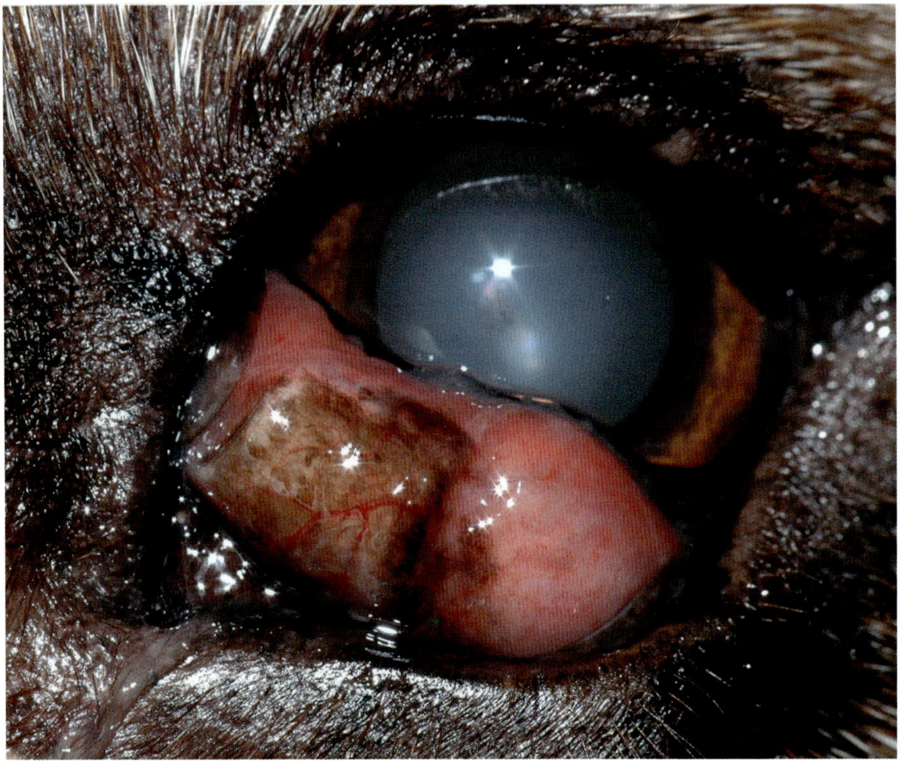

Nine-year-old Irish Setter with cartilage eversion of the nictitating membrane (NM) since four months of age. Chronic exposure of the internal conjunctiva of the NM is confirmed by melanin deposition.

Breed predisposition

The most predisposed breeds are the Great Dane, Neapolitan Mastiff, Shar Pei, Saint Bernard, and Weimaraner.

Cartilage eversion

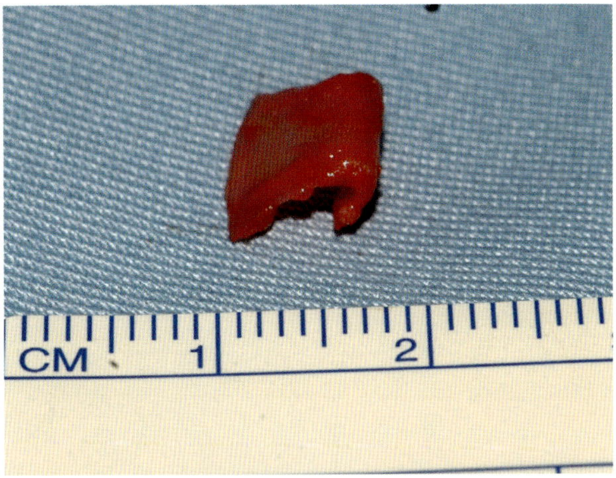

Portion of affected cartilage from the patient above. Close-up of the scrolled cartilage.

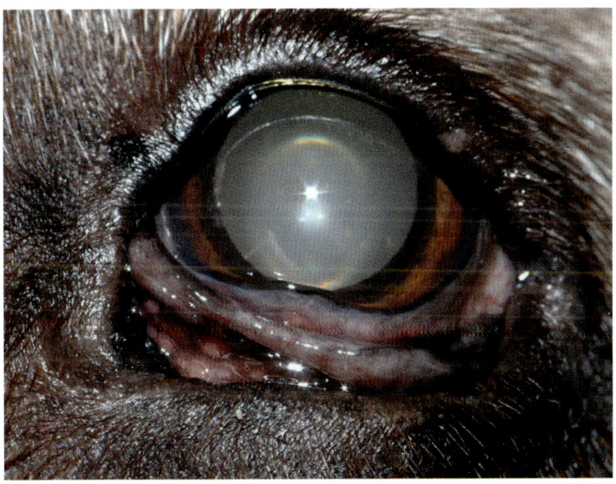

Physiological position of the nictitating membrane once the eversion is corrected.

Surgical technique

- Approach the cartilage via the internal surface of the nictitating membrane.
- Do NOT suture the surgical defect.

Plasmoma

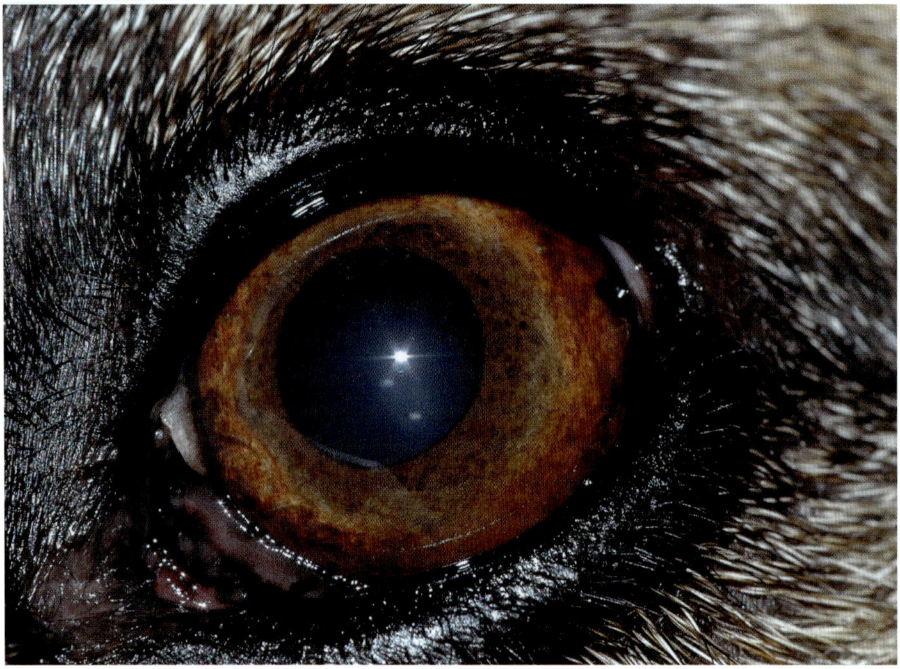

Plasmoma in a five-year-old German Shepherd. Note the prominent areas of depigmentation on the external surface of the NM.

Lymphoplasmacytic infiltration of the NM.

Important notes

- Immune-mediated.

Breed predisposition

- Mainly described in the German Shepherd, Belgian Tervuren, and mixes of these breeds.

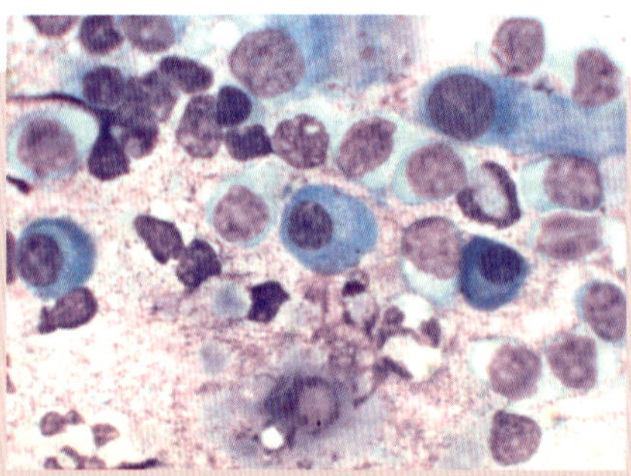

Lymphoplasmacytic infiltration (100× immersion). Image courtesy of Cristina Fernández Algarra.

Plasmoma

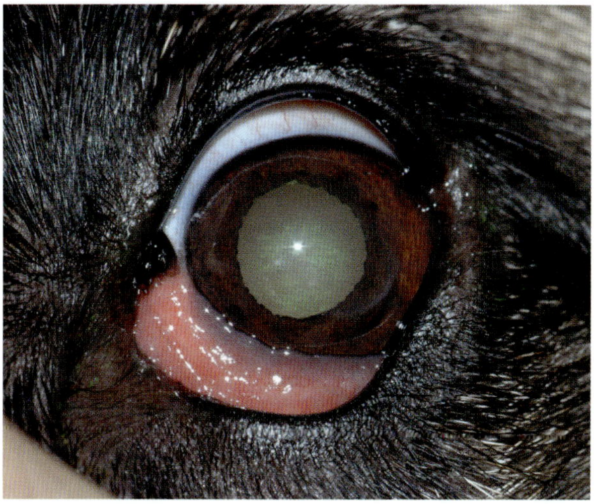

Lymphoplasmacytic infiltration in a five-year-old German Shepherd.
Close-up of the depigmentation and severe inflammation.

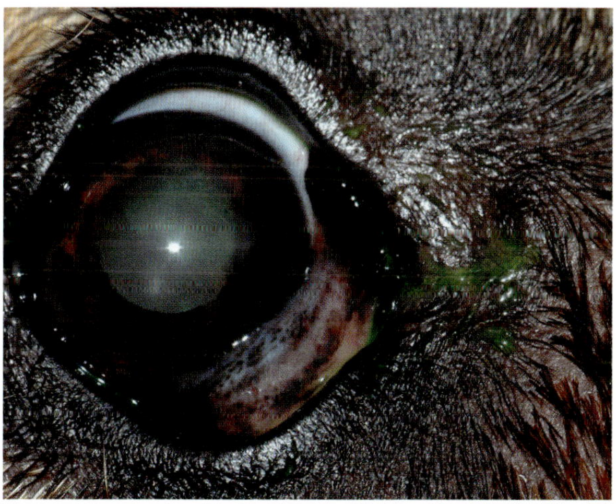

Seven-year-old German Shepherd with plasmoma. Note the rough external surface of the NM and the depigmentation.

Treatment

- Medical treatment is based on the use of topical corticosteroids (dexamethasone) and topical cyclosporine.
- Treatment should be long-term because recurrence is common.

Plasmoma

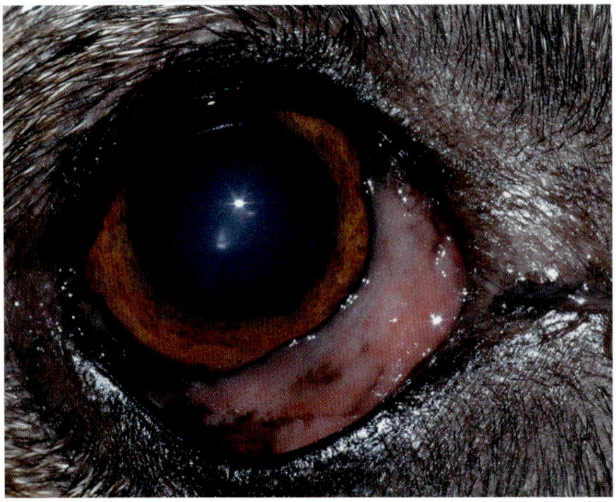

Plasmoma in a four-year-old German Shepherd.

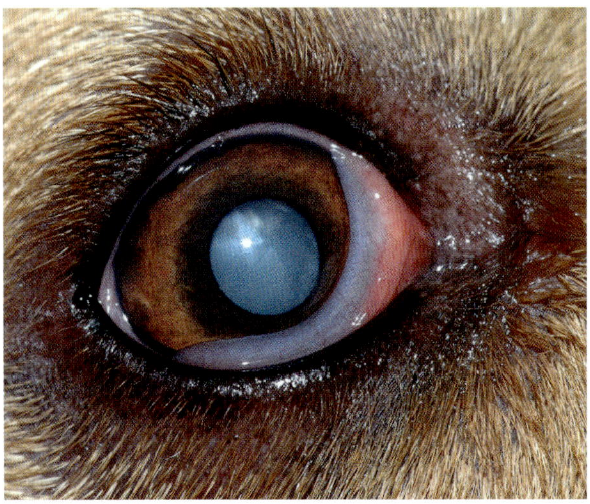

Depigmentation of the free edge of the NM in a two-year-old Beagle.

Important notes

DO NOT CONFUSE lymphoplasmacytic infiltration with depigmentation of the free edge of the NM.

Follicular conjunctivitis

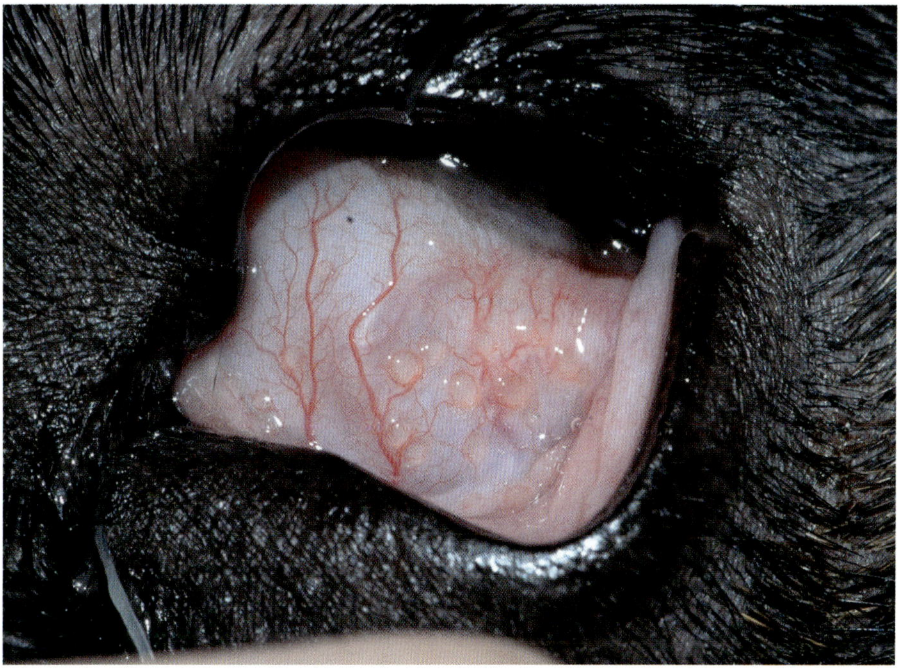

Follicular conjunctivitis in a 10-month-old Boxer.

Conjunctival inflammation accompanied by lymphoid follicle hyperplasia. This can affect both the internal and external surfaces of the nictitating membrane.

Prior antigenic stimulation is required for this condition to develop.

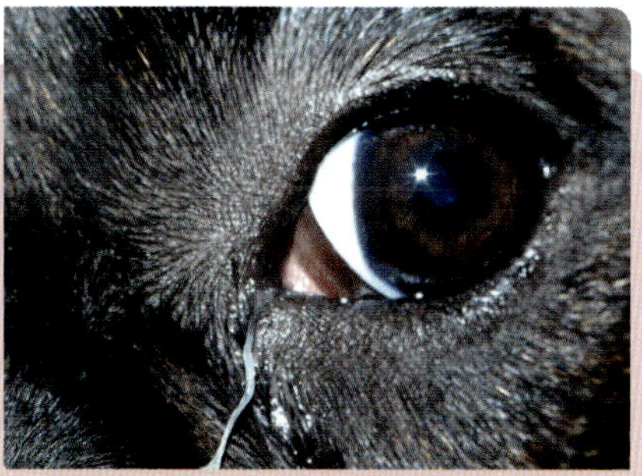

Patient pictured above. Follicular conjunctivitis is generally accompanied by a mucoid ocular discharge.

Follicular conjunctivitis

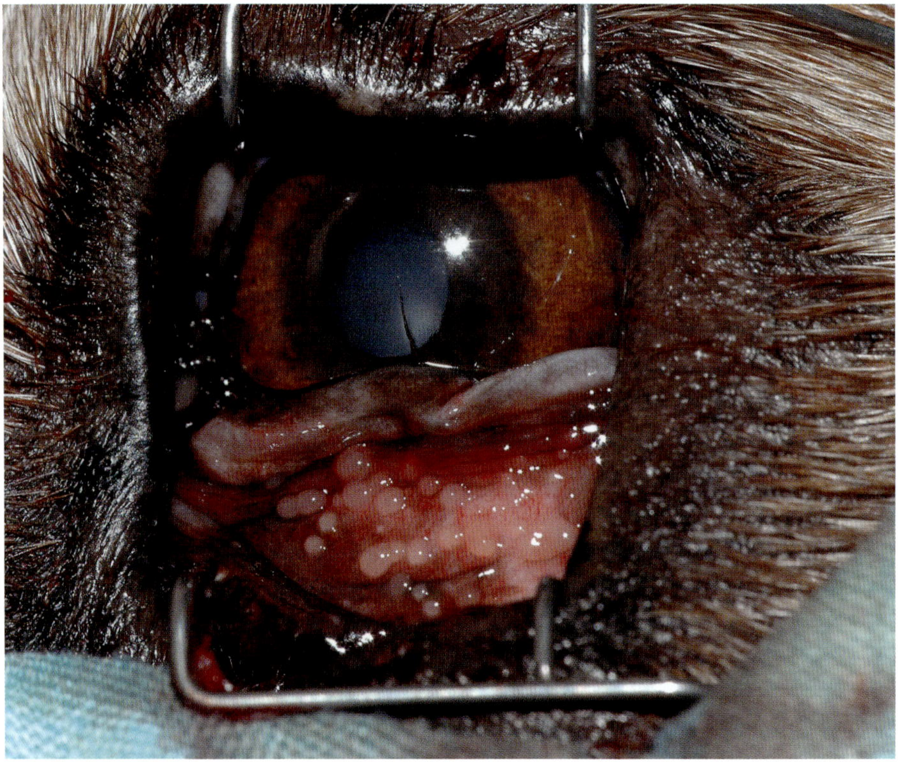

Follicular conjunctivitis. Close-up of the hyperplastic lymphoid follicles.

Treatment

- Topical corticosteroids can be used in mild cases.
- A follicle scraping and medical treatment are recommended in severe cases.

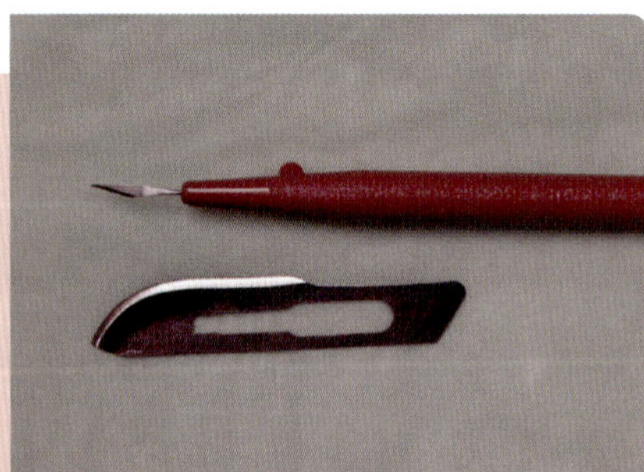

Scalpel blade and slit knife.

Leishmania-induced granulomas

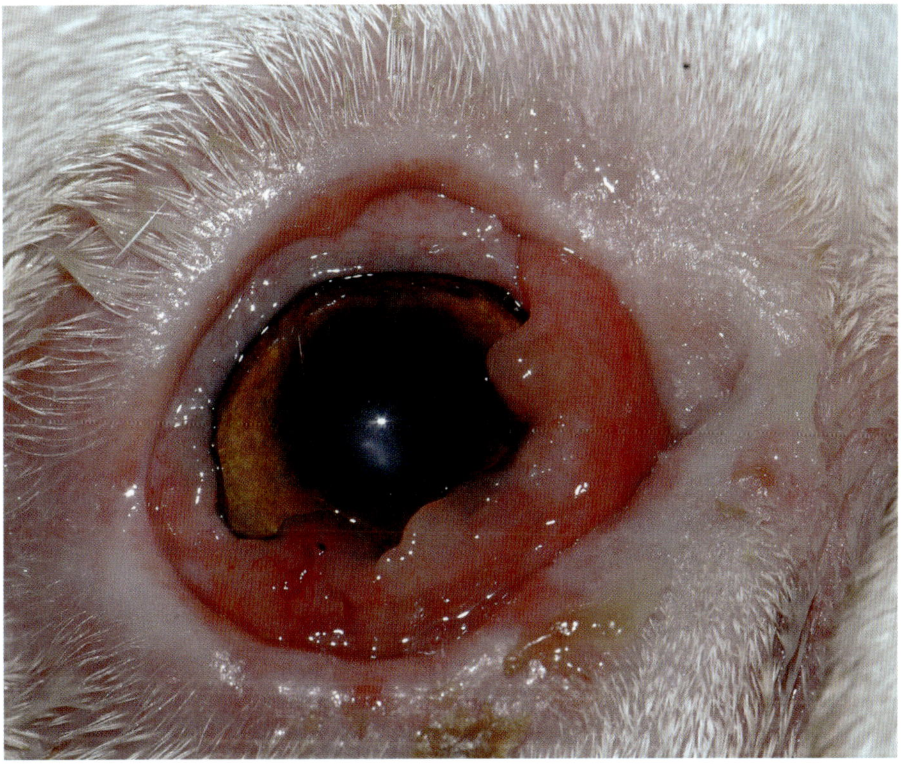

Lesions of the nictitating membrane caused by *Leishmania* in a white Boxer. Close-up of the granulomas on the nictitating membrane and the eyelids.

Interesting notes

Consider cytology and/or biopsy of the conjunctiva in these cases.

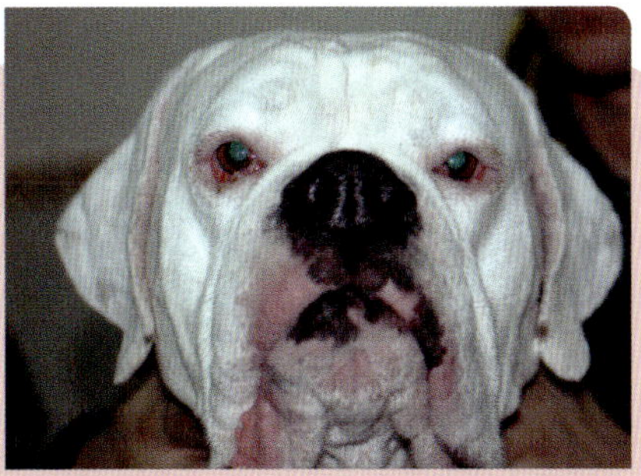

Patient pictured above. Bilateral lesion.

Lacerations/tears

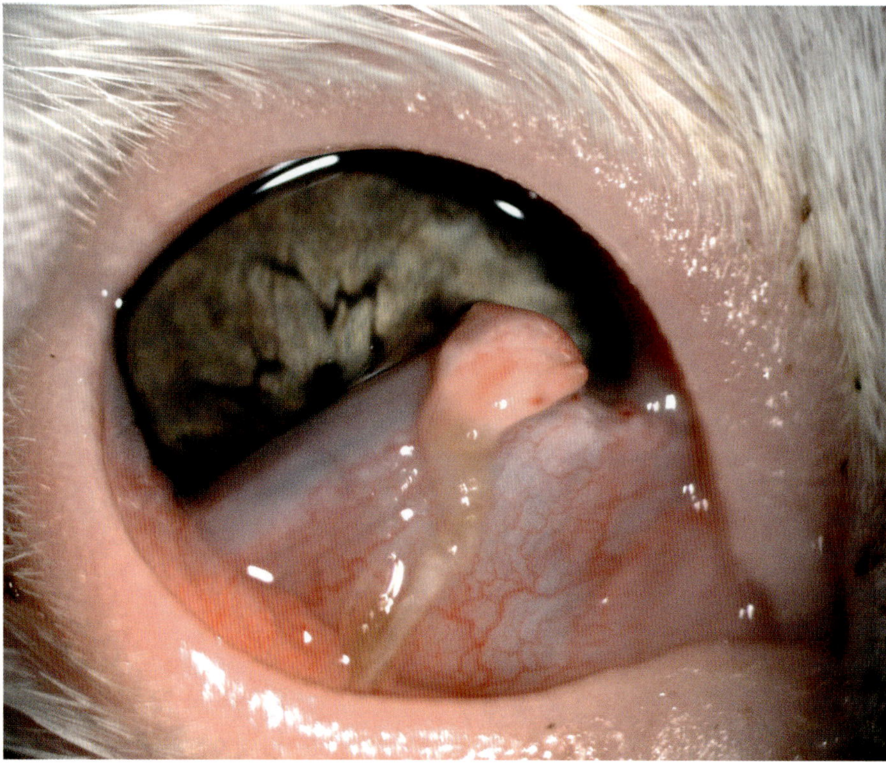

Tear in a cat's nictitating membrane caused by a scratch from another cat during a fight.

i These are acute injuries that require a detailed examination of the other ocular structures, since they are sometimes accompanied by corneal perforations.

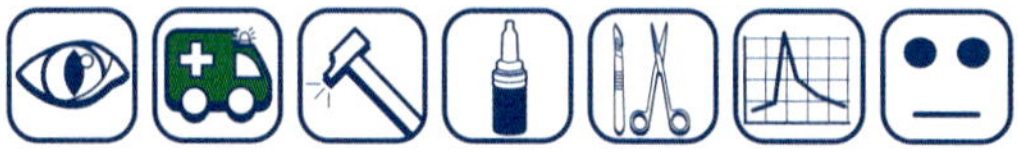

Lacerations/tears

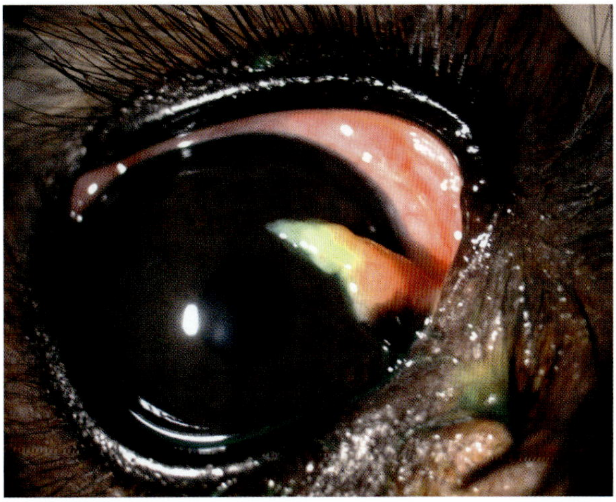

Laceration of the nictitating membrane in a two-year-old Yorkshire Terrier after a fight with a cat.

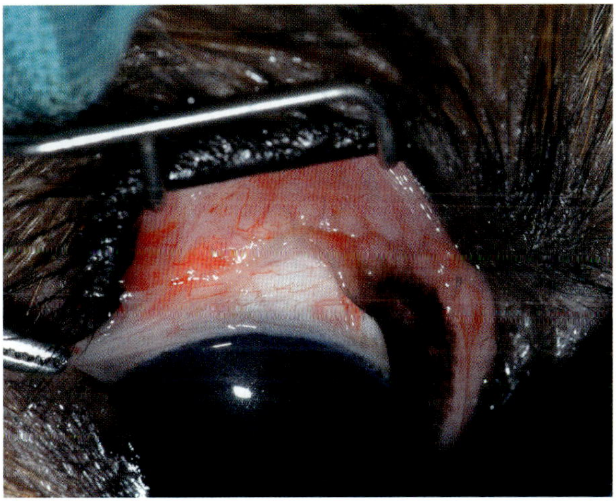

Surgical reconstruction of the free edge of the nictitating membrane of this patient.

Surgical technique

- If the laceration affects the nictitating membrane cartilage, and thus its function, surgical reconstruction is advised.
- If the cartilage damage is not full-thickness, or in case of a mild conjunctival tear, surgery is not necessary.

Lacerations/tears

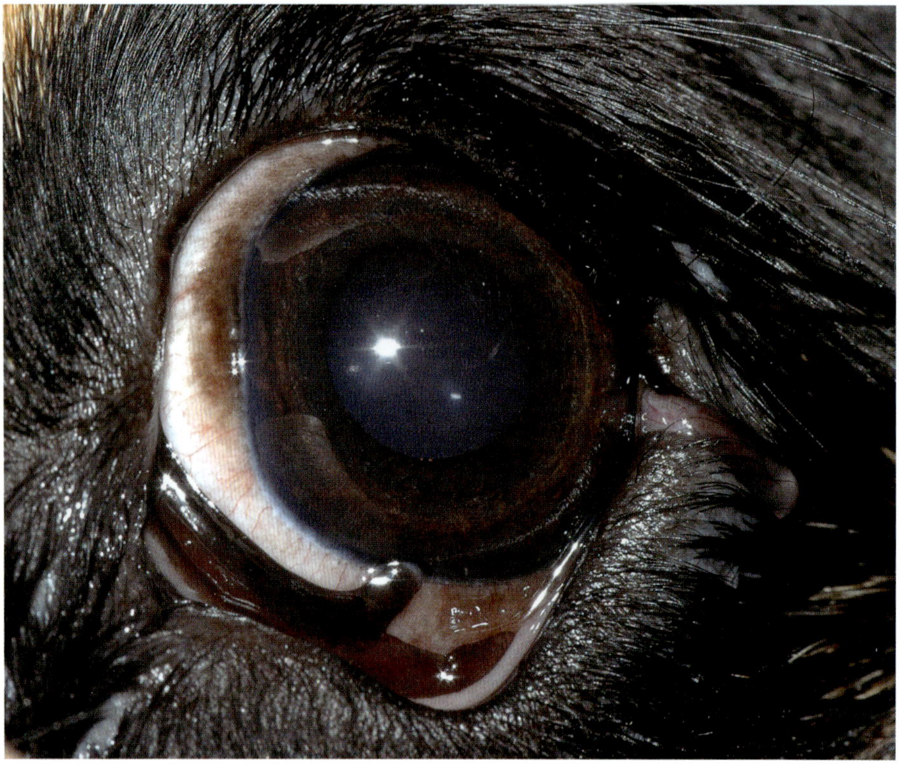

Mild laceration of the nictitating membrane in a dog.
Note the defect in the free edge of the NM. The wound has caused a partial loss of cartilaginous tissue without affecting the motion of the NM.
Cause: cat scratch.

- Lesion five days after it occurred.
- Surgery was not performed on the nictitating membrane. Only a small remnant of palpebral conjunctiva was removed from the lateral canthus area.

Protrusion of the nictitating membrane

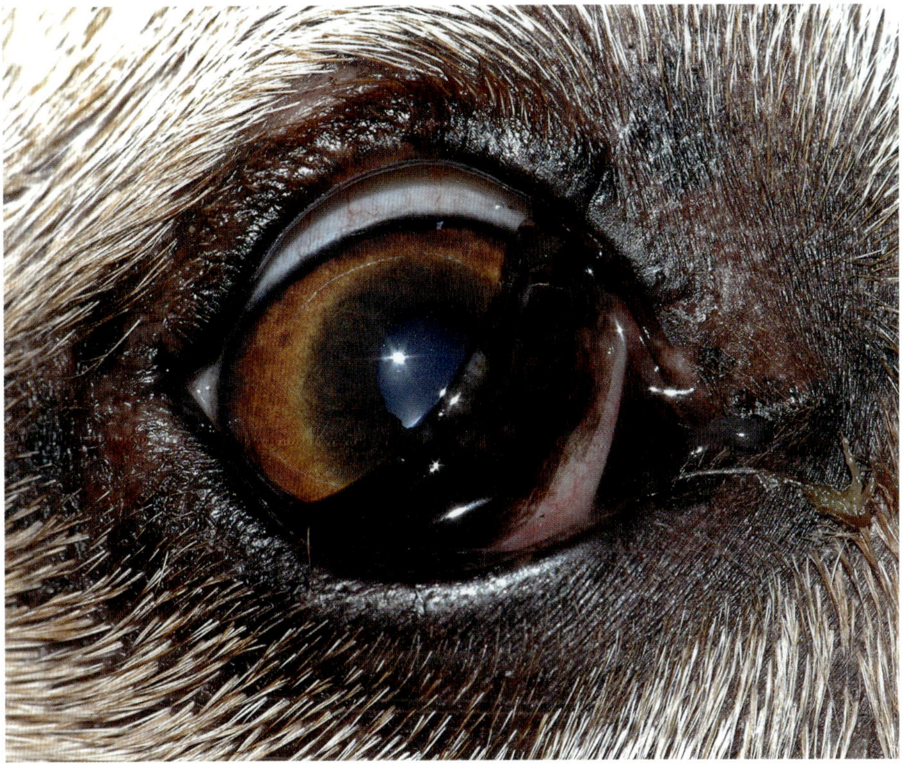

Unilateral protrusion of the nictitating membrane in a dog.

This is an upward displacement of the nictitating membrane, covering the cornea partly or fully.

It is also known as prolapse.

It may be unilateral or bilateral.

Protrusion of the nictitating membrane

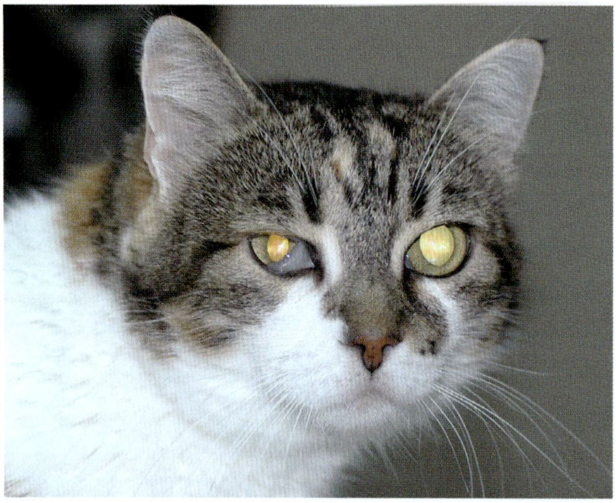

Cat with a protruding nictitating membrane due to Horner's syndrome.

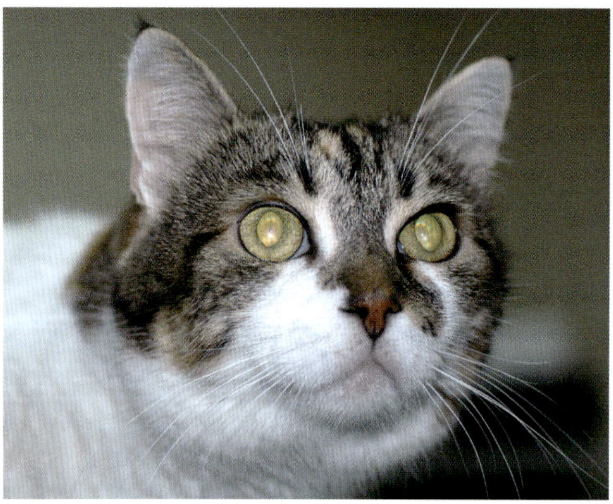

Patient pictured above after recovery.

i Horner's syndrome involves an interruption of the sympathetic innervation. The clinical signs noted include miosis, protrusion of the nictitating membrane, palpebral ptosis, and enophthalmos.

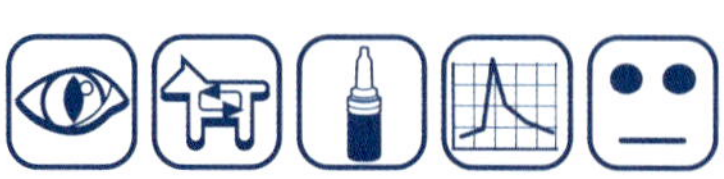

Protrusion of the nictitating membrane

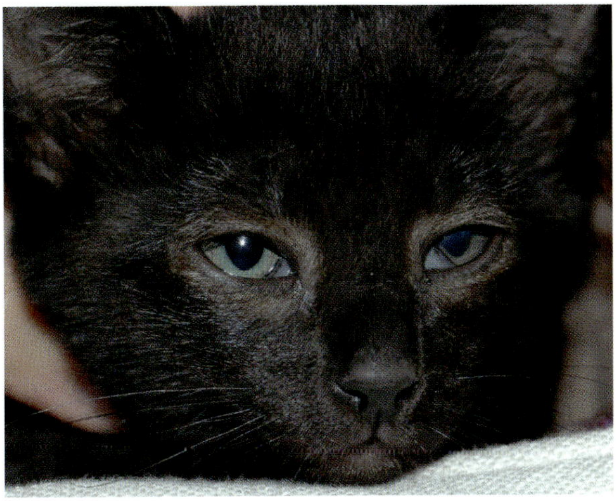

Bilateral protrusion of the nictitating membrane in a six-month-old kitten with haws syndrome.

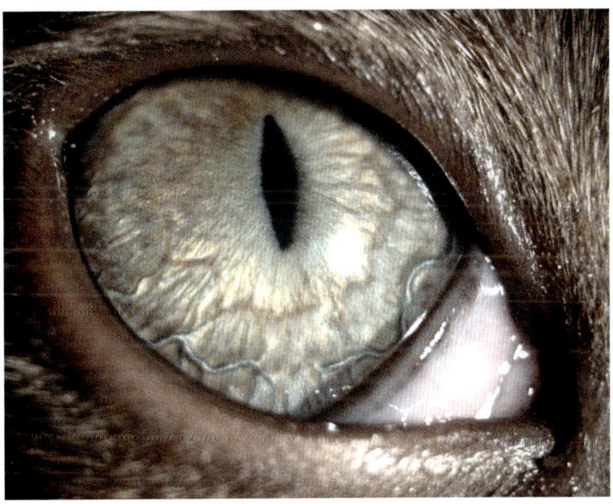

Close-up of the protrusion of the nictitating membrane of the patient's right eye.

Haws syndrome is caused by postganglionic sympathetic denervation and tends to affect young cats (under two years old). It generally resolves spontaneously.

Protrusion of the nictitating membrane

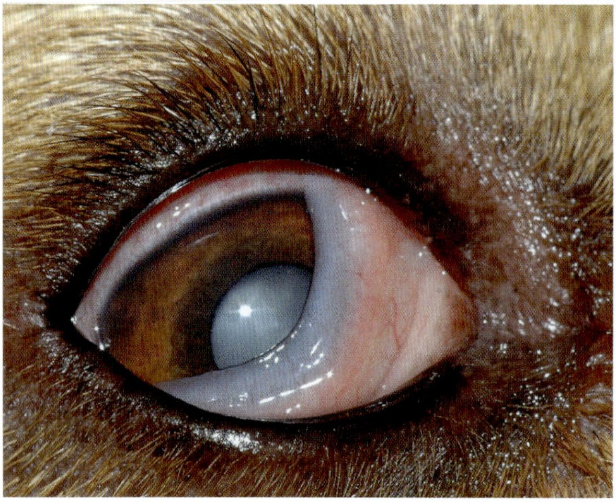

Protrusion of the nictitating membrane in a Beagle with lens-induced uveitis.

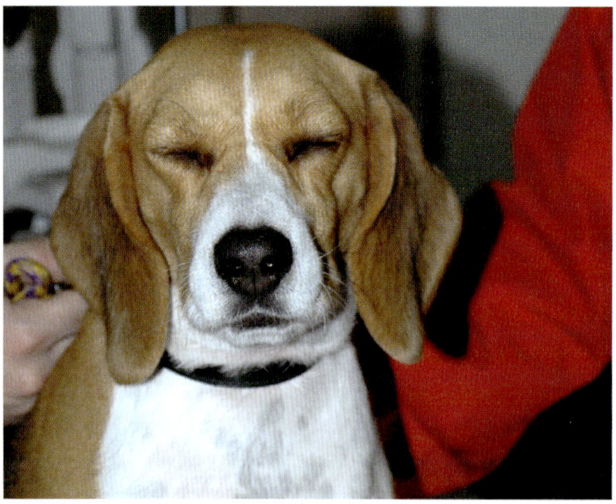

Close-up of the blepharospasm caused by uveitis.

The protrusion of the nictitating membrane and enophthalmos are common clinical signs of painful conditions (uveitis and corneal ulcers).

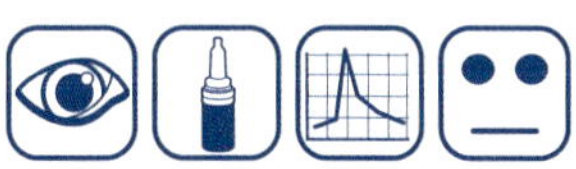

Protrusion of the nictitating membrane

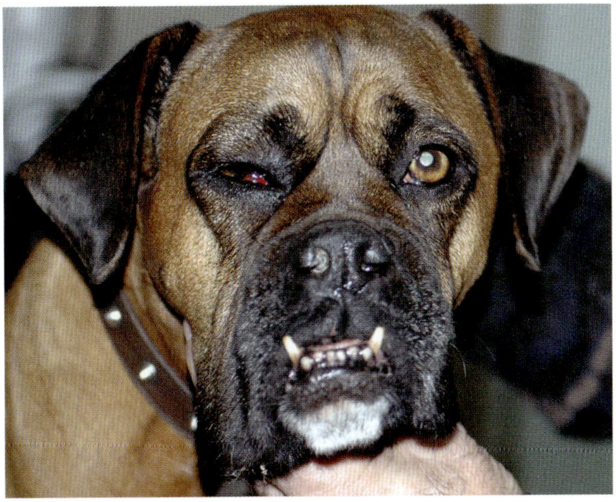

Protrusion of the nictitating membrane in a Boxer with orbital disease.

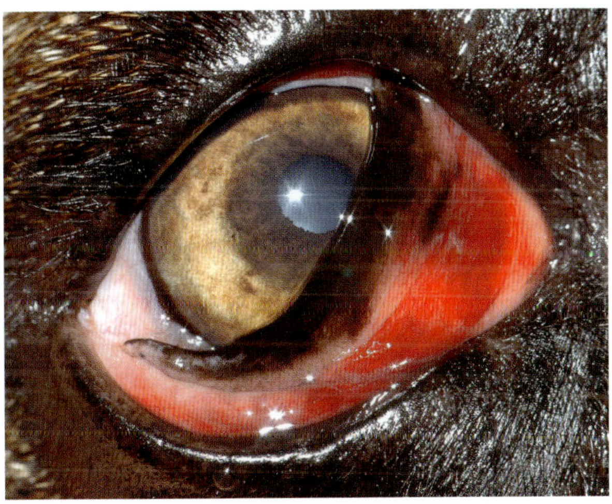

Close-up of the nictitating membrane protrusion in this Boxer. This patient had orbital osteosarcoma.

i | Neoplasms, retrobulbar abscesses, and cellulitis are often accompanied by protrusion of the nictitating membrane.

Neoplasms

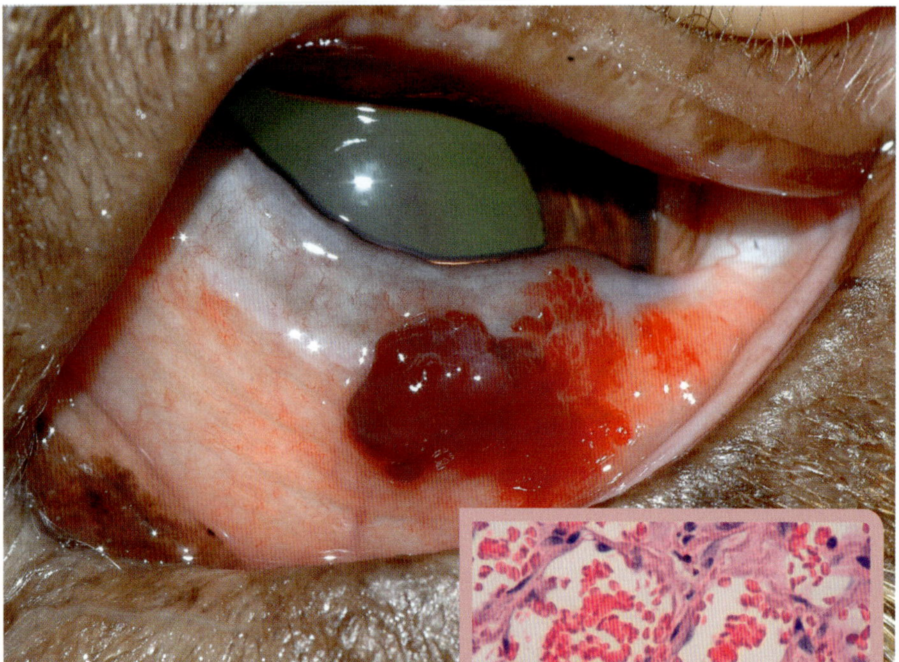

Haemangiosarcoma.
Seven-year-old male Spanish Mastiff.
Time since onset: six months.
Rapid progression.
Surgical treatment: excision.

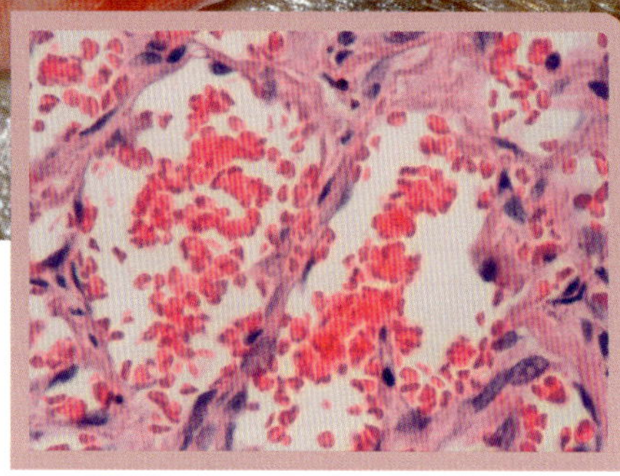

Histological image courtesy of Dr Elena Alonso Fernández-Aceytuno.

Important notes

- Preoperative ultrasound examination (liver, heart, and spleen) and chest radiographs.
- Monitor for recurrence.

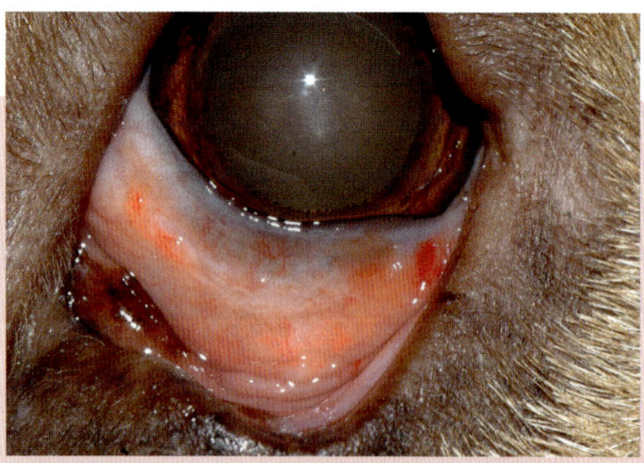

Patient five months after treatment.

Neoplasms

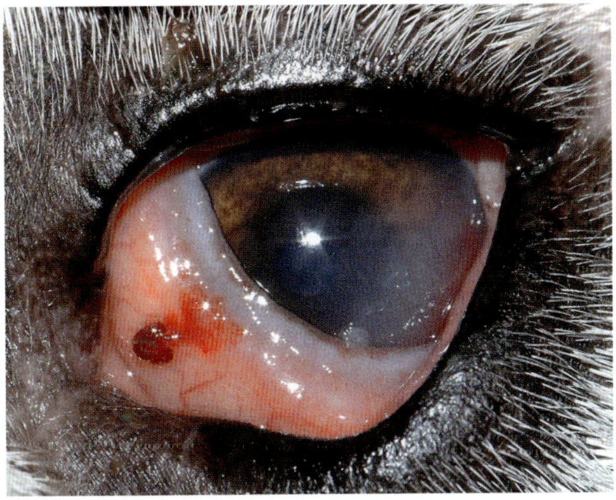

Haemangioma in the nictitating membrane of a nine-year-old Boxer.

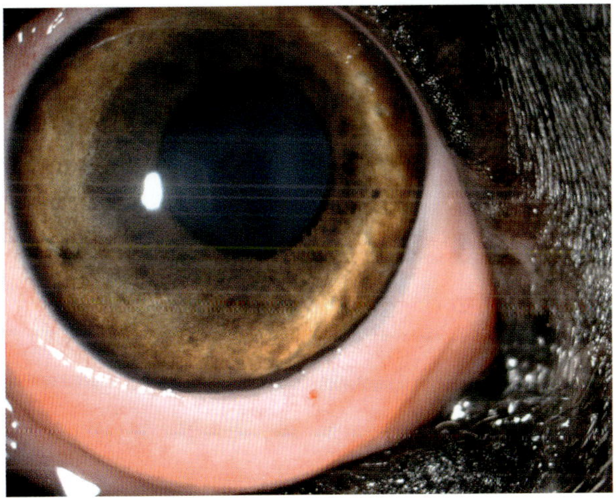

Haemangioma seven days after appearance in the nictitating membrane of a Boxer.

i | Haemangioma and haemangiosarcoma of the nictitating membrane are rare in dogs. Solar radiation (UV) seems to be a risk factor.

Neoplasms

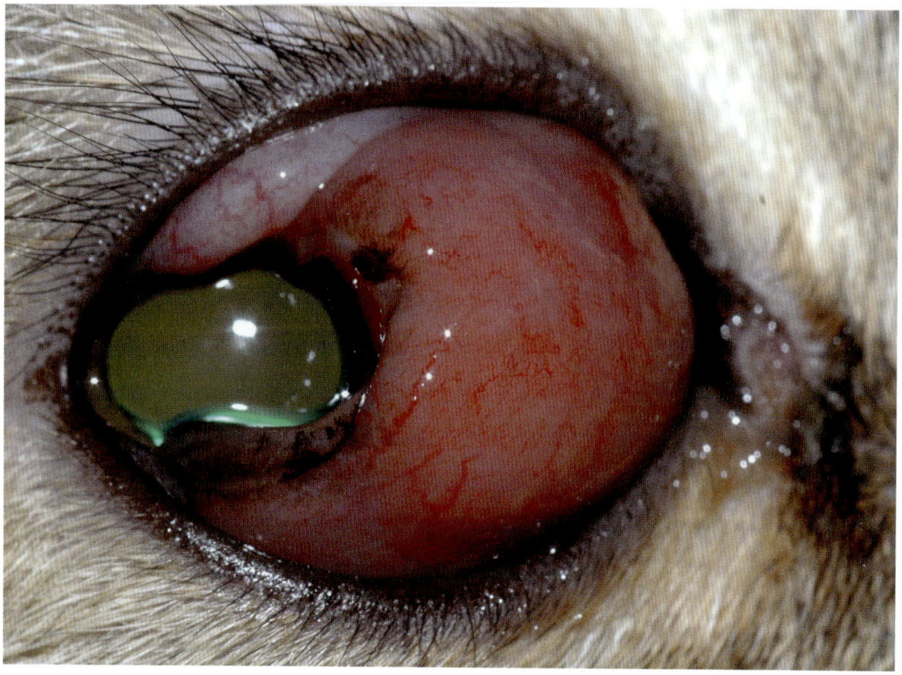

Lymphosarcoma in the nictitating membrane of a 13-year-old domestic cat.

The most common neoplasms of the nictitating membrane are adenocarcinomas, squamous cell carcinomas, melanomas, haemangiomas, haemangiosarcomas and lymphosarcomas.

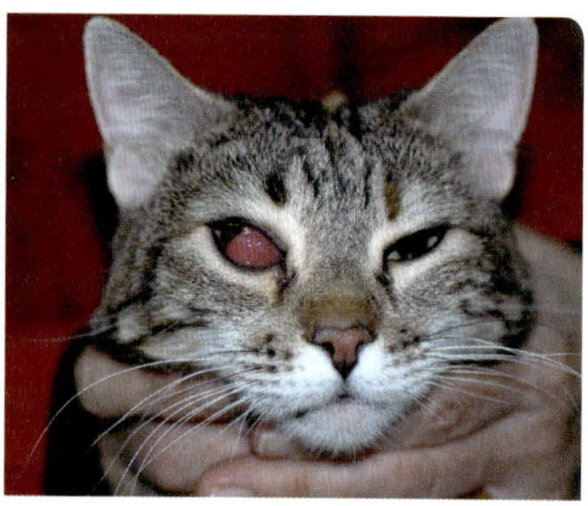

Patient pictured above.

Neoplasms

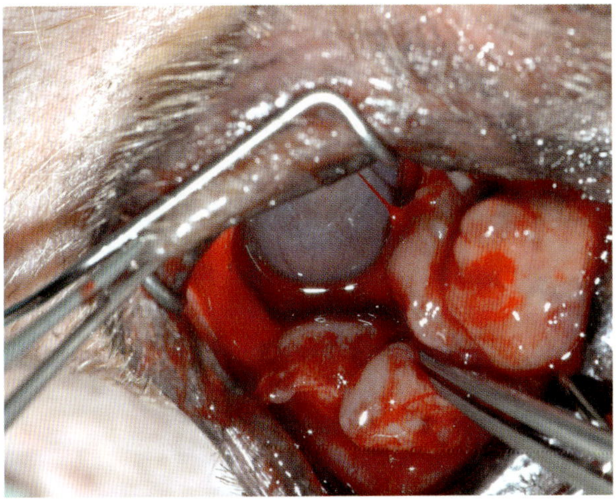

NMG adenocarcinoma in a 15-year-old Yorkshire Terrier.

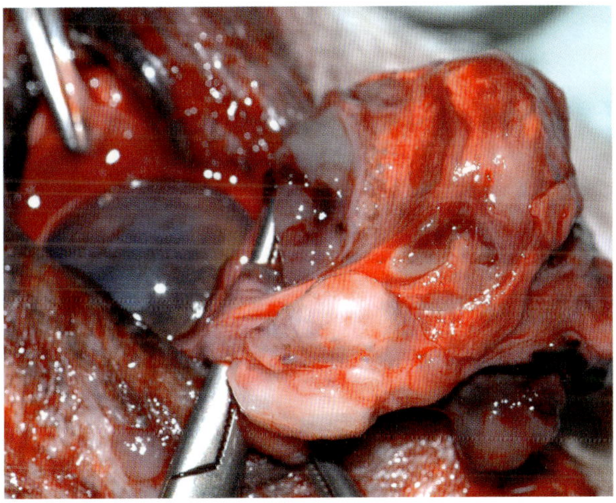

Surgical excision of the patient's adenocarcinoma.

Adenocarcinoma of the NMG is the most common tumour (bearing in mind that NMG tumours have a low incidence).

It may be primary or metastatic.

Foreign bodies

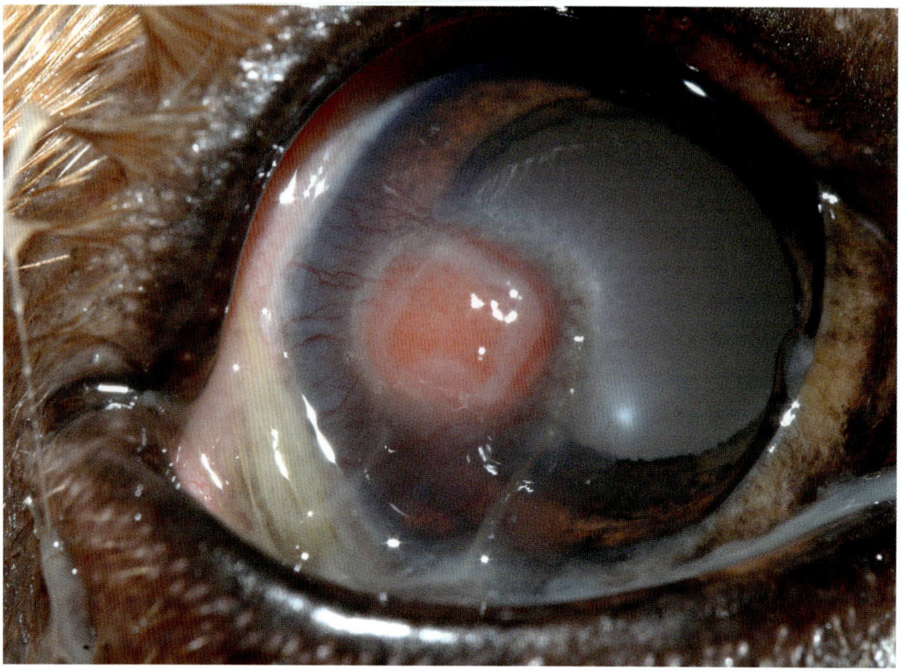

Grass awn underneath the nictitating membrane. Close-up of the grass awn (temporal area) and corneal lesion it has induced.

Interesting notes

- A purulent ocular discharge may signify the presence of a plant foreign body.
- The degree of blepharospasm is quite variable.

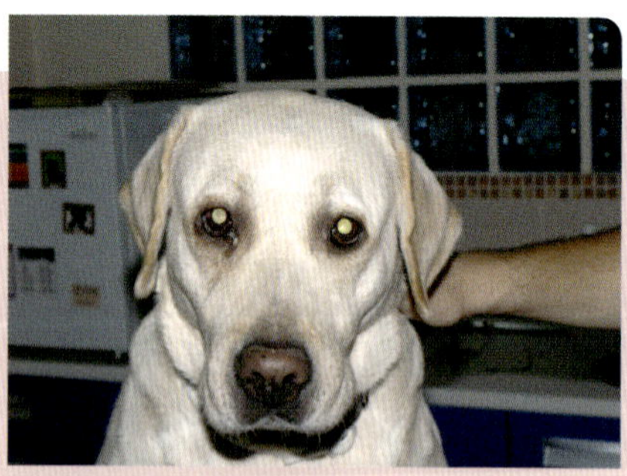

Our patient six days later.

Foreign bodies

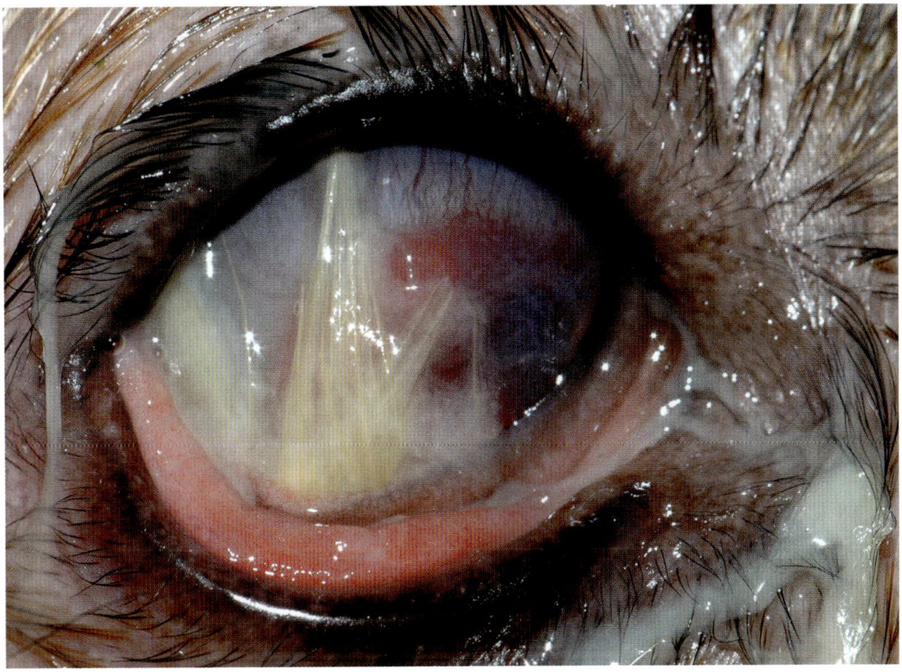

Grass awn underneath the nictitating membrane.
Time since injury: 15 days.
Severe corneal damage.

Important notes

- Removal of a grass awn lodged in the internal conjunctiva should be performed under sedation.

Contraindicated

- NEVER PULL A GRASS AWN FROM ONE END.
  There is a risk of corneal perforation.

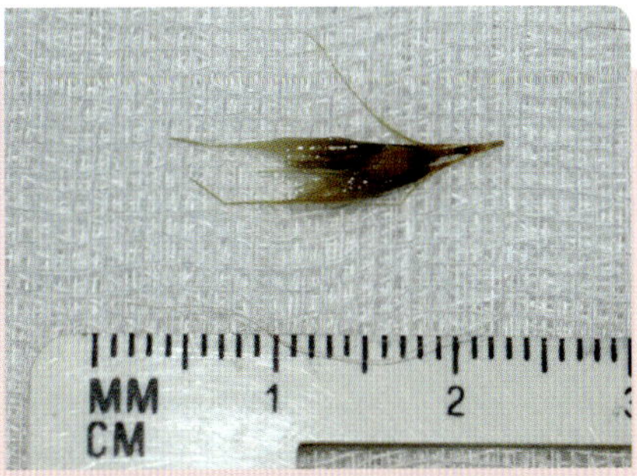

Grass awn removed from the patient's eye.

Foreign bodies

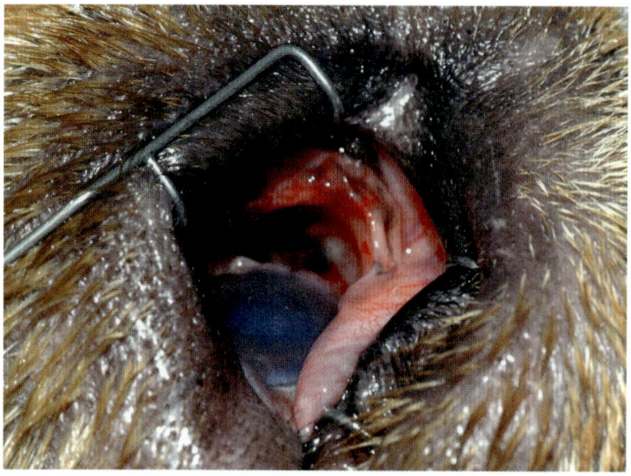

Eversion of the nictitating membrane with a clamp may reveal the foreign body.

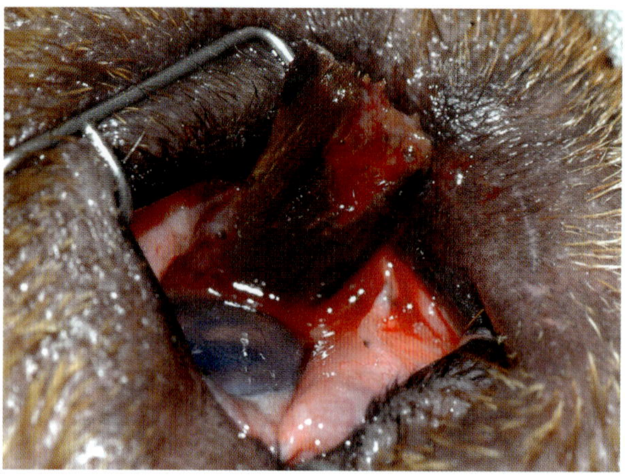

Removal of a foreign body (rockrose twig) from underneath the nictitating membrane. Patient under general anaesthesia.

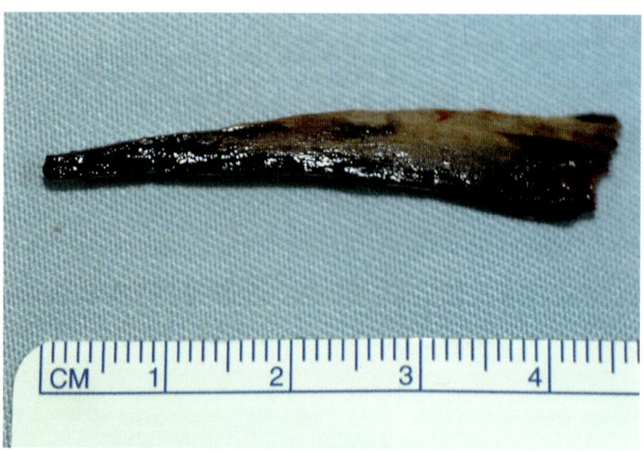

Foreign body.

Depigmentation of the free edge of the nictitating membrane

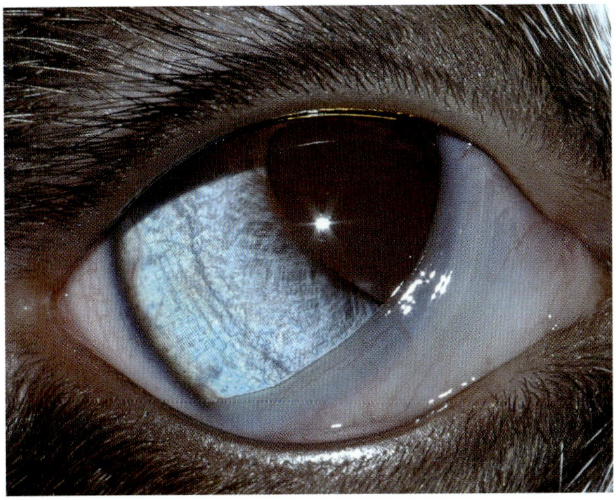

Depigmentation of the free edge of the NM of a cat.

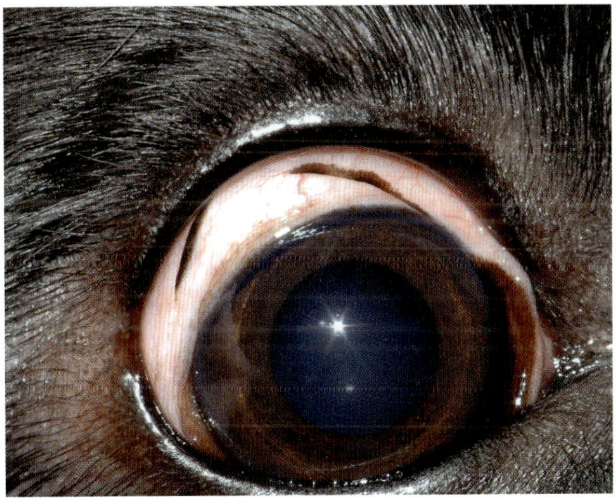

Nictitating membrane of a Cocker Spaniel. Close-up of the pigmentation of the free edge of the nictitating membrane and its dorsal extension (characteristic of this breed).

Interesting notes

- Depigmentation of the free edge of the NM is not considered pathological.
- It may be unilateral or bilateral.
- It affects both cats and dogs and is related to coat colour and age.

Conjunctiva

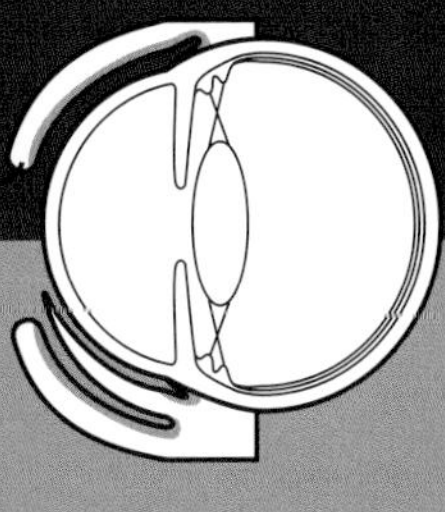

Conjunctival dermoid

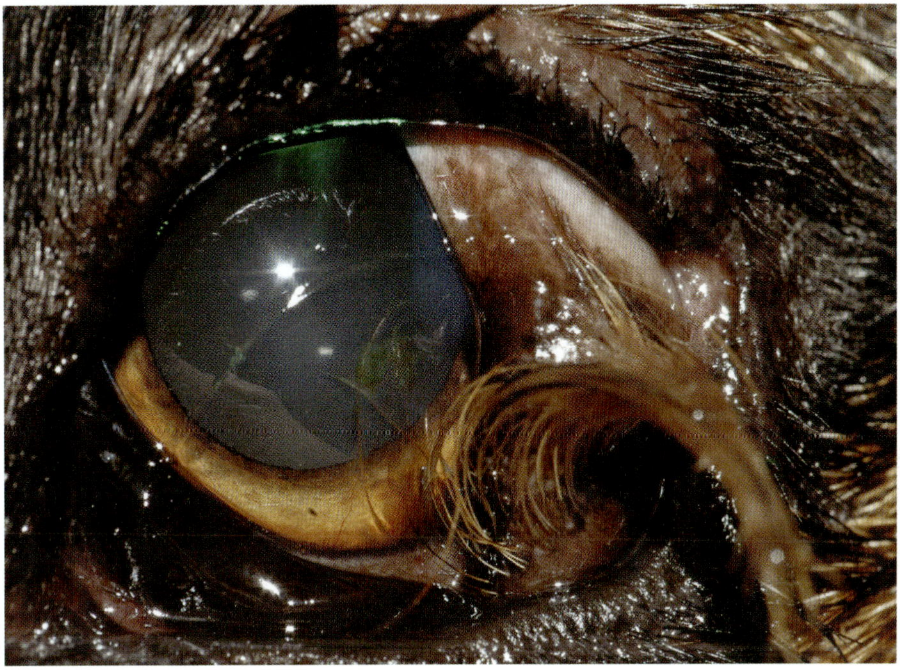

Thirteen-month-old German Shepherd with a dermoid cyst in the lower palpebral conjunctiva. Note the corneal damage.

i | Conjunctival and corneal dermoids are the most common.

Interesting notes

Large areas of conjunctiva must be removed to avoid recurrence.

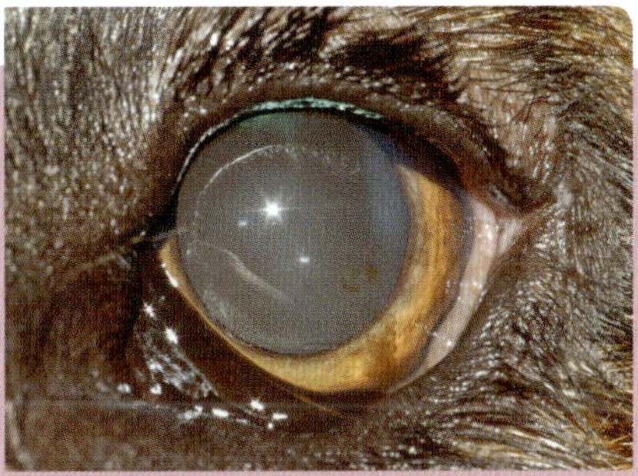

Surgical excision.
Our patient two months later.

Conjunctival dermoid

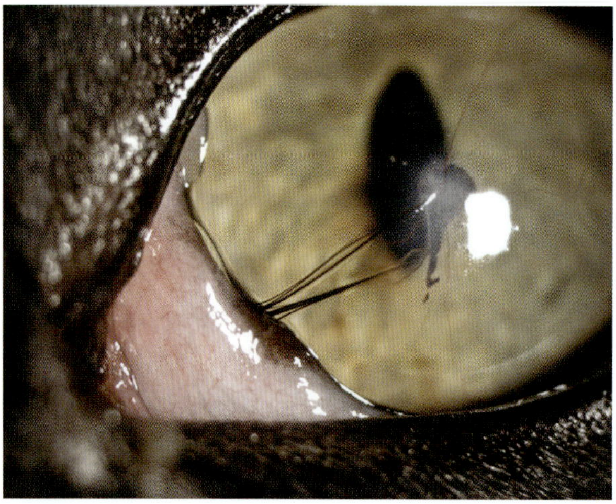

Eight-month-old Burmese cat with chronic ocular discomfort. Note the hairs emerging from behind the nictitating membrane.

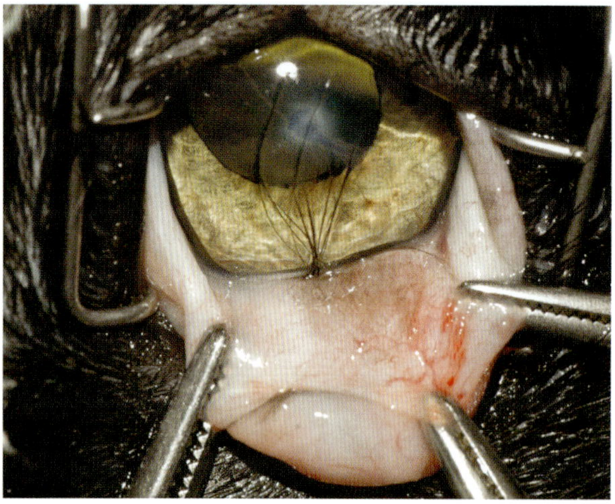

Eversion of the nictitating membrane under general anaesthesia reveals a dermoid cyst.
It is located in the bulbar conjunctiva, adhered to the limbus.

i

Dermoid cysts are less common in cats but have been reported in the Burmese, Birman, and Shorthair breeds.

The treatment is the same (excision).

Conjunctival cysts

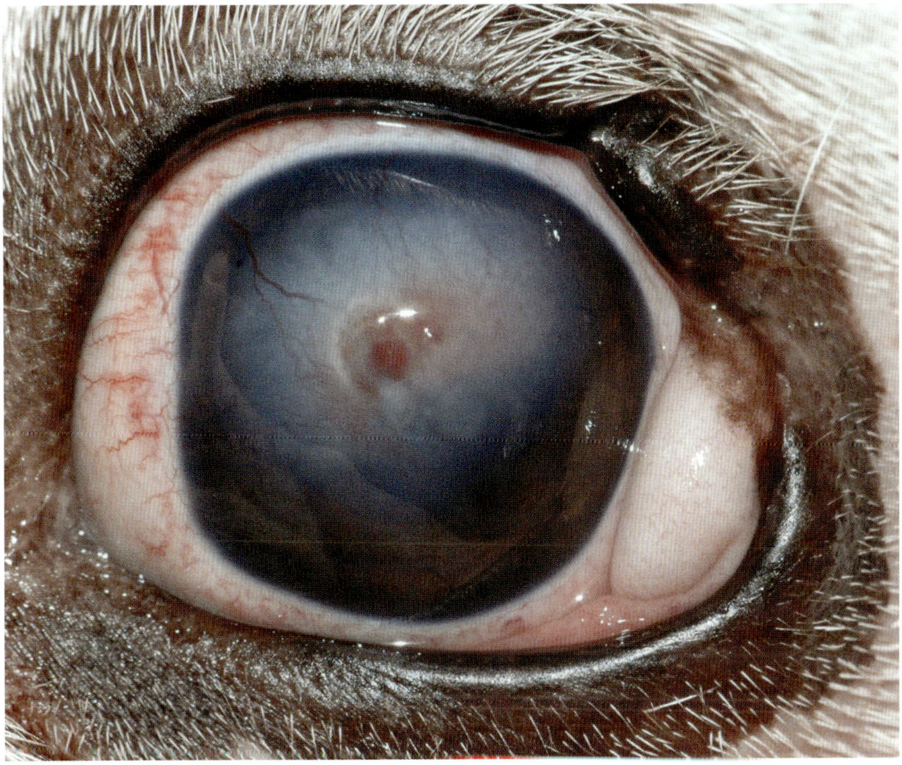

Seven-month-old French Bulldog with a conjunctival cyst.
Bulbar and palpebral lesion.
The corneal damage is secondary to an ectopic cilium.

i Conjunctival cysts are fluid-filled epithelial formations.

- They may affect the palpebral or bulbar conjunctiva, as well as that of the nictitating membrane.
- The treatment is surgical excision.

Conjunctivitis

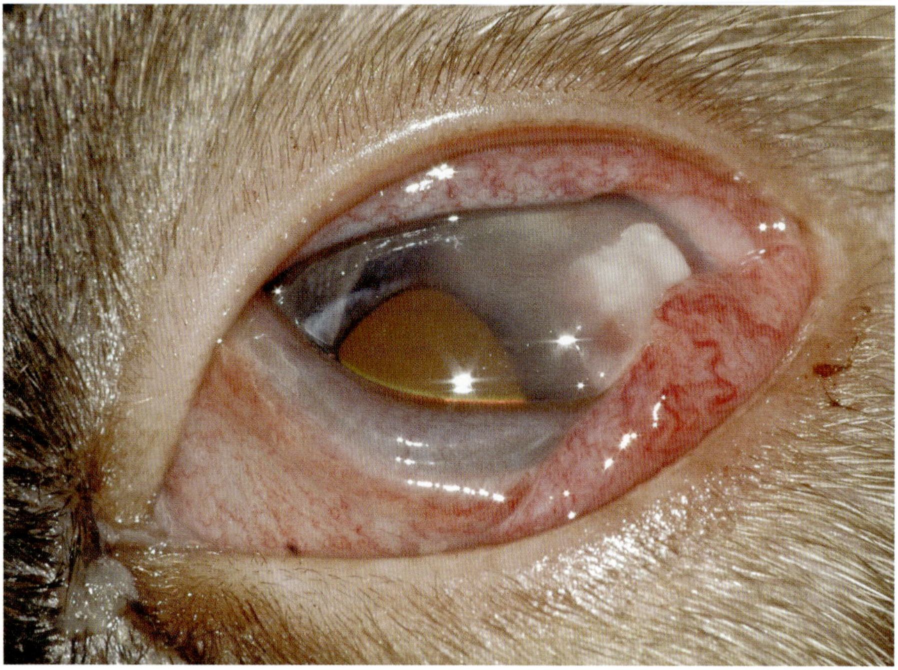

Feline eosinophilic conjunctivitis.
Time since onset: 45 days.
Severe conjunctival hyperaemia and hypertrophy.

Interesting notes

- The aetiology of this corneal conjunctival disease is unclear. It may be immune-related. Feline herpesvirus type I has been isolated from affected cats.

Treatment

- Topical corticosteroids and/or cyclosporine.

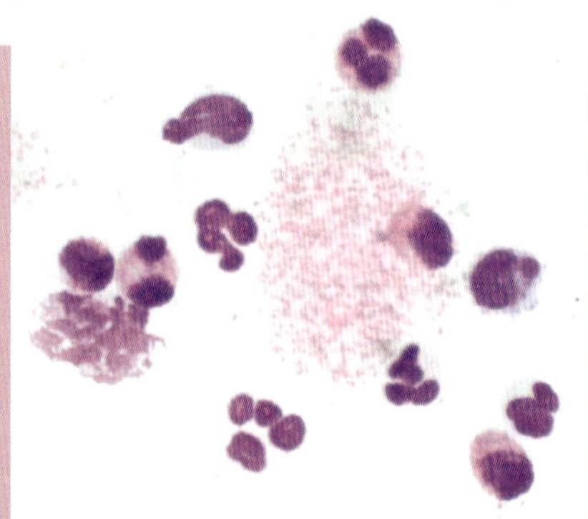

Eosinophils in feline eosinophilic conjunctivitis (100× immersion). Image courtesy of Cristina Fernández Algarra.

Conjunctivitis

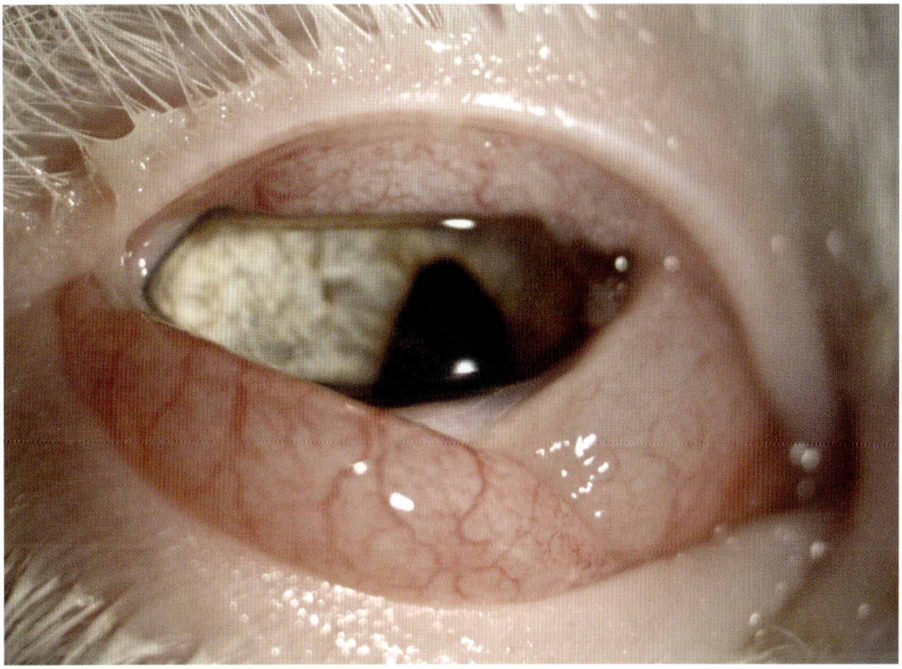

Acute conjunctivitis due to chlamydia in a one-year-old cat.
Time since onset: two days.
Close-up of chemosis and conjunctival hyperaemia.

Important notes

- In the acute phase, it may present unilaterally and occur with ocular discomfort and epiphora.
- Chemosis is pathognomonic.

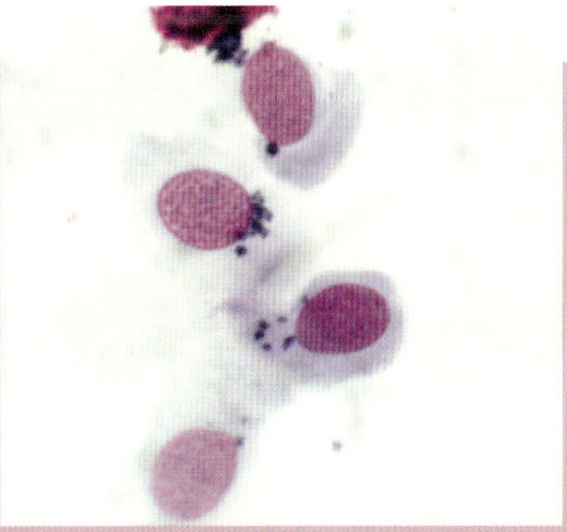

Intracytoplasmic inclusions in chlamydial conjunctivitis (100× immersion). Image courtesy of Cristina Fernández Algarra.

Conjunctivitis

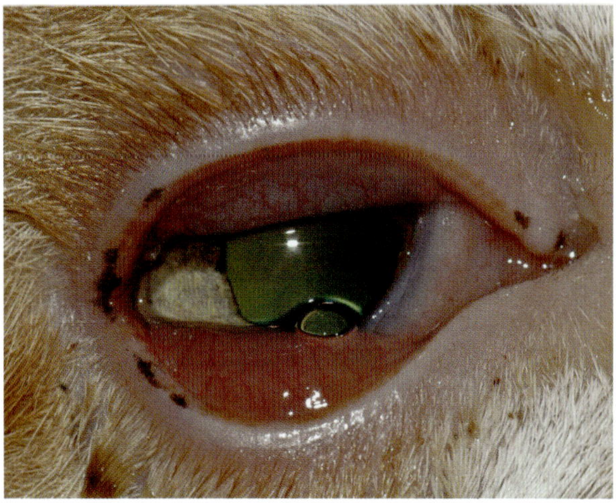

Right eye of a cat with *Chlamydophila felis* conjunctivitis.
Note the conjunctival congestion, chemosis, and protrusion of the nictitating membrane.

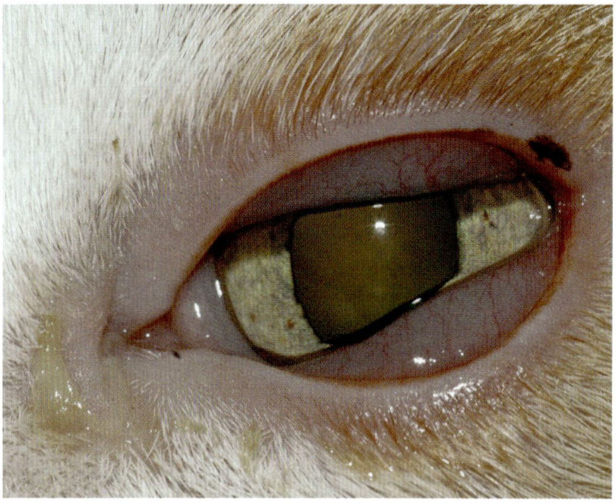

Left eye of the patient six days following appearance of the right eye lesion.

- In advanced stages, the disease may present bilaterally. This tends to occur 5–8 days following the unilateral lesion.
- It may be accompanied by a mild respiratory illness.
- The treatment of choice is topical tetracycline.

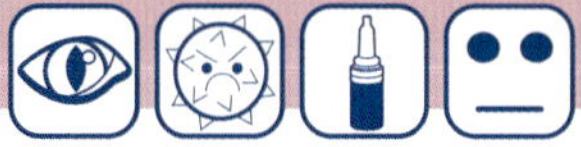

Conjunctivitis

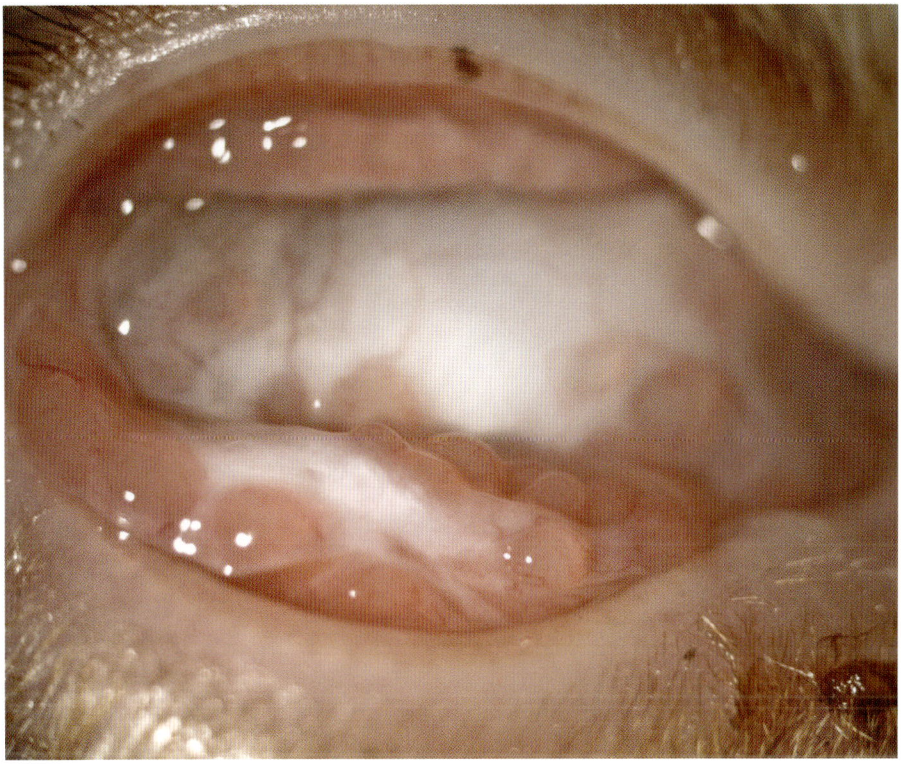

Fourteen-month-old domestic shorthair cat with chlamydial conjunctivitis.
Time since onset: 18 days.

The appearance of the follicles and the conjunctival hypertrophy indicate chronicity.

Treatment

- Topical tetracyclines applied 4–6 times daily will improve the clinical condition.
- Perform a lymphoid follicle scraping only in cases refractory to medical treatment.

Conjunctivitis

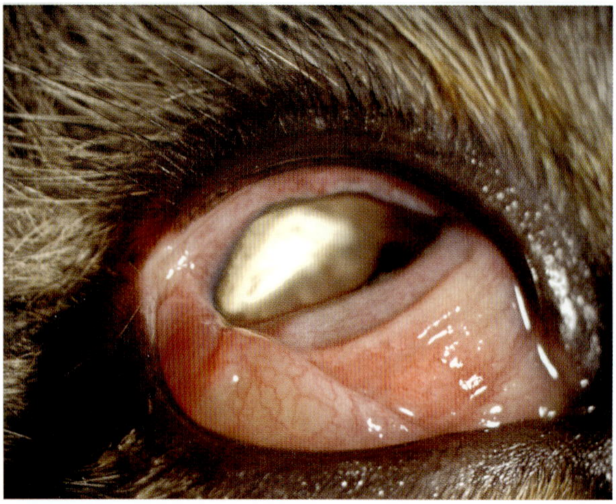

Mycoplasma conjunctivitis in a cat.
Time since injury: eight days.
Unilateral presentation.

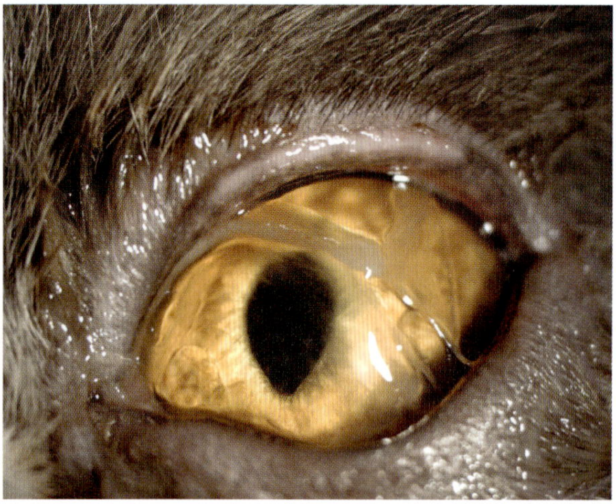

Chronic conjunctivitis due to *Mycoplasma felis* in a Persian cat.

Interesting notes

- Acute phases are characterised by conjunctival thickening and hyperaemia.
- Chronic phases involve mucopurulent or pseudomembranous secretions.

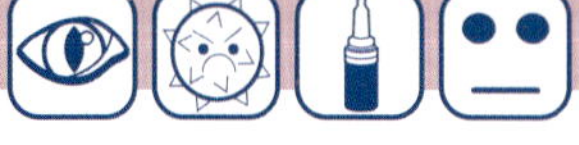

Conjunctivitis

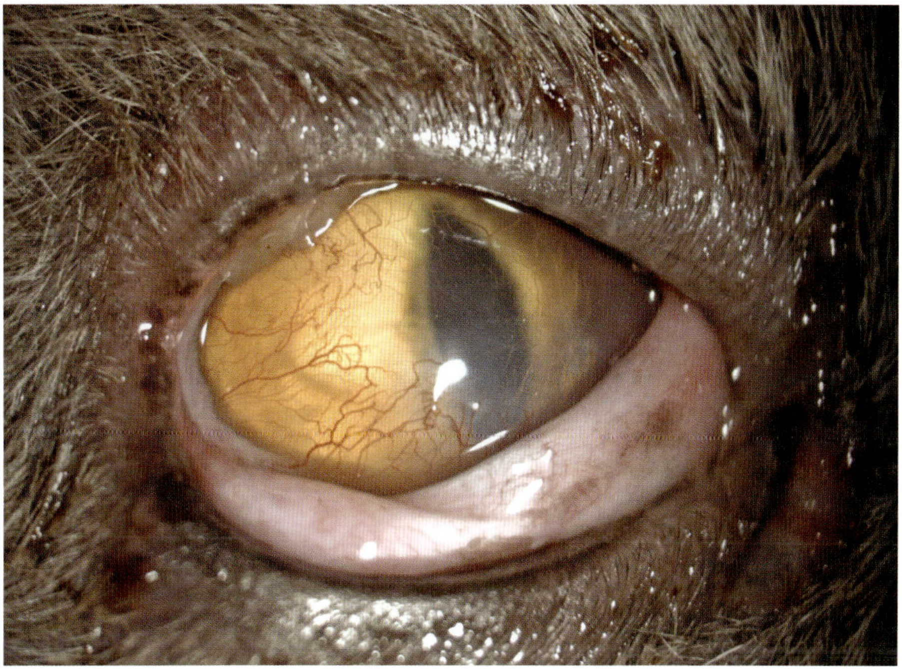

Feline herpesvirus conjunctivitis.
Time since onset: two months.
Conjunctival hyperaemia, protrusion of the nictitating membrane, and ocular discharge.

Important notes

- Feline herpesvirus type 1 is responsible for most cases of feline conjunctivitis.
- It may occur with severe respiratory illness in young animals.

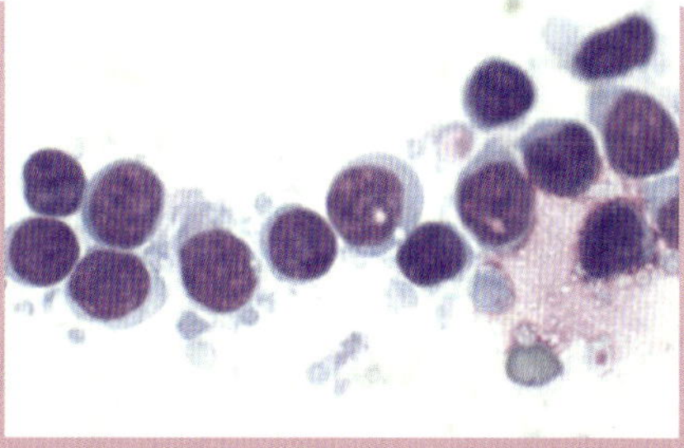

Increased lymphoid response in viral conjunctivitis. Common in herpesvirus (100× immersion). Image courtesy of Cristina Fernández Algarra.

Conjunctivitis

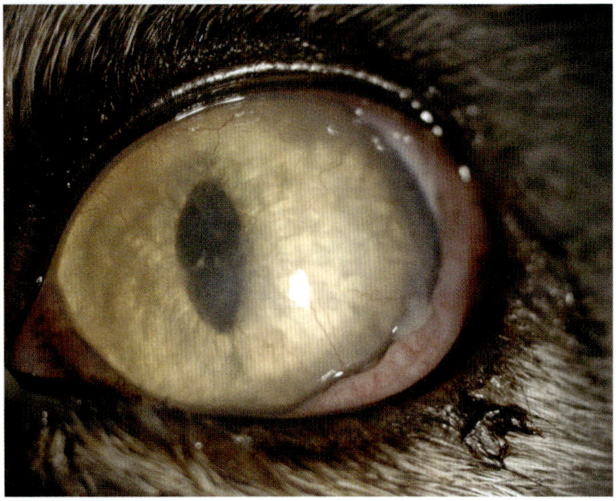

Domestic shorthair cat with herpesvirus conjunctivitis. Close-up of the ocular discharge and conjunctival hypertrophy.
Corneal neovascularisation is indicative of keratitis.

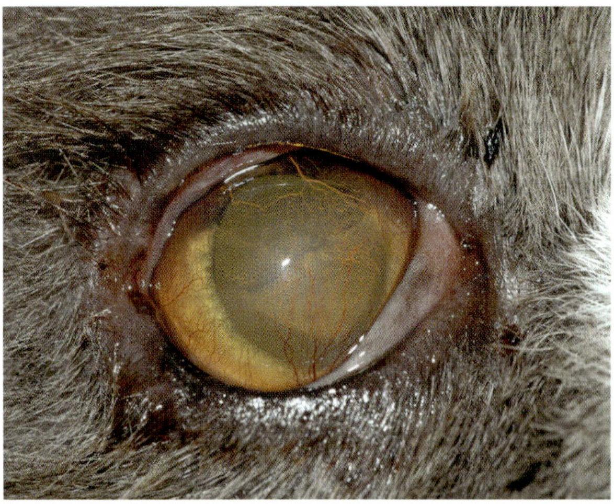

Chronic herpes conjunctivitis. Time since onset: seven months.

Interesting notes

- In any case of a cat with conjunctivitis and associated keratitis that are poorly responsive to treatment, consider feline herpesvirus type 1.

Conjunctivitis

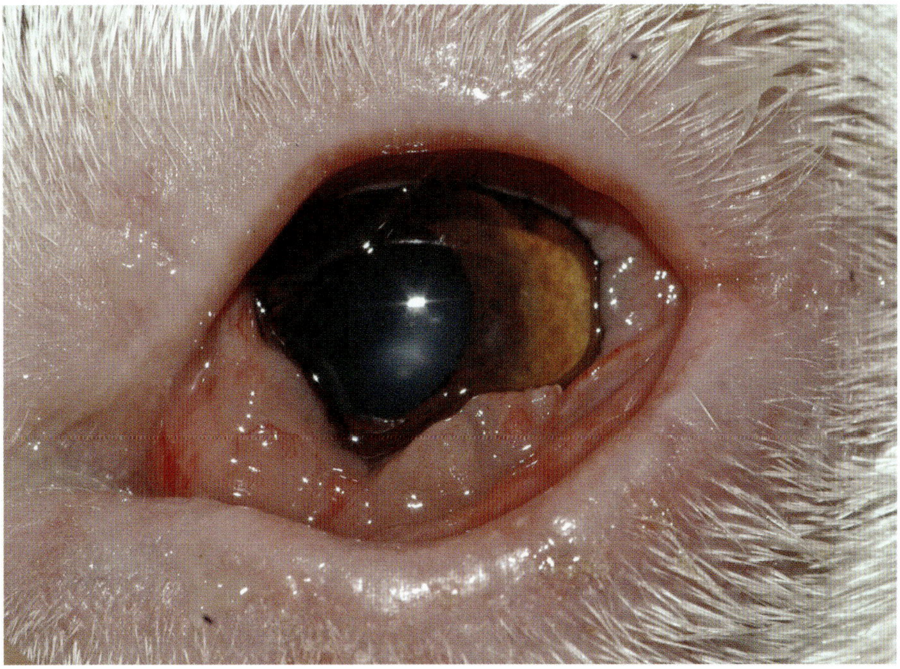

Conjunctivitis due to *Leishmania* in a dog.
Hyperaemia and conjunctival hypertrophy, along with granulomas, characterise this parasitic disease.

In this case, cytology and/or biopsy are required to reach a diagnosis. It may be confused grossly with squamous cell carcinoma.

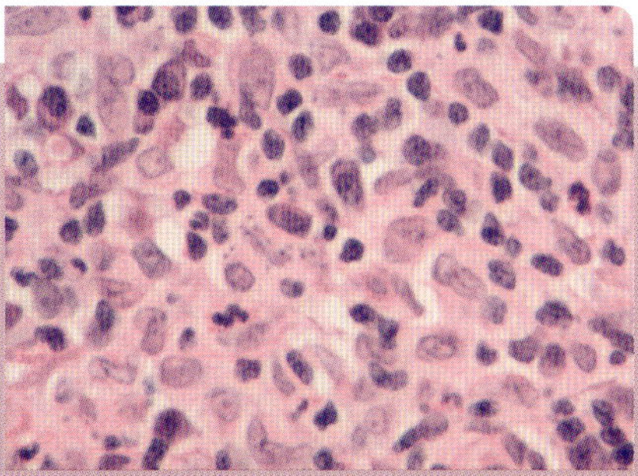

Leishmania amastigotes in a conjunctival biopsy. Image courtesy of Dr Elena Alonso Fernández-Aceytuno.

Keratoconjunctivitis sicca

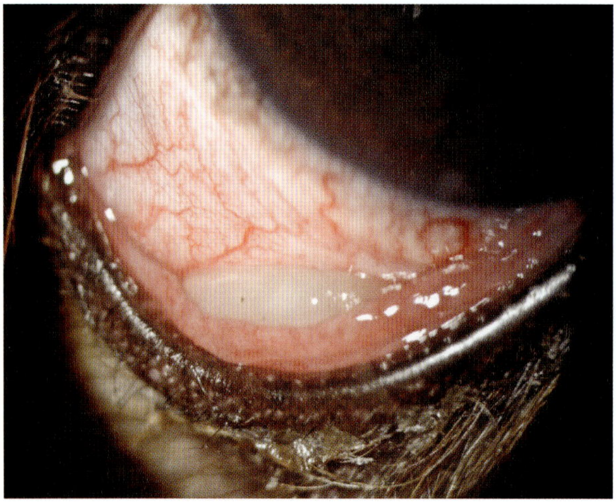

Dog with keratoconjunctivitis sicca (KCS).
Conjunctival hyperaemia and mucus are the most common clinical signs of this disease.

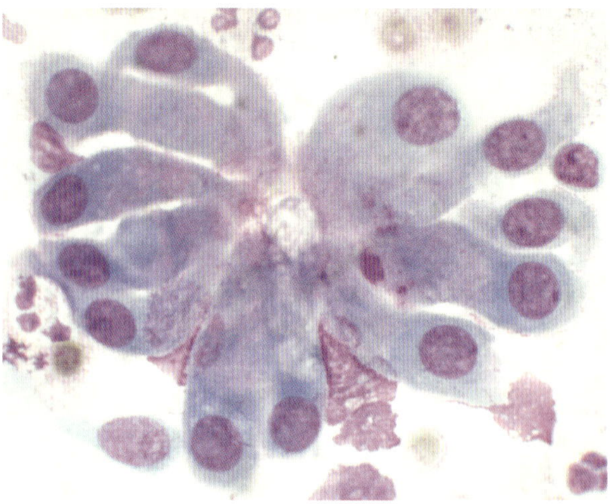

KCS, mucus-producing cells (100× immersion). Image courtesy of Cristina Fernández Algarra.

Interesting notes

- Conjunctivitis related to a defect in tear production is always accompanied by MUCUS.
- Do not confuse it with a purulent secretion.

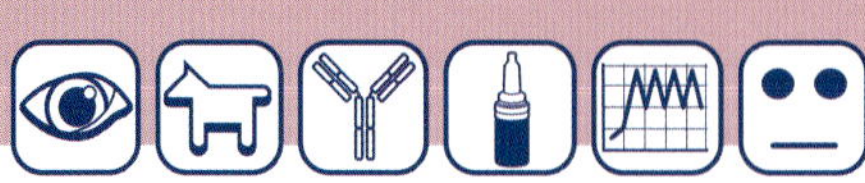

Keratoconjunctivitis sicca

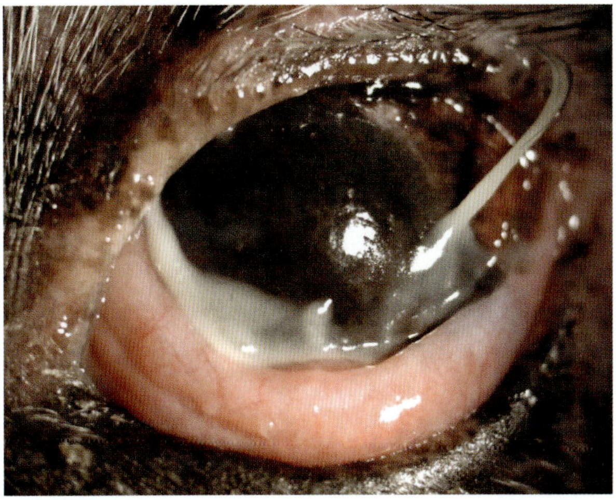

Chronic keratoconjunctivitis sicca (KCS) in a dog. Close-up of the mucus and conjunctival hypertrophy.

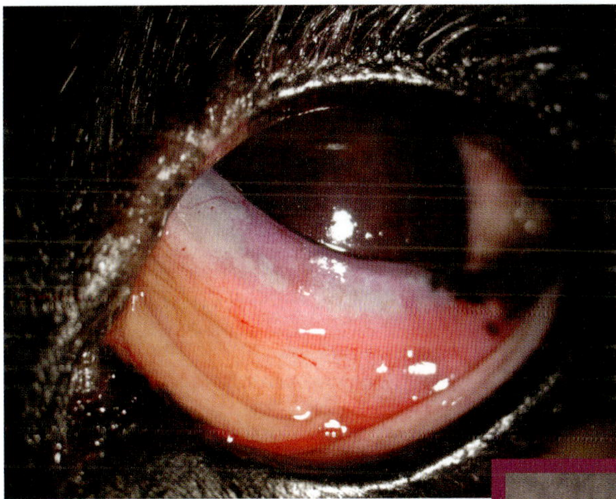

Rose bengal is a vital stain that helps to identify the degenerating cells in the conjunctiva. Patient with KCS.

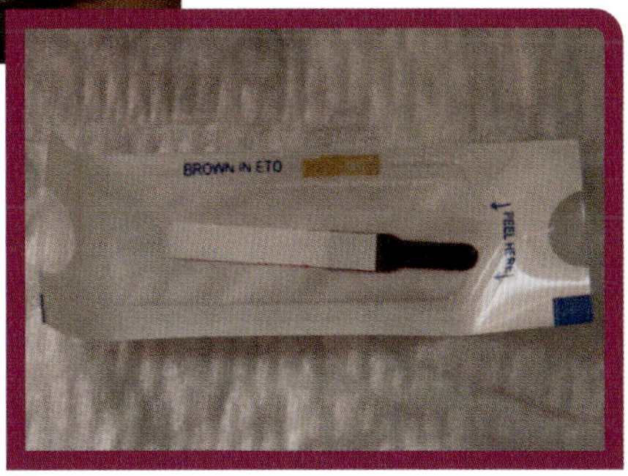

Single-use rose bengal strips, which are used for early diagnosis of KCS.

Symblepharon

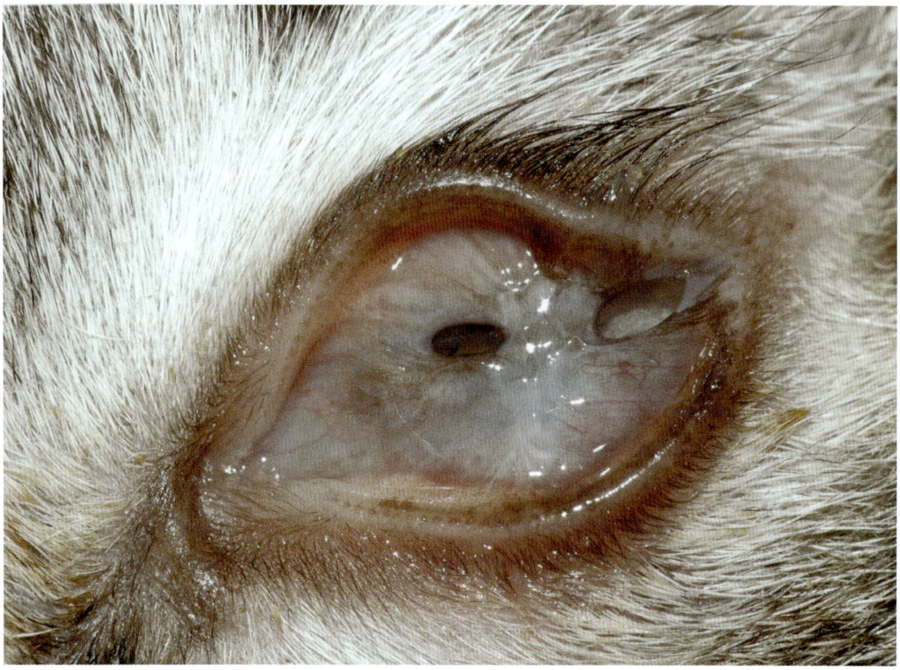

Five-month-old domestic shorthair kitten with symblepharon.
The cornea is visible through the gaps in the conjunctiva.

This is an adhesion of the conjunctiva to the cornea or between different sections of the conjunctiva.

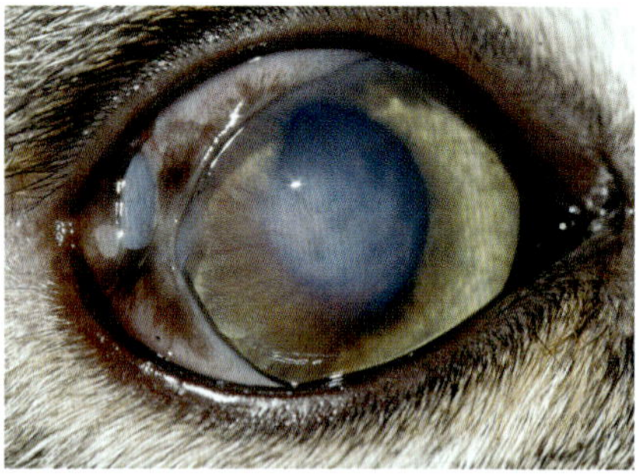

Symblepharon in the temporal region.

Symblepharon

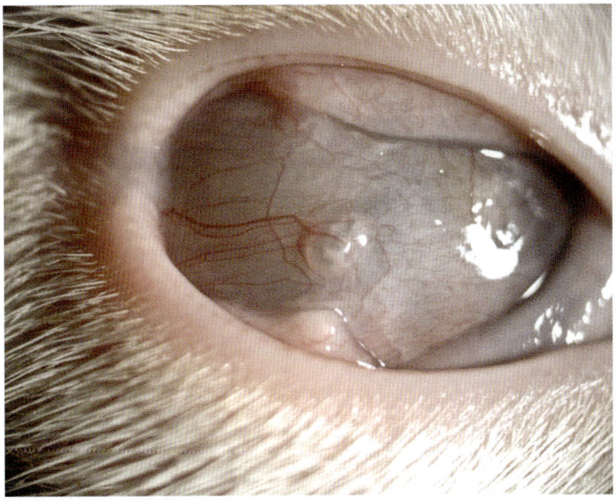

Six-month-old cat with symblepharon.
The conjunctiva and cornea adhere closely to one another.

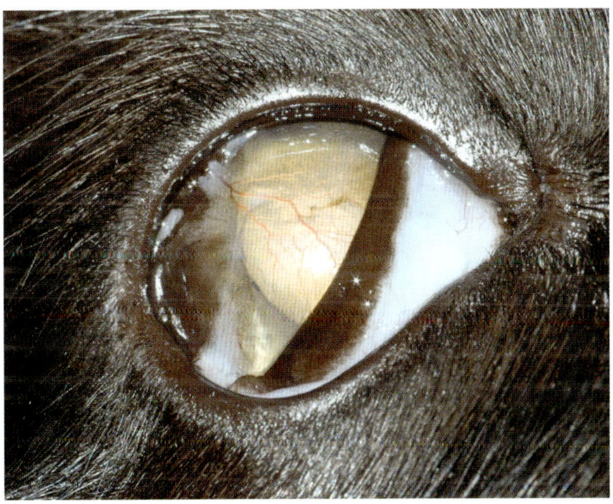

Pigmentation of a symblepharon signifies chronicity.

Important notes

- Most cats with symblepharon have feline herpesvirus type 1.
- This is difficult to treat. Recurrence after surgery is common.

Drug plaques

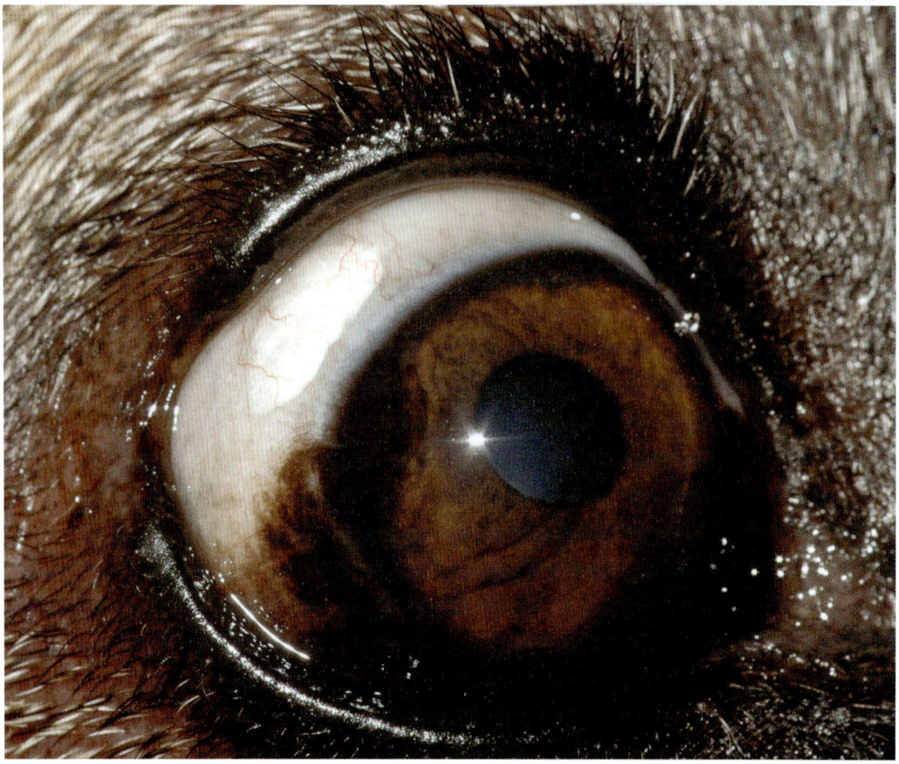

Drug plaque in a dog, six months after a subconjunctival injection of methylprednisolone acetate.

i In some cases, subconjunctival deposits of drugs can leave remnants under the bulbar conjunctiva.

Mucinosis

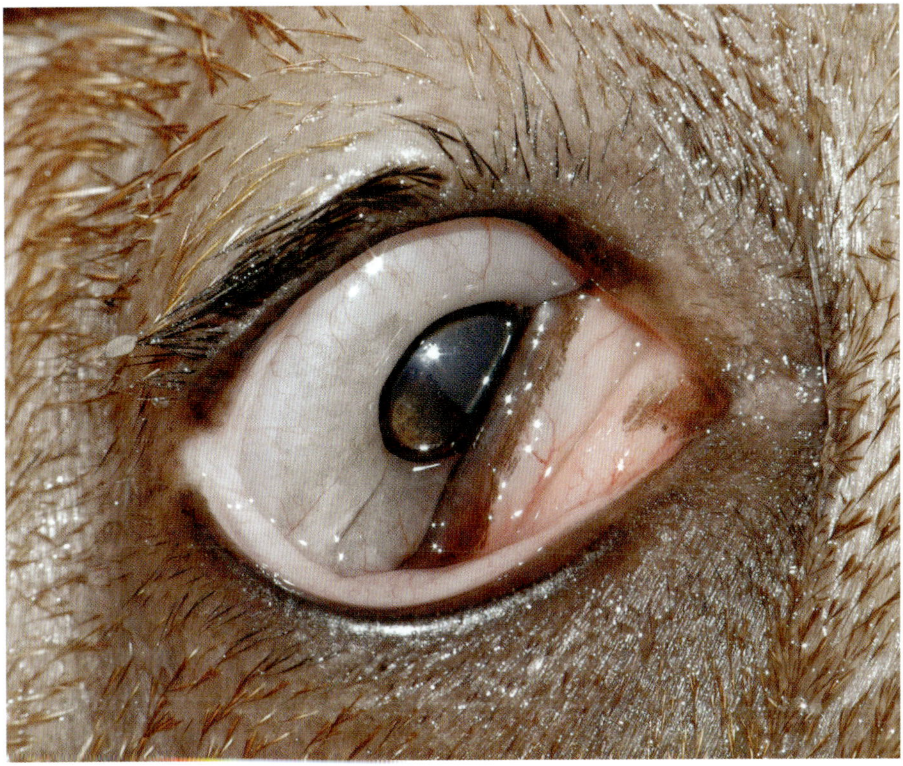

Conjunctival mucinosis in a Shar Pei puppy.

Important notes

- Do not confuse this with conjunctival chemosis.
- Due to the high mucin concentration in this breed.
- It tends to resolve with age.

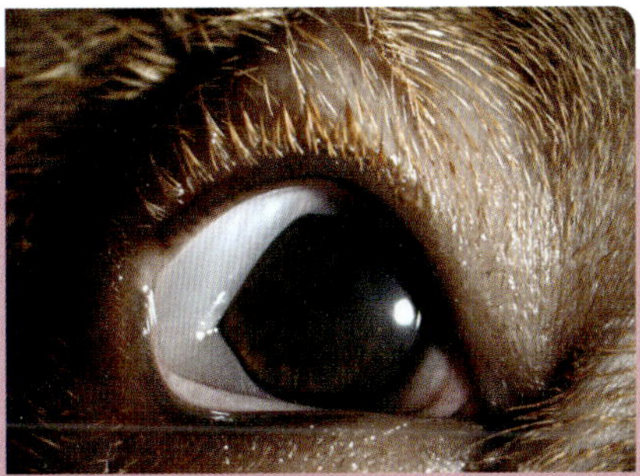

Conjunctival mucinosis is characteristic of the Shar Pei.

Haemorrhages

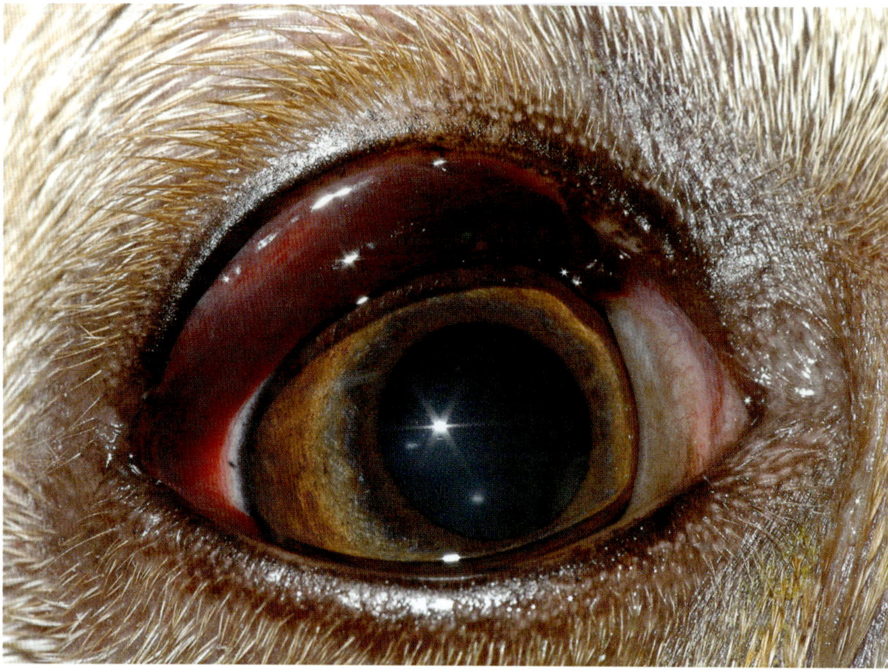

Subconjunctival haemorrhage in a dog that was hit in the face with a ball.
Time since onset: 30 minutes.

- Post-traumatic subconjunctival haemorrhages resolve spontaneously.
- Examine the intraocular structures and the sclera carefully.

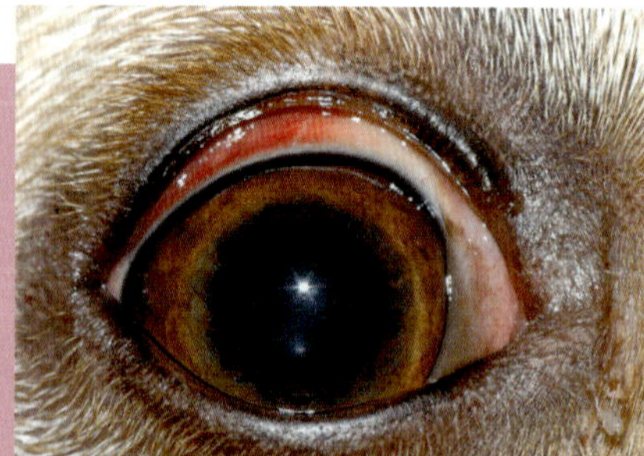

Patient three days later.

Haemorrhages

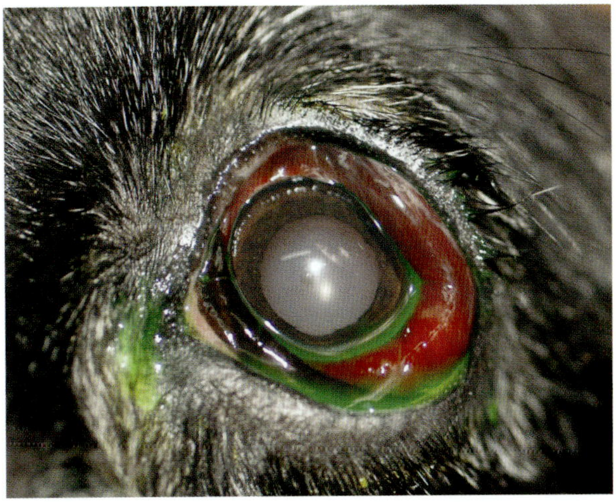

Profuse subconjunctival haemorrhage in a lymphoma patient.

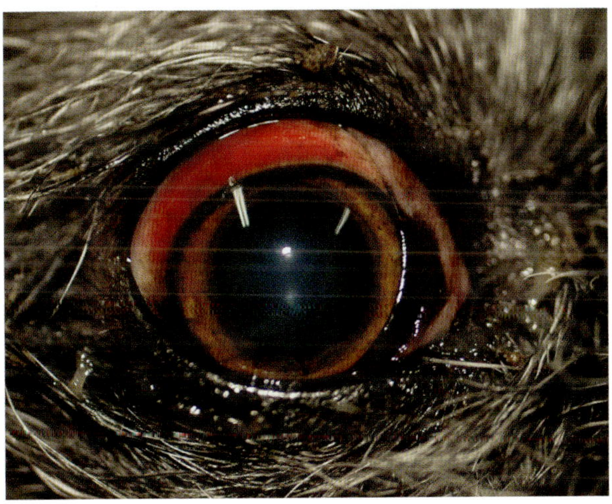

Subconjunctival haemorrhage in a patient with ehrlichiosis.

Important notes

- Conjunctival haemorrhages are often linked to systemic processes.
- It is crucial to distinguish between parasitic diseases, liver diseases, alterations in coagulation, and neoplasms.

Chemosis

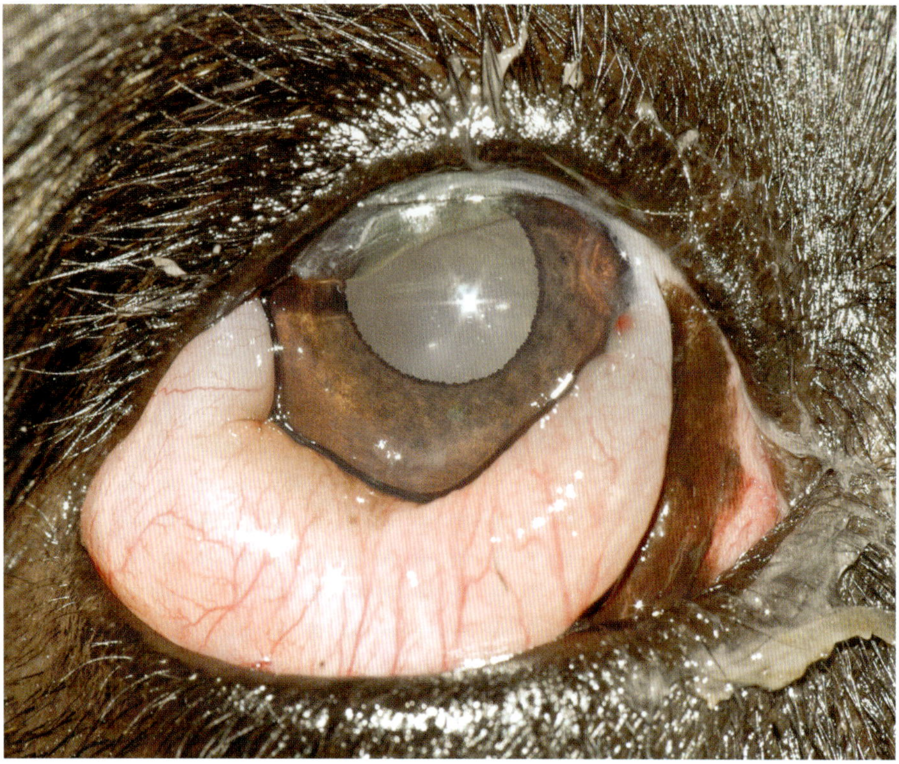

Acute conjunctival chemosis in a Boxer with orbital disease (neoplasm).
Time since onset: 24 hours.

i | Conjunctival oedema. Mainly linked to inflammatory processes.

Other causes of chemosis

- Anaphylaxis.
- Parasitosis (*Toxocara, Leishmania*).
- Trauma.
- Infections (*Staphylococcus, Streptococcus*).
- Associated with uveitis.

Chemosis

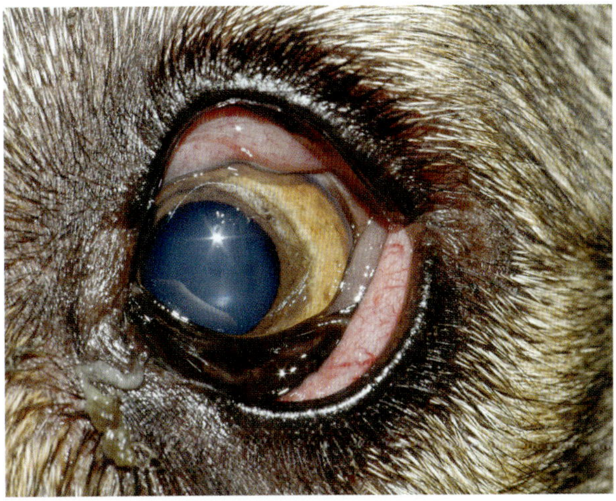

Unilateral conjunctival oedema in a dog with an insect bite.

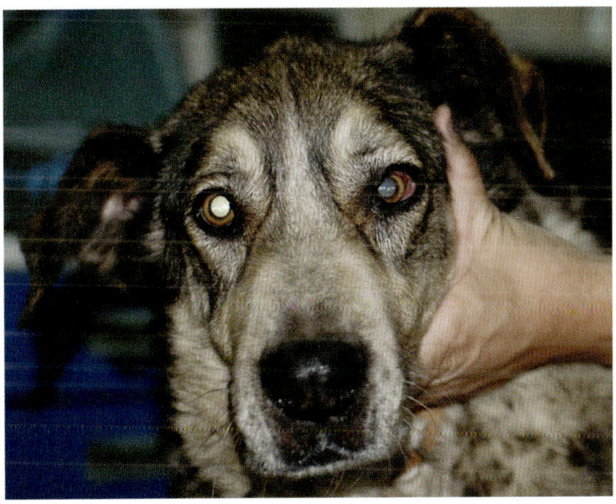

Picture of the patient.

i | Facial allergic reactions tend to involve conjunctival chemosis (bulbar and/or palpebral).

Treatment

Begin treatment with systemic corticosteroids. If necessary, topical corticosteroids can be added.

Wounds

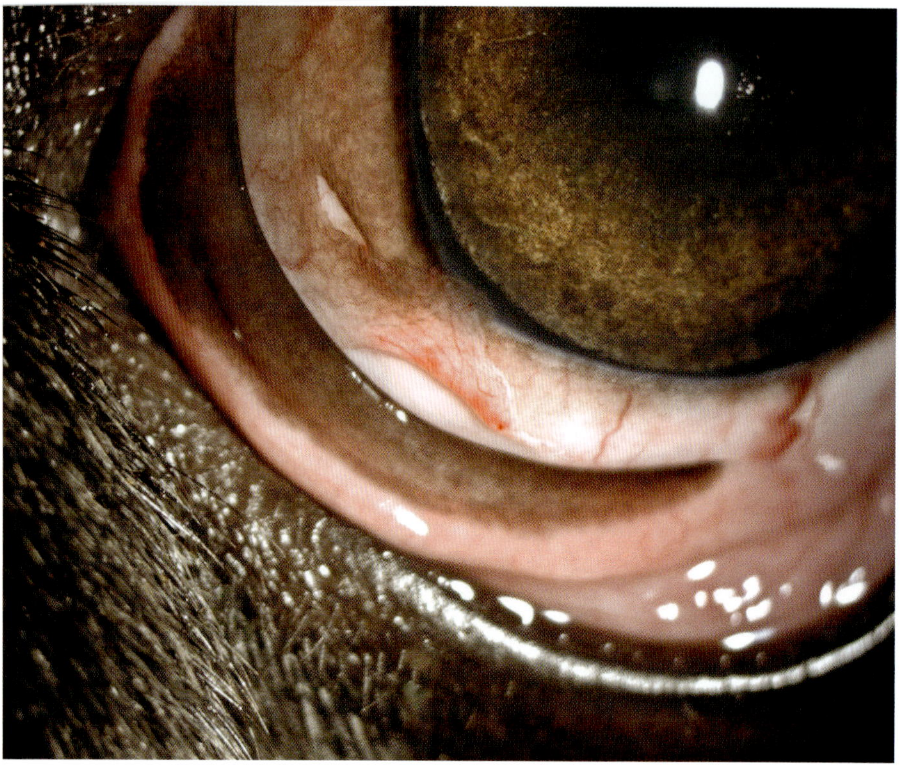

Laceration of the bulbar conjunctiva from a cat scratch in a French Bulldog.
Time since onset: two hours.

Contraindicated

- Small conjunctival tears do not require surgical reconstruction. The conjunctiva scars well.

Important notes

- In extensive conjunctival tears, the necrotic tissue should be removed and the conjunctiva reconstructed with absorbable material. Sutures must never rub on the cornea.

Neoplasms

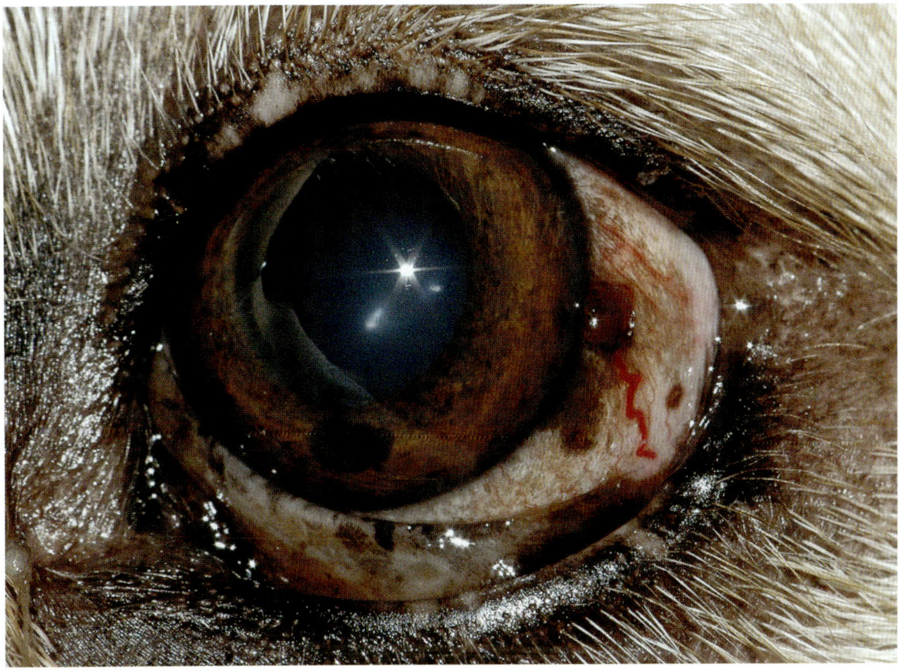

Conjunctival haemangioma in an 11-year-old dog. They tend to be elevated, vascular red masses.

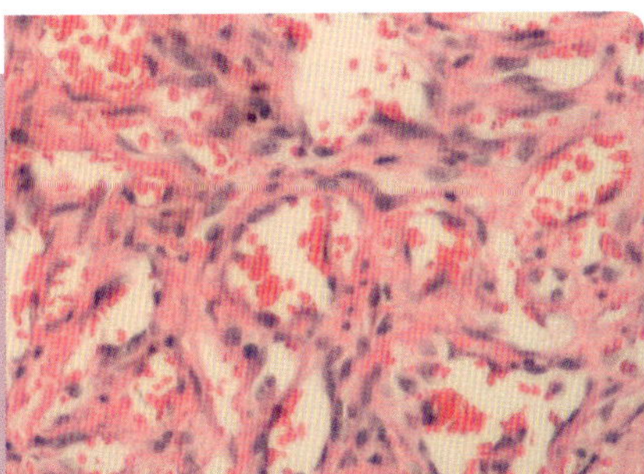

Histopathological image of the conjunctival haemangioma in the patient pictured above. Image courtesy of Dr Elena Alonso Fernández-Aceytuno.

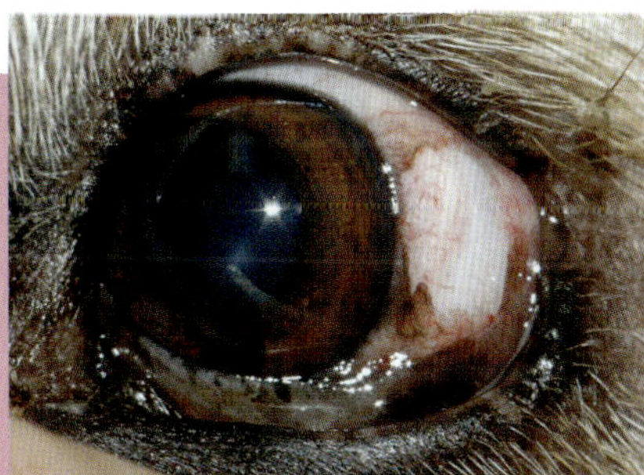

Our patient immediately after surgery.

- Conjunctival tumours are most often treated surgically.
- Laser or cryotherapy may be indicated in some cases.

Neoplasms

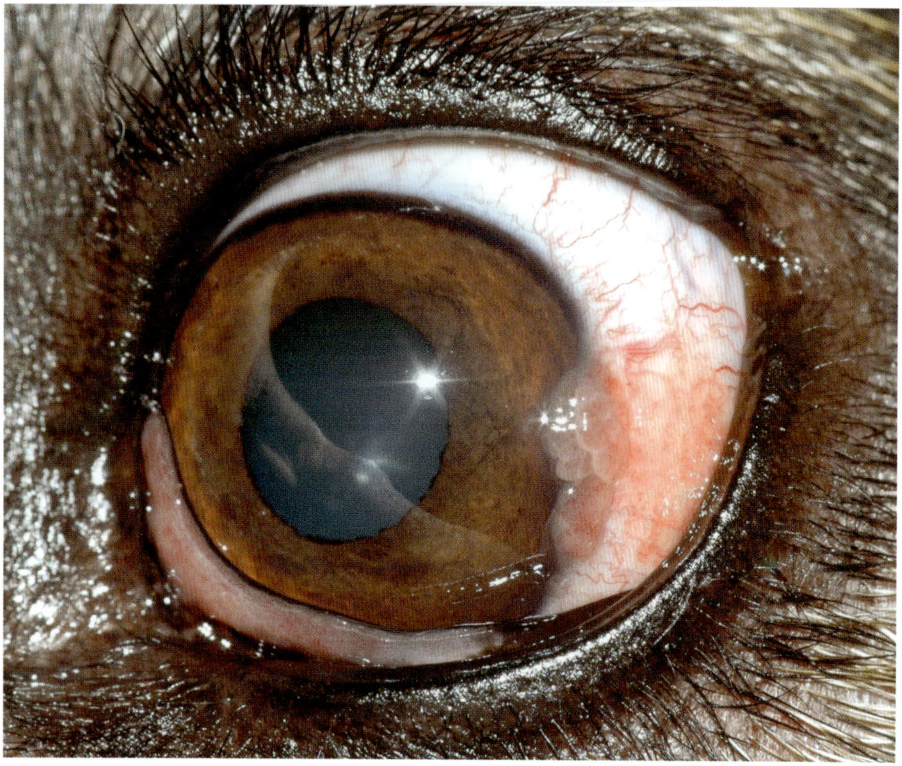

Conjunctival squamous cell carcinoma involving the limbus in a German Shepherd.
Time since onset: four months.

Interesting notes

- The most common conjunctival tumours are haemangiomas, haemangiosarcomas, squamous cell carcinomas, and melanomas.
- Mastocytomas, papillomas, and fibrosarcomas (among others) have also been reported.

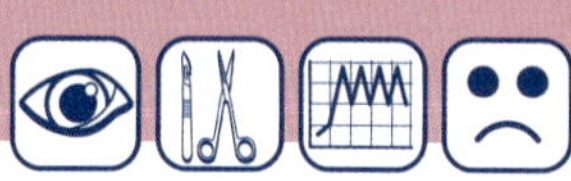

Cornea and sclera

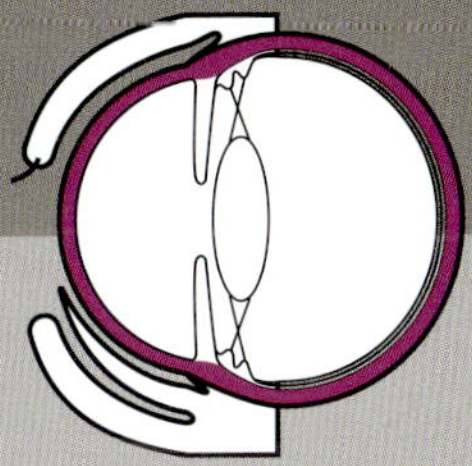

Superficial corneal ulcer

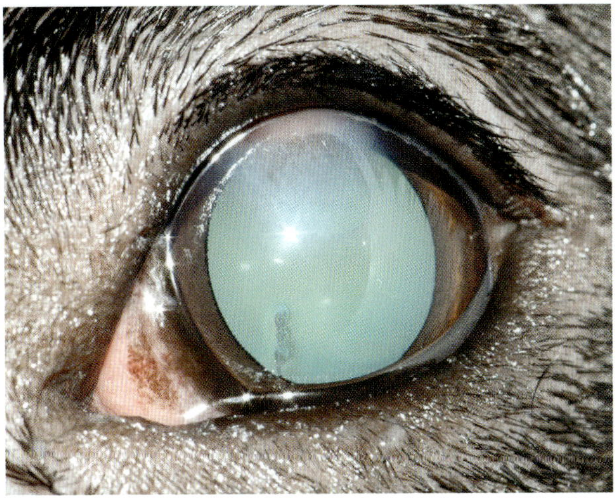

Superficial corneal ulcer located dorsally in a French bulldog.
Time since onset: four days.
Cause: ectopic cilium on the upper eyelid.

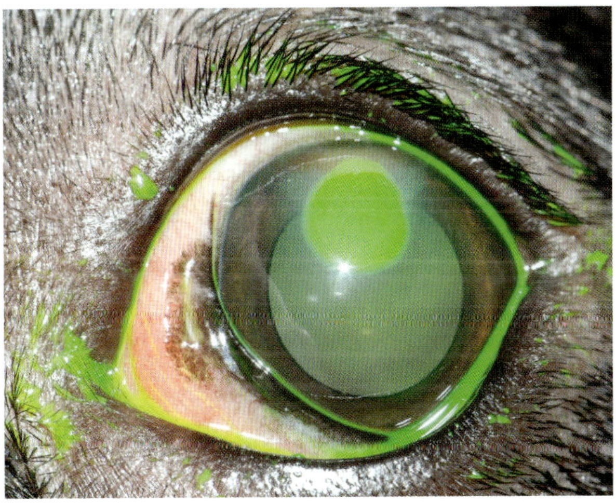

Fluorescein uptake in the corneal stroma. Same eye as above.

Superficial ulcerative keratitis is an inflammation of the corneal surface (epithelium and superficial stroma) linked to insufficient epithelial tissue.

Important notes

- The use of fluorescein is critical to diagnosis.
- The uptake of fluorescein (a hydrophilic stain) by the corneal stroma (a hydrophilic environment) demonstrates the loss of corneal epithelium (which is hydrophobic).

Superficial corneal ulcer

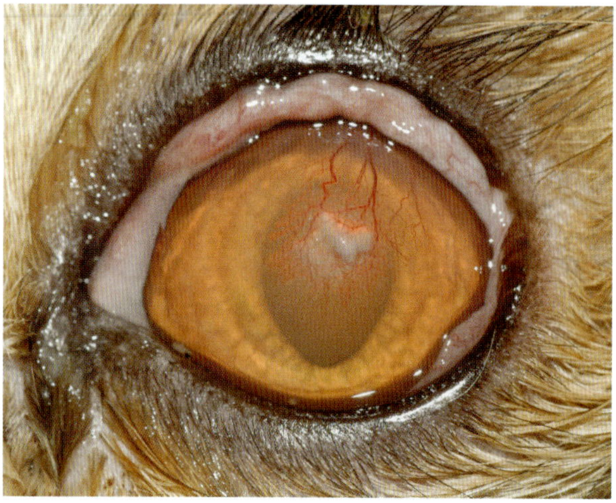

Superficial corneal ulcer in a cat with herpes keratitis. Close-up of the neovascularisation. The lack of transparency suggests a corneal ulcer.

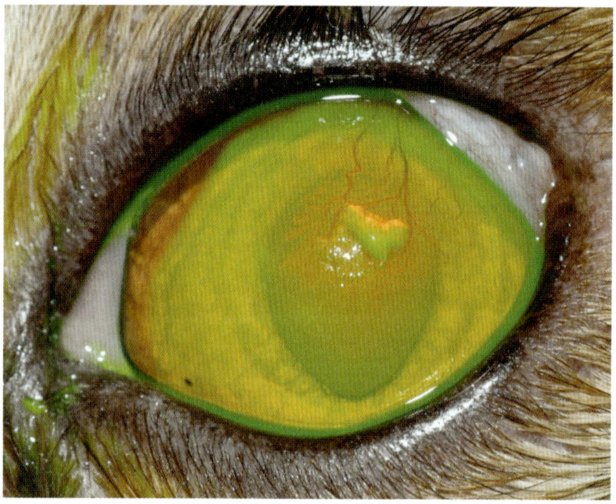

Conjunctival chemosis is more appreciable in feline corneal ulcers than in canine ones. Extensive fluorescein uptake.

Contraindicated

- As a general rule, DO NOT USE TOPICAL CORTICOSTEROIDS in corneal ulcers.

Superficial corneal ulcer

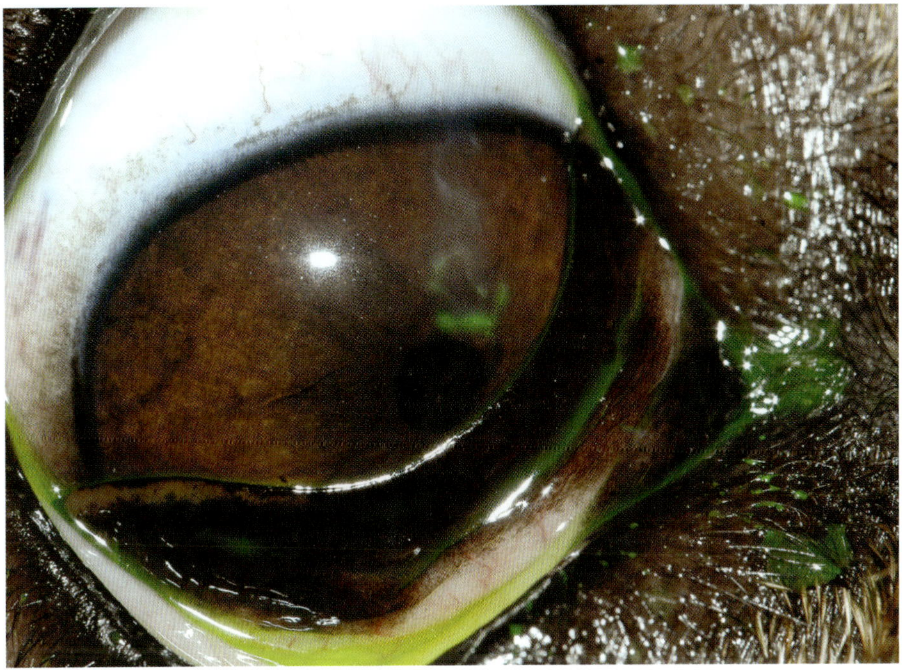

Superficial corneal ulcer due to a plant foreign body in a dog.
Time since onset: three days.

Always select the treatment that is best suited to the cause of the ulcer.

Treatment

The most common topical antibiotics to treat superficial ulcerative keratitis are chloramphenicol and tobramycin.

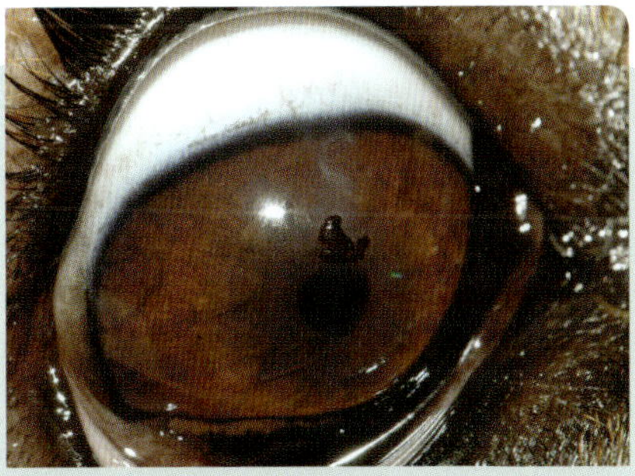

Close-up of a foreign body adhered to the cornea, just prior to removal.

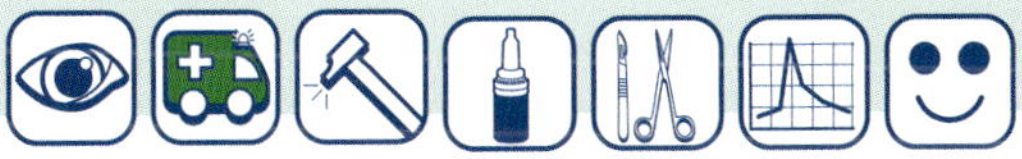

Superficial corneal ulcer

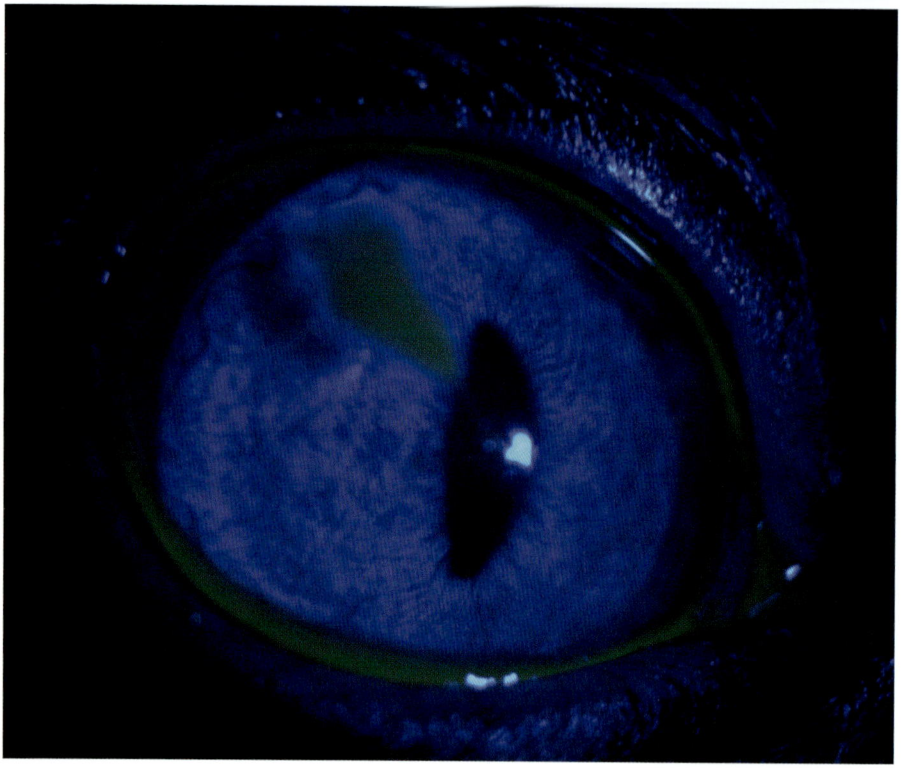

Traumatic corneal ulcer in a cat as seen through a cobalt blue filter.

i | A cobalt blue filter is very useful to highlight fluorescein uptake in superficial ulcers.

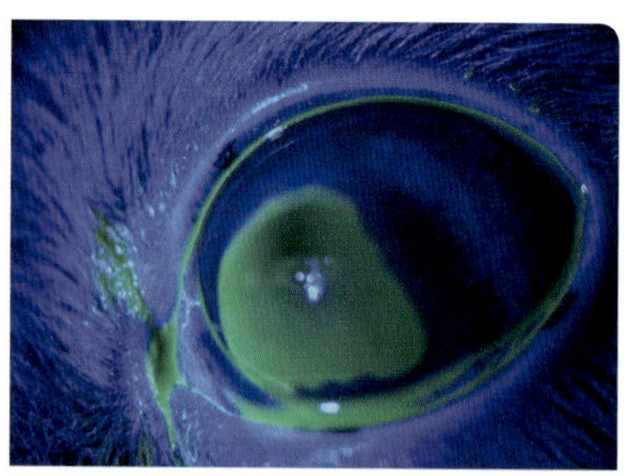

Superficial corneal ulcer associated with feline corneal degeneration in a Persian cat.

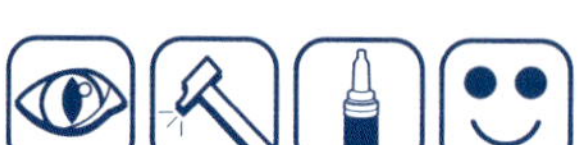

Refractory corneal ulcer

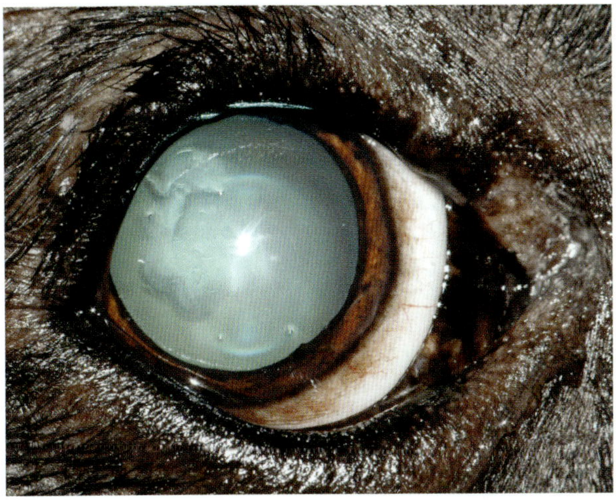

Corneal ulcer with free edges in a nine-year-old Boxer. Note the "loose lip" of nonadherent epithelial tissue.

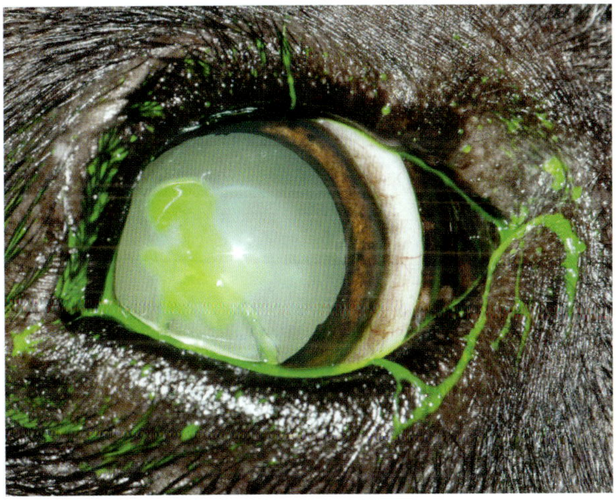

Fluorescein goes underneath the ulcer edges, outlining the extent of the lesion.

i | Refractory, or indolent, superficial ulcers are named for their general resistance to medical treatment.

Important notes

They are mainly due to poor adhesion between the basal epithelial cells and the underlying stroma.

Refractory corneal ulcer

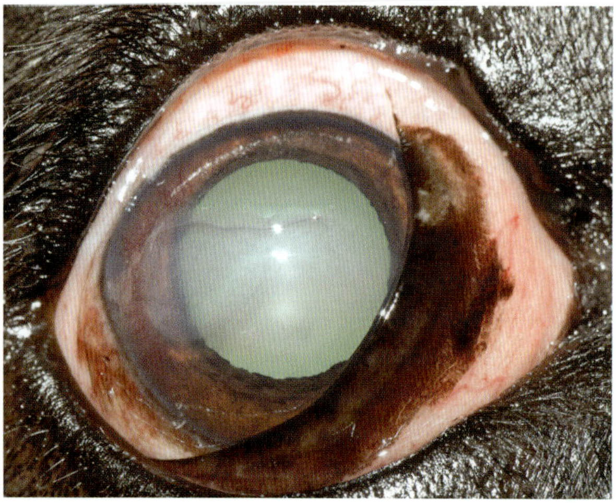

Refractory corneal ulcer in a seven-year-old Boxer.
Time since onset: 30 days.
The neovascularisation is a sign of chronicity.

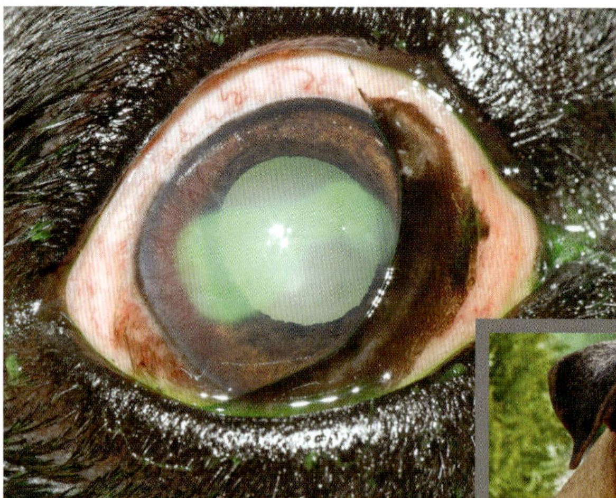

Fluorescein uptake in the cornea of the patient pictured above.

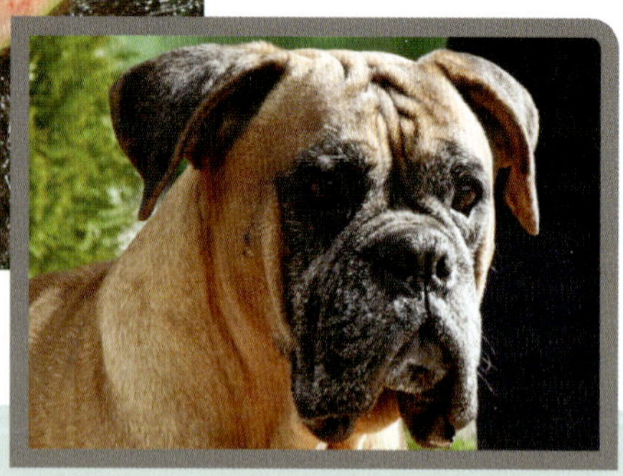

Boxers are the breed most predisposed to this type of ulcer.

Interesting notes

- Boxers are the breed most predisposed to this type of ulcer; hence, it is also referred to as a "Boxer ulcer".
- It is more common in older than younger animals.

Refractory corneal ulcer

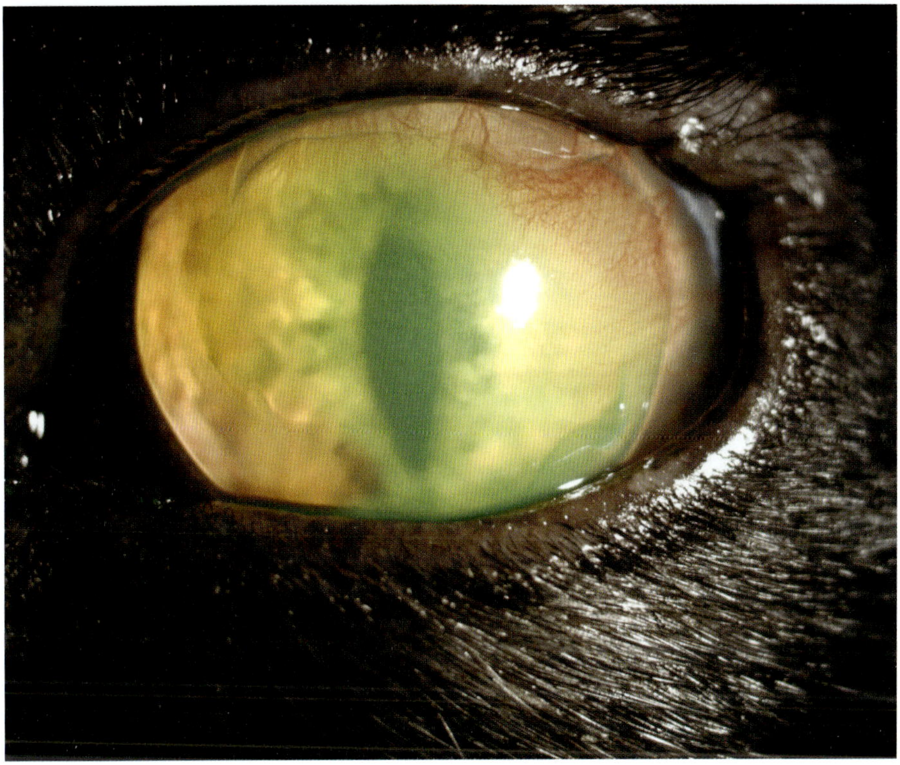

Ulcer with free edges in a cat's cornea.
Close-up of the loose epithelial edges.

This type of refractory ulcer is less common in cats than in dogs, and most cases are associated with feline herpesvirus type 1.

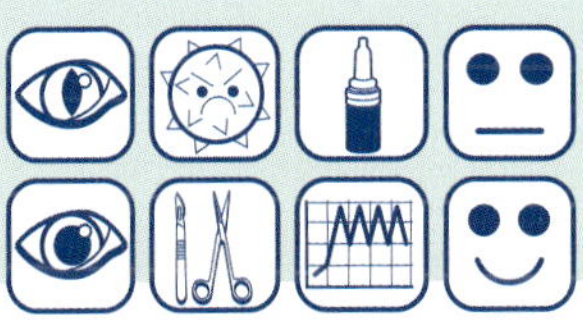

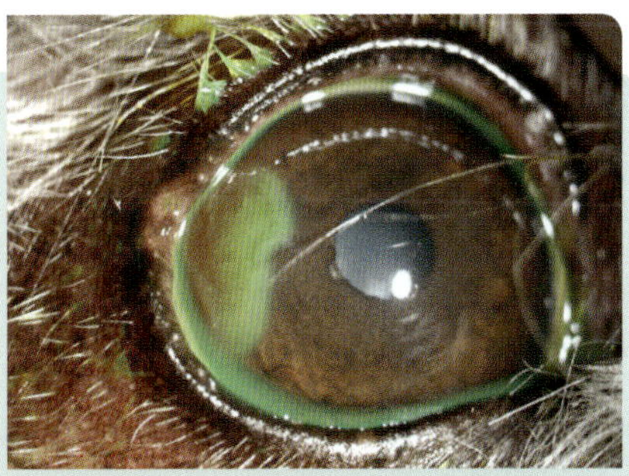

Refractory corneal ulcer in the temporal area of the eye in a West Highland Terrier. Close-up of the fluorescein stain underneath the loose epithelial edges.

Refractory corneal ulcer

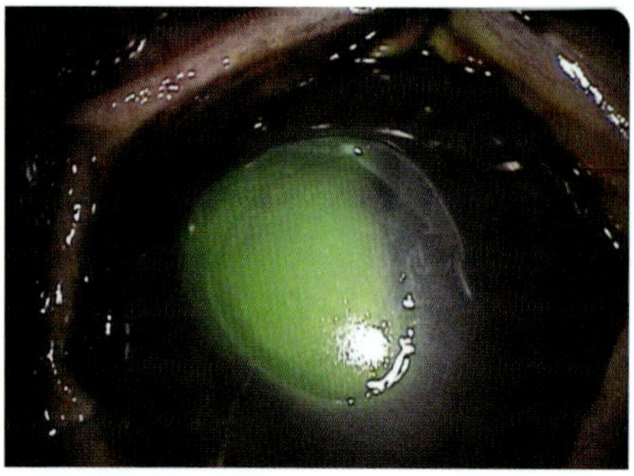

Refractory ulcer in a Boxer. Preoperatively.

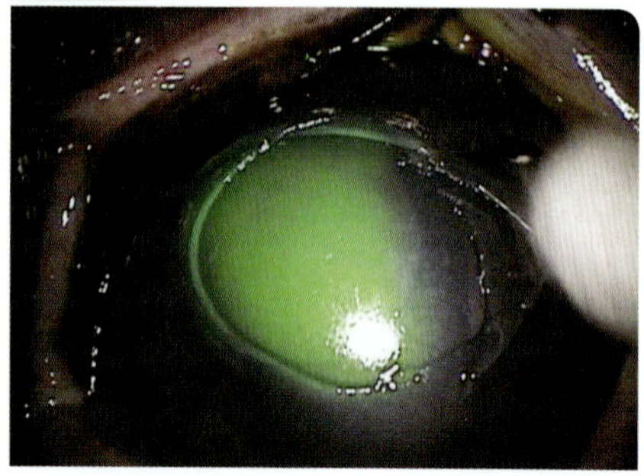

Debriding of the loose corneal epithelium using a cotton swab (under general anaesthesia).

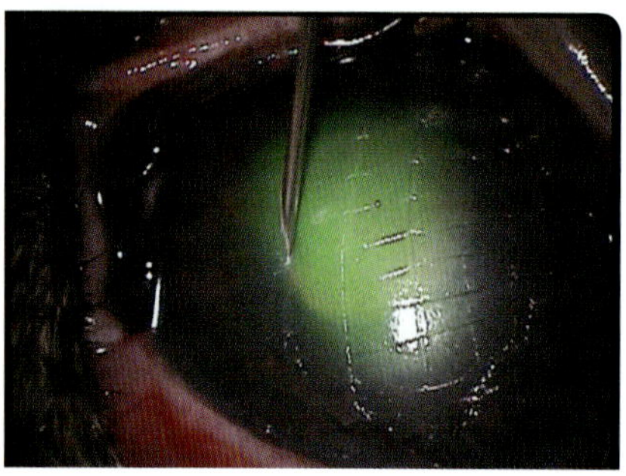

Grid keratotomy with a 25-gauge needle.

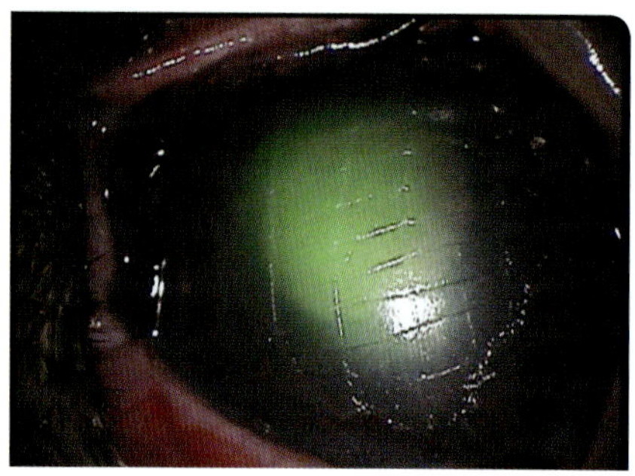

After surgery.

Contraindicated

Do not perform keratotomies in cats because corneal sequestra may result. Simply debride the loose epithelium.

Stromal ulcer

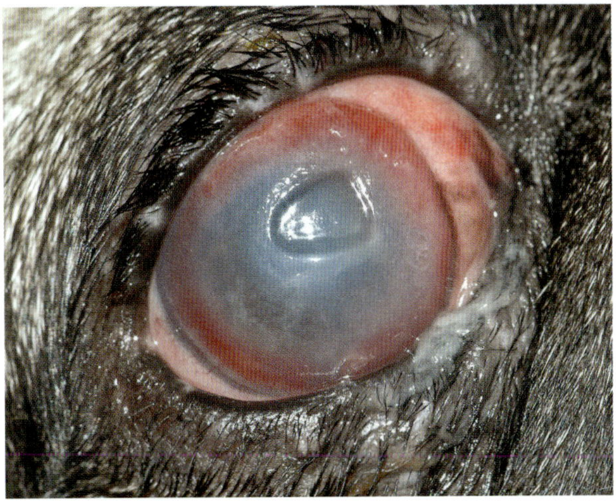

Stromal ulcerative keratitis in a two-year-old Pug. Close-up of the tissue defect, corneal oedema, and generalised inflammatory response of the cornea.
Time since onset: 14 days.

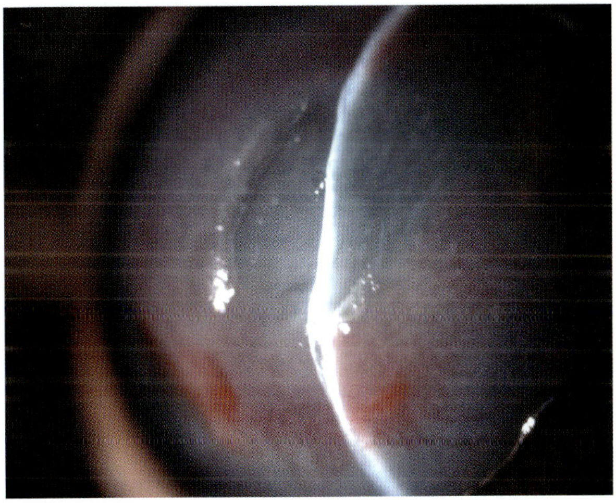

Slit-lamp picture of the patient pictured above. Note the defect in the corneal curvature, which indicates the midstromal damage.

Important notes

Stromal ulcers are generally accompanied by a severe inflammatory uveal response. Uveitis secondary to corneal damage is characteristic of this type of ulcer.

Stromal ulcer

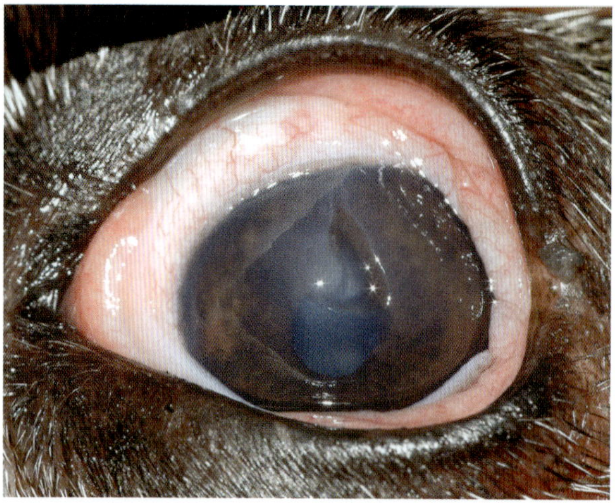

Stromal ulcer in a dog after six hours.
A cat scratch has damaged one-half of the corneal stroma.
A few hours later, corneal oedema and uveitis appear.

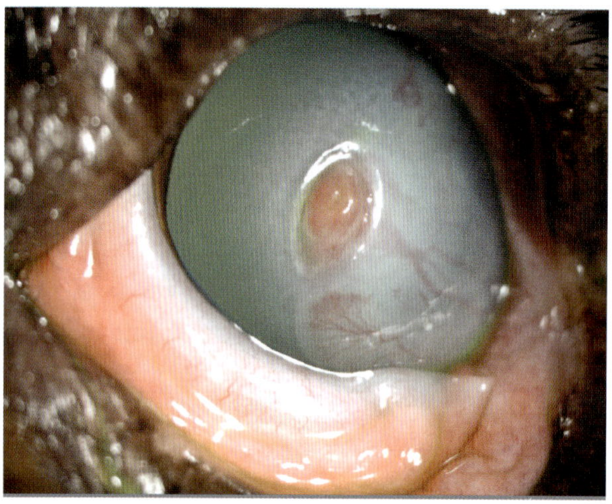

Stromal ulcerative keratitis, in the process of scarring, in an English Bulldog. The ulcer was caused by entropion of the lower eyelid.

If medical treatment begins promptly and is frequent (every 1–2 hours to start), and the ulcer is not deep, scarring may be achieved.

If progress is not favourable in the first 24 hours, consider corneal surgery.

Stromal ulcer

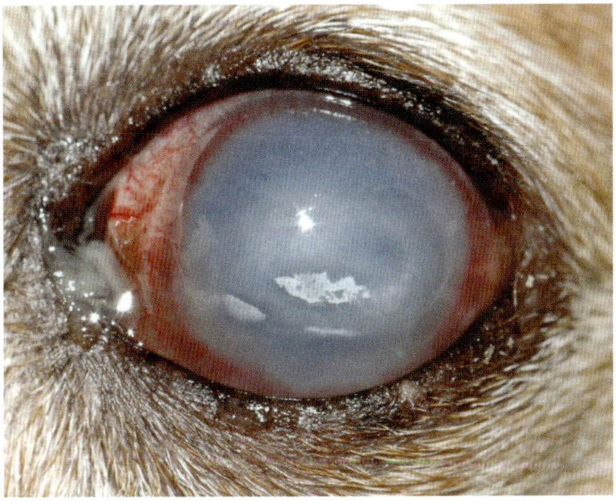

Stromal ulcerative keratitis in a six-year-old Shih-Tzu. Time since onset: 35 days. Close-up of the pericorneal ring and corneal oedema associated with uveitis. Aetiology: stromal ulcer due to exposure.

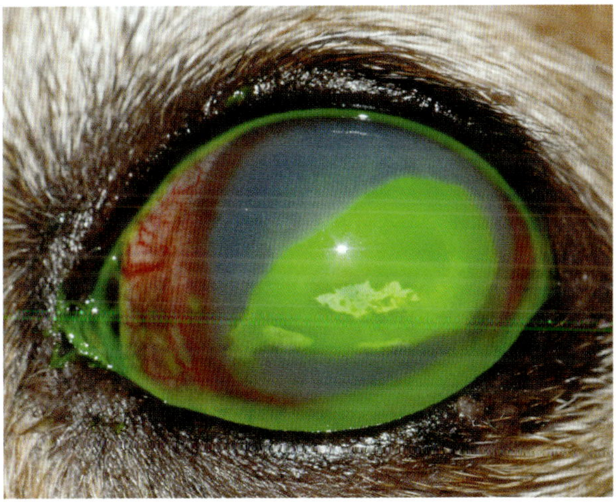

Fluorescein vital staining outlines the extent of the stromal damage in a cornea with generalised oedema.

Interesting notes

In order to promote corneal regeneration, consider using autologous serum, hyaluronic acid, or chondroitin sulphate (in addition to topical antibiotics) in the medical treatment of this type of ulcer.

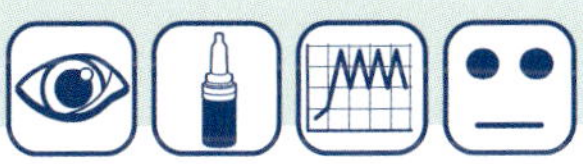

Stromal ulcer

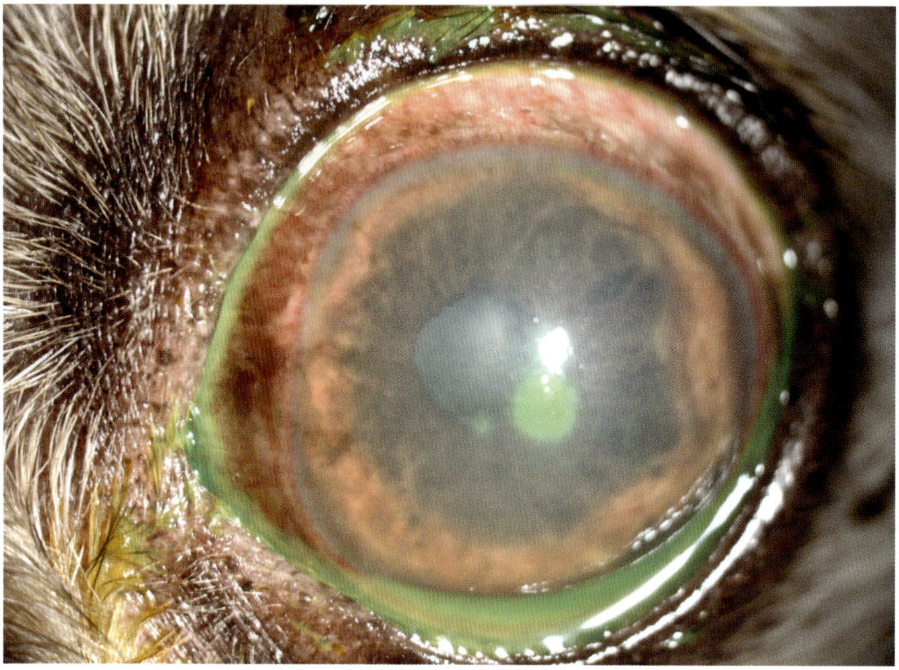

Central stromal ulcer in a three-year-old Shih-Tzu.
Time since onset: 24 hours.

Important notes

- Central stromal ulcers in brachycephalic dog breeds (Pug, Shih-Tzu, Lhasa Apso, Pekingese, French Bulldog, etc.) should be closely monitored, even daily, due to the high risk of rapid progression to a deep corneal ulcer in a matter of hours.

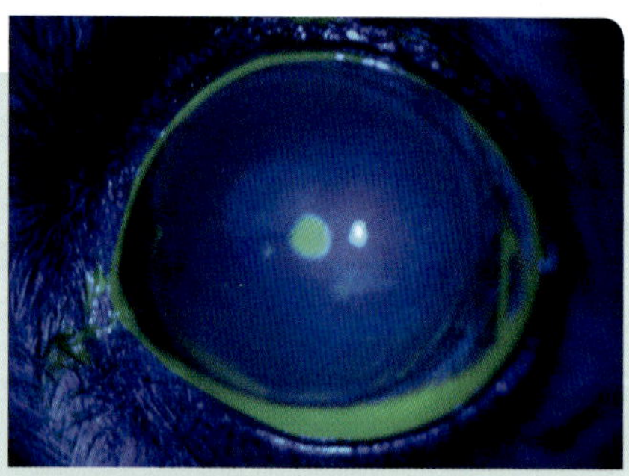

Close-up of the patient's lesion using fluorescein and a cobalt blue filter.

Deep corneal ulcer

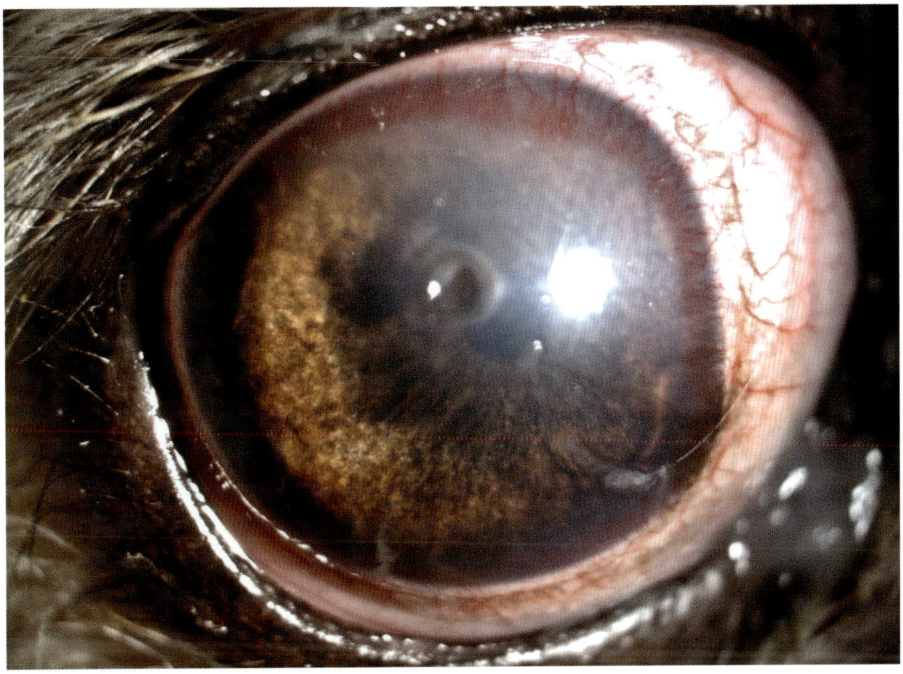

A deep corneal ulcer, central, in a two-year-old Lhasa Apso.
Time since onset: two days.
This animal exhibited photophobia and blepharospasm.

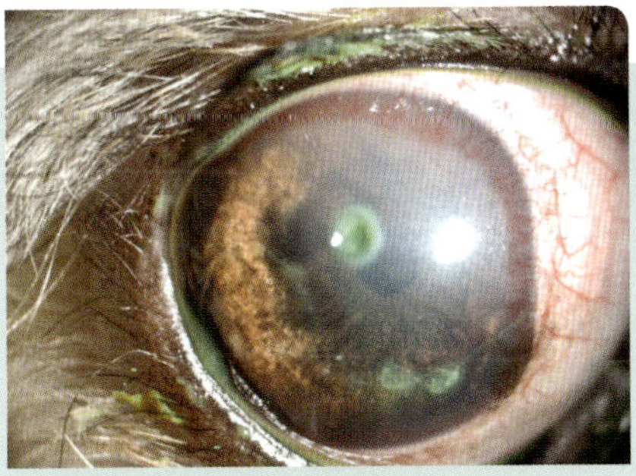

Fluorescein uptake in the deep corneal stroma.

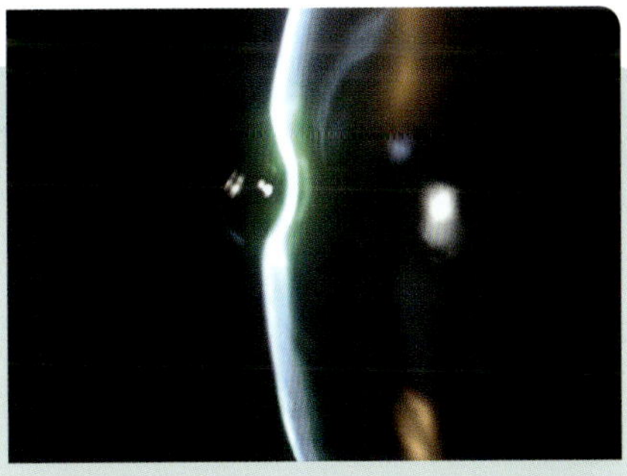

The slit-lamp examination confirms that the corneal defect extends $^2/_3$ of the thickness of the stroma.

We can attempt medical treatment in such cases, but most will require corneal surgery.

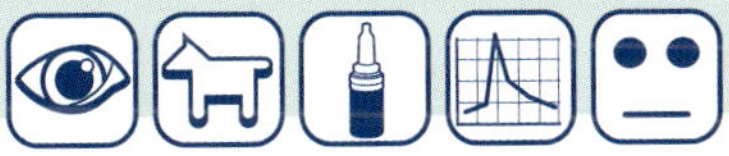

Deep corneal ulcer

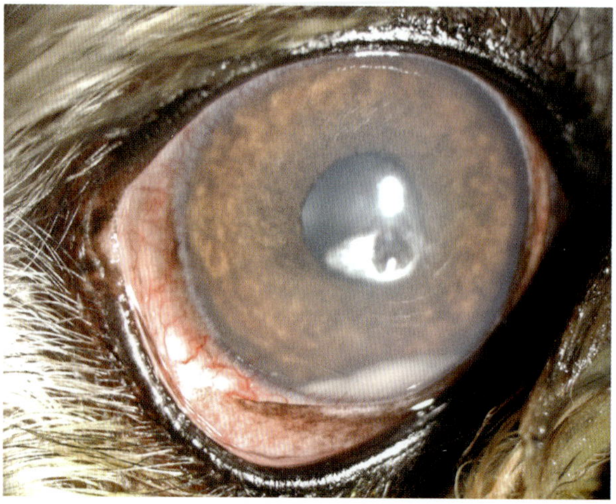

Deep corneal ulcer in a brachycephalic patient. The uveal inflammatory reaction becomes more severe as the corneal damage progresses. Hypopyon and corneal oedema are present.

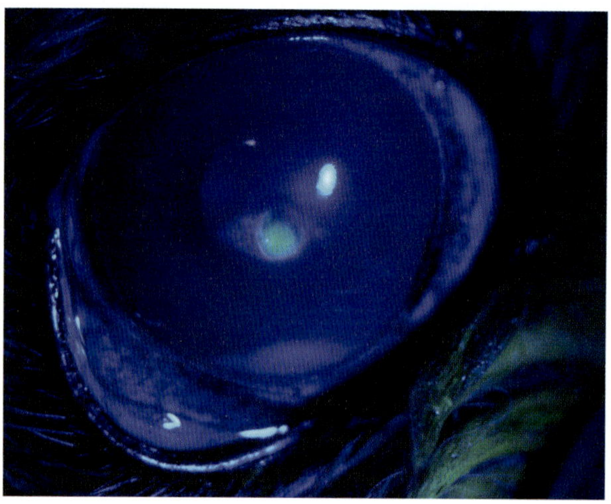

Close-up of the corneal lesion of the patient pictured above. Note the corneal dystrophy in the area surrounding the ulcer.

Important notes

Uveitis becomes more severe as the corneal damage progresses. Hypopyon may be sterile or nonsterile (in case of bacterial contamination).

Deep corneal ulcer

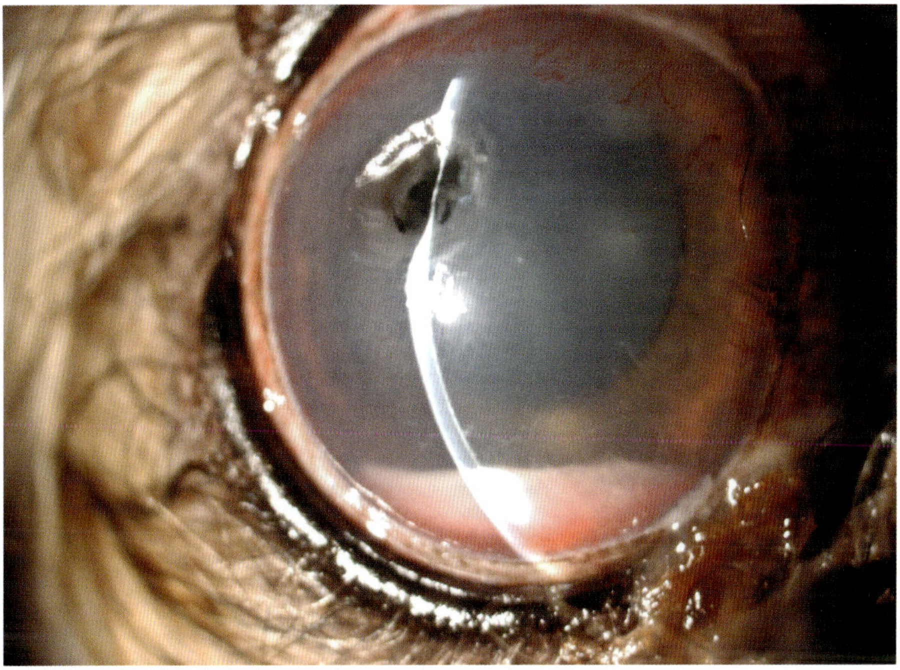

Slit-lamp picture of the patient pictured above. Close-up of the depth of the ulcer (predescemetic) and the hypopyon in the anterior chamber.

Emergency

These ulcers require emergency surgery due to the risk of imminent worsening and perforation.

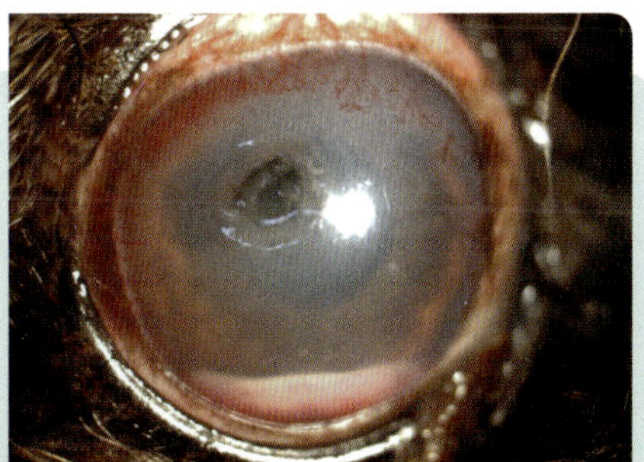

Deep ulcer after 36 hours.
Severe intraocular damage (uveitis).

Deep corneal ulcer

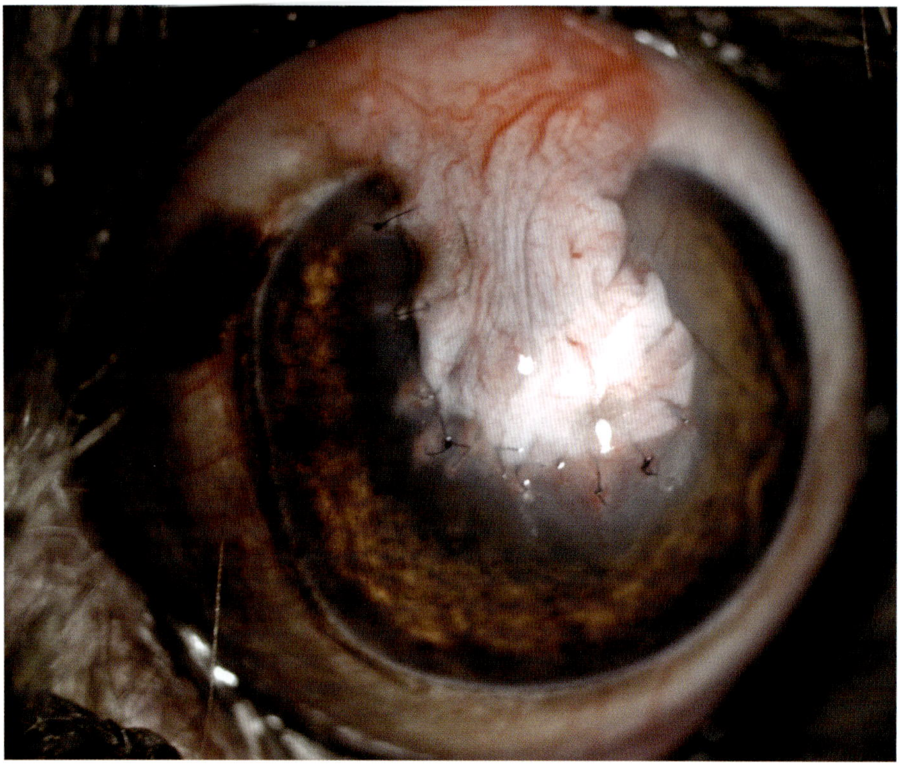

A flap of bulbar conjunctiva is sutured to the cornea to treat a deep corneal ulcer. Twenty days postoperatively. Nylon 9-0 suture, simple interrupted pattern.

Important notes

- The preferred surgical technique to treat deep corneal ulcers depends on the surgeon's microsurgical proficiency and the state of the cornea.
- Treatment may involve a conjunctival flap (pedicle, bridge, or 360º), a corneal scleral conjunctival transposition, or the use of biomaterials (porcine intestinal submucosa, fresh or frozen cornea, etc.).

Descemetocoele

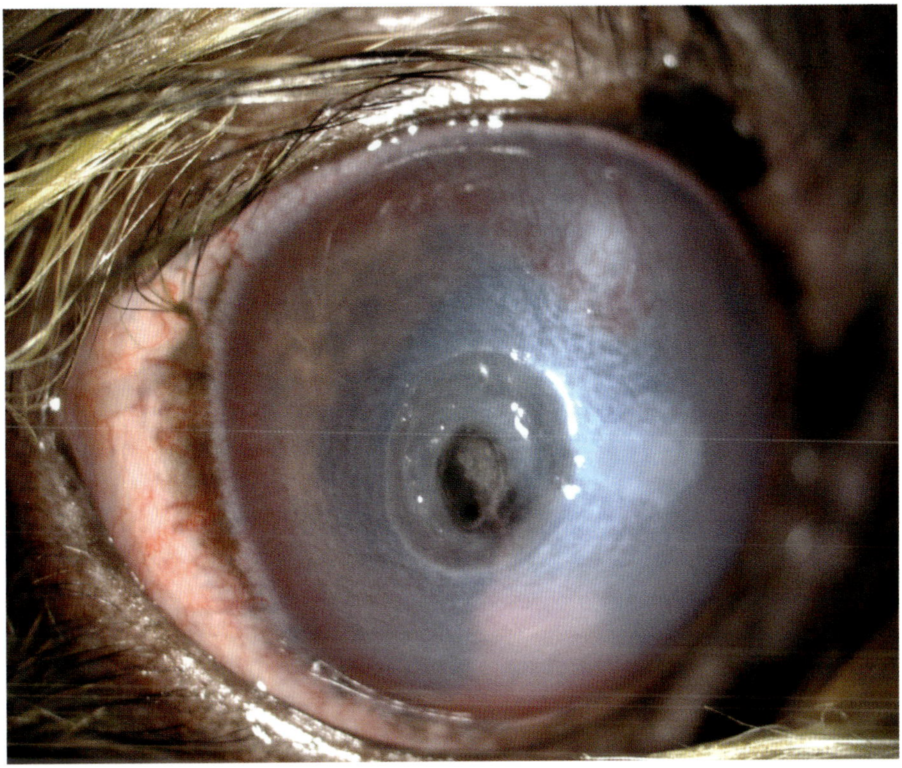

Descemetocoele in a dog's cornea. Note the loss of corneal stroma in the ulcer defect. The visible layer is Descemet's membrane.

This is the deepest type of corneal ulcer, seen prior to perforation.

Due to the nearly complete lack of nerve endings in this part of the cornea, these lesions tend to be less painful than superficial ulcers.

Emergency

Surgical treatment is imperative.

Descemetocoele

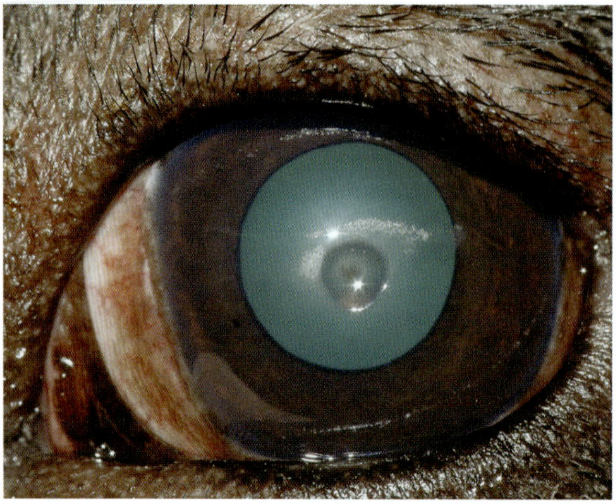

Descemetocoele in a three-year-old French Bulldog. Total loss of stroma in the central part of the deep ulcer.
Time since onset: two days.

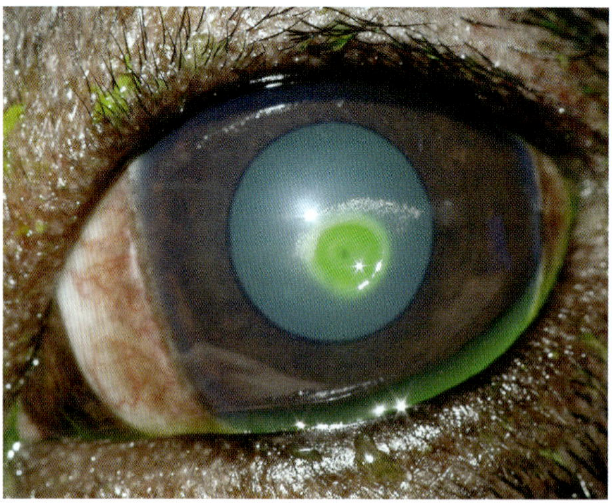

Fluorescein is absorbed into the stroma only, so the centre of the ulcer is not stained (descemetocoele).

Interesting notes

Fluorescein (hydrophilic stain) is not taken up into Descemet's membrane (basement membrane of the corneal endothelium) because it is hydrophobic.

Corneal perforation

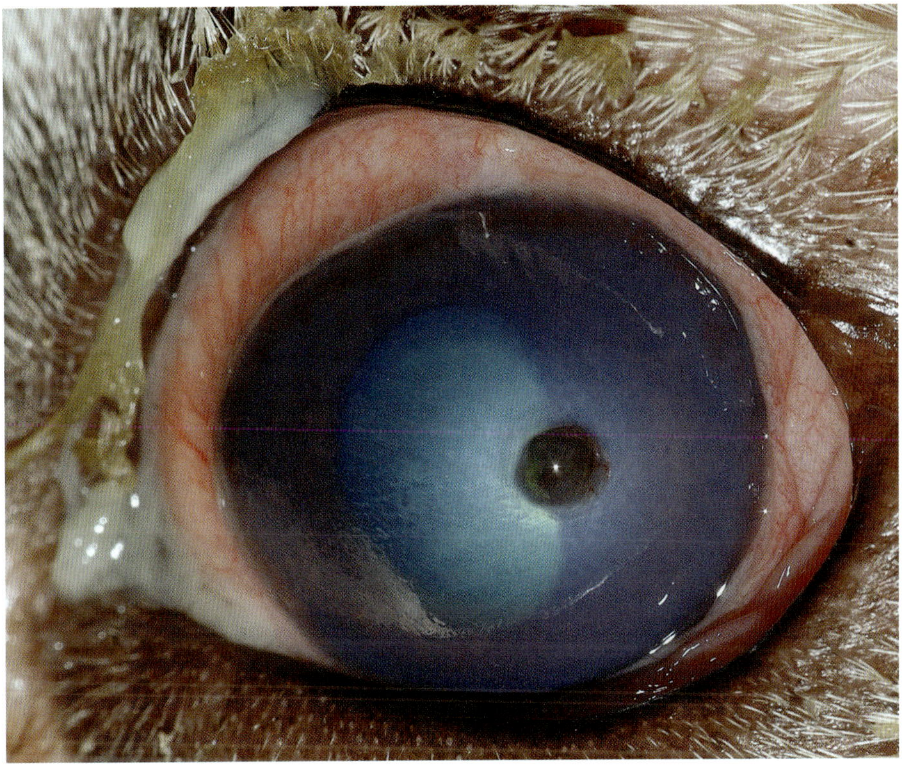

Traumatic corneal perforation in a dog.
The hernia in the iris is visible through the corneal defect.

Interesting notes

The irregular shape of the pupil helps in diagnosis.

Corneal perforation

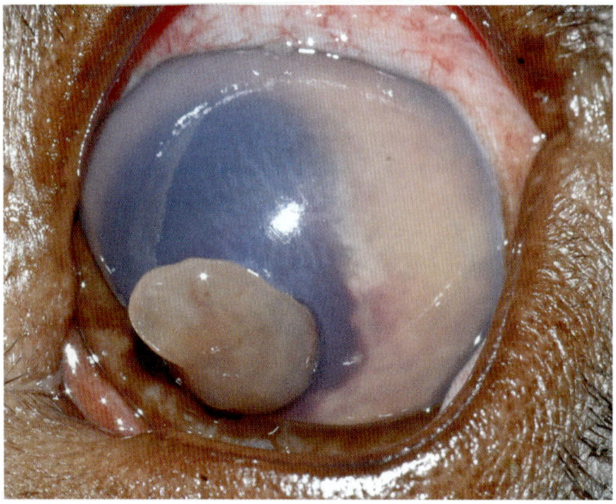

Corneal perforation in a Pointer after a day of hunting. Close-up of the fibrin plug that covers the hernia of the iris.
Time since onset: 12 hours.

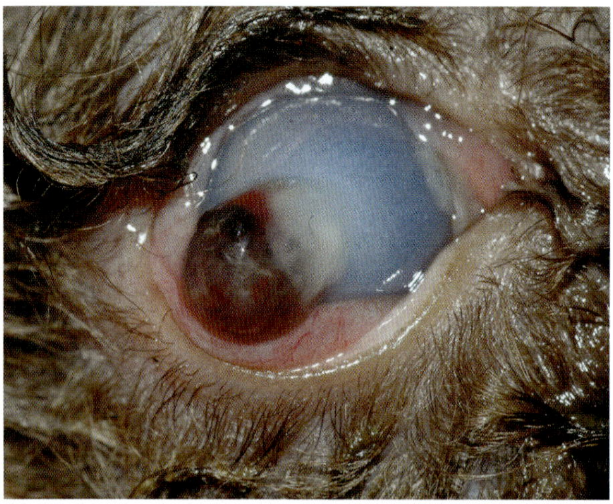

Corneal perforation after 24 hours. Severe intraocular damage and loss of uveal tissue occur through the wound. Cat scratch.

i The most common causes of corneal perforations are direct traumas: shotgun pellets, sticks, and cat scratches.

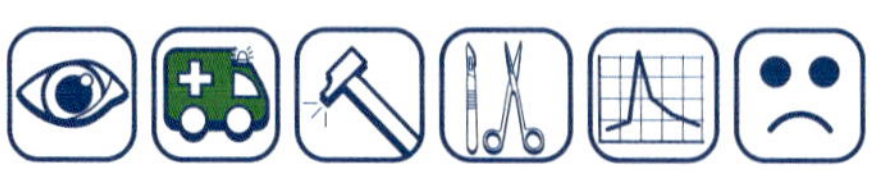

Corneal perforation

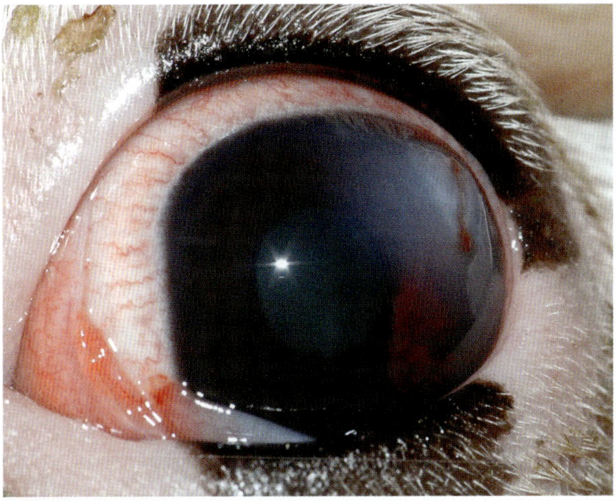

Corneal perforation due to a vertical cat scratch in a French Bulldog.
Blood in the anterior chamber (hyphaema) is indicative of the extent of the intraocular damage.

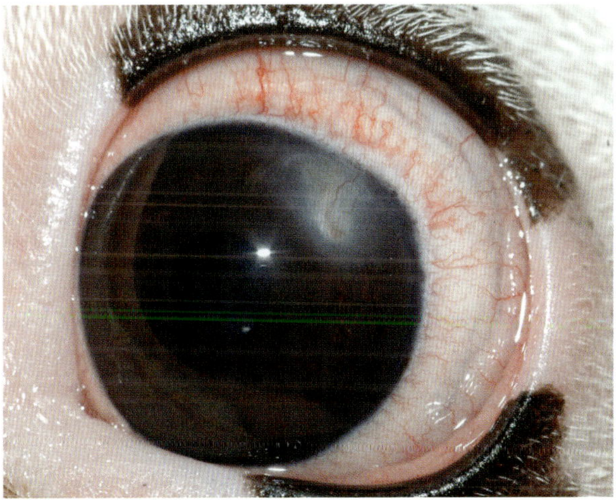

Patient's eye 25 days later.

In corneal perforations without iris prolapse, start with medical treatment. A fibrin plug usually forms at the site of the perforation and prevents the loss of aqueous humour.

Important notes

- Use of tropicamide minimises the risk of synechiae.

Corneal perforation

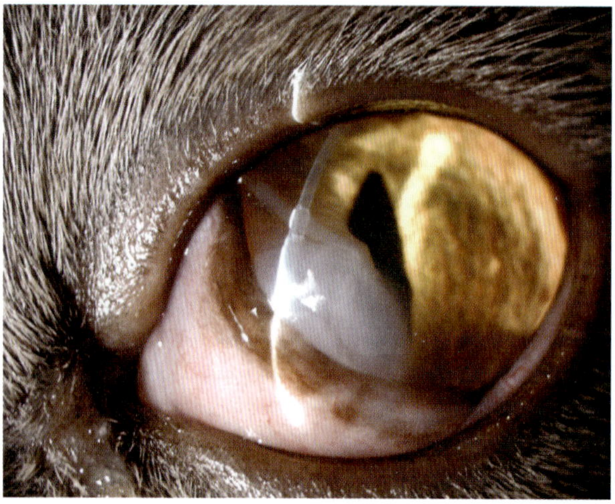

Corneal perforation due to a horizontal scratch.
Common lesion in cat fights.

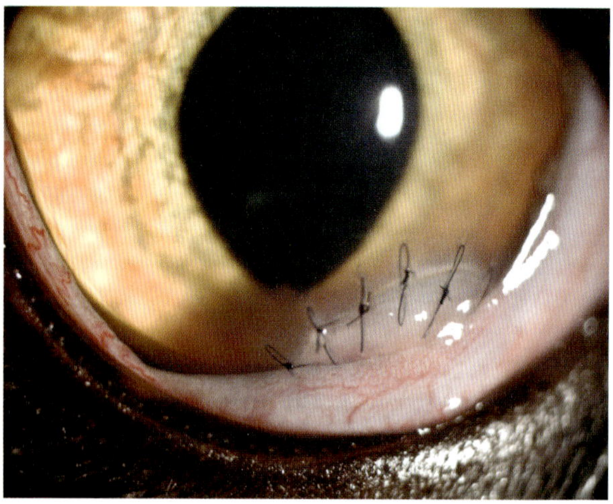

Surgical reconstruction of a feline corneal perforation similar to that pictured above.

Surgical technique

- When suturing the cornea, NEVER CROSS THE CORNEAL ENDOTHELIUM (include 2/3 of the corneal thickness).
- Always use viscoelastic material.
- Test the viability of prolapsed tissue.

Corneal perforation

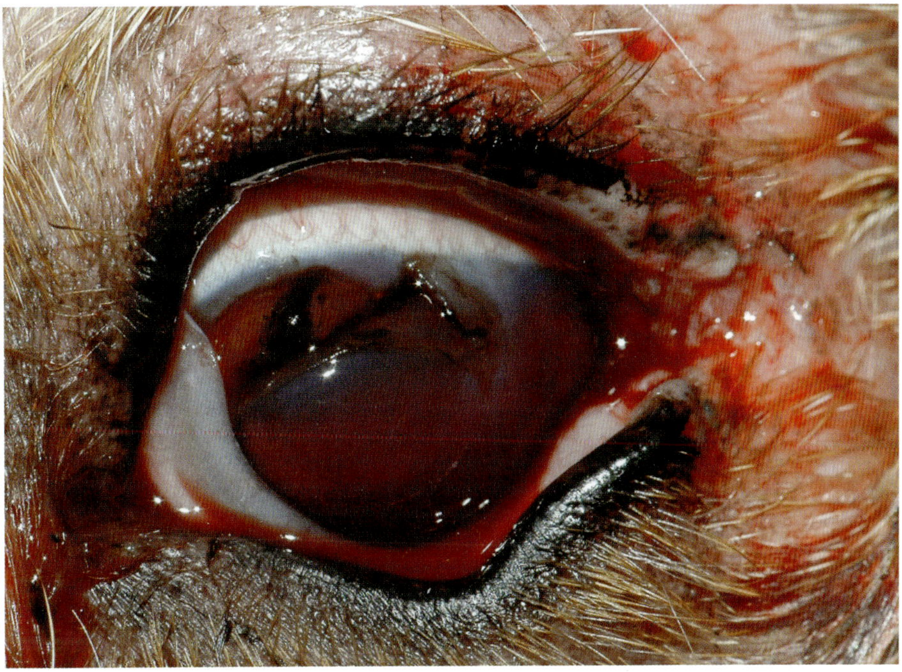

Corneal perforation with iris hernia and severe intraocular haemorrhage.
Cause: pellet wound. Note the burn in the palpebral margin (temporal area) caused by the pellet.

Important notes

In corneal perforations, carefully evaluate the intraocular damage before considering reconstructive surgery.

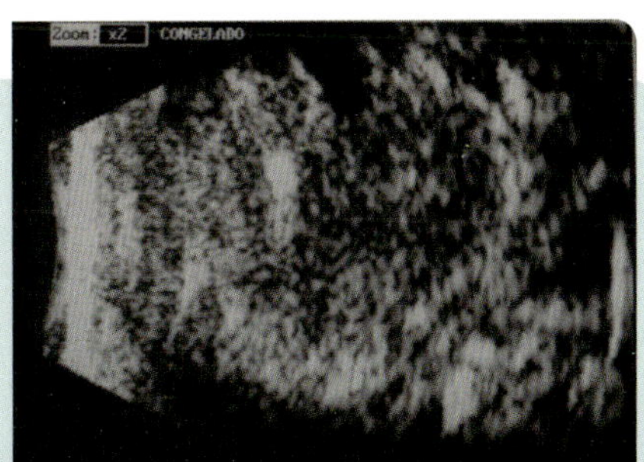

Ocular ultrasound of the patient's eye. Severe tissue destruction. Vitreal haemorrhage.

Melting corneal ulcer

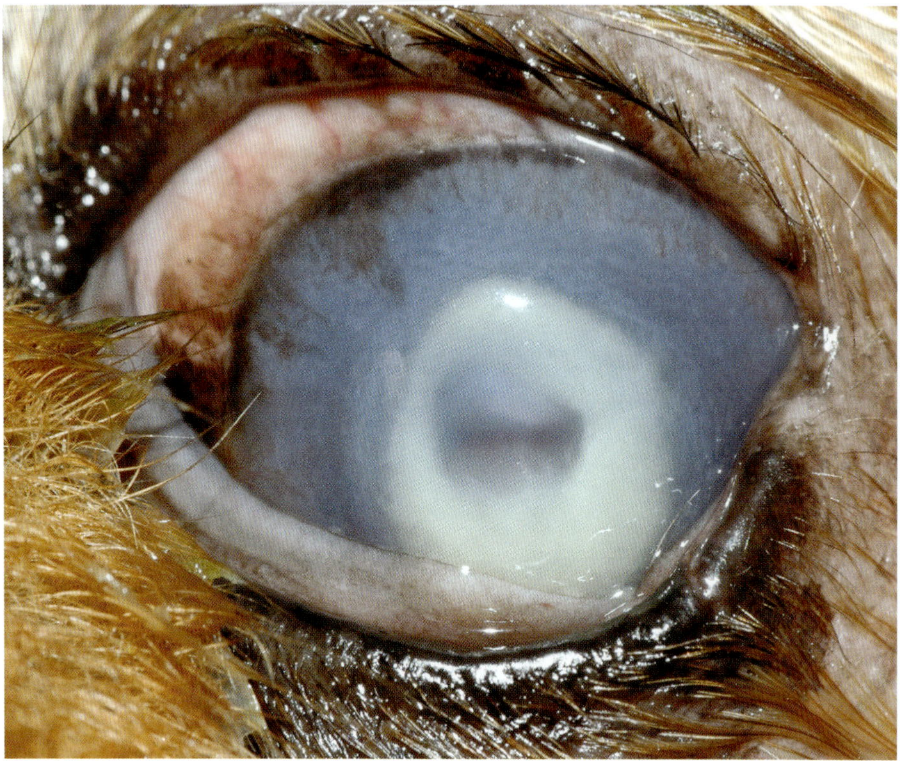

Complicated melting corneal ulcer in a Pekingese.
Characteristic appearance of liquefied corneal stroma.

The proteases and collagenases (enzymes that can degrade the corneal stroma) cause rapid destruction of the corneal collagen fibres. *Pseudomonas* is often found in these cases.

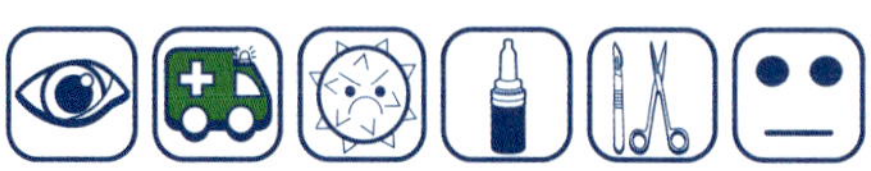

Melting corneal ulcer

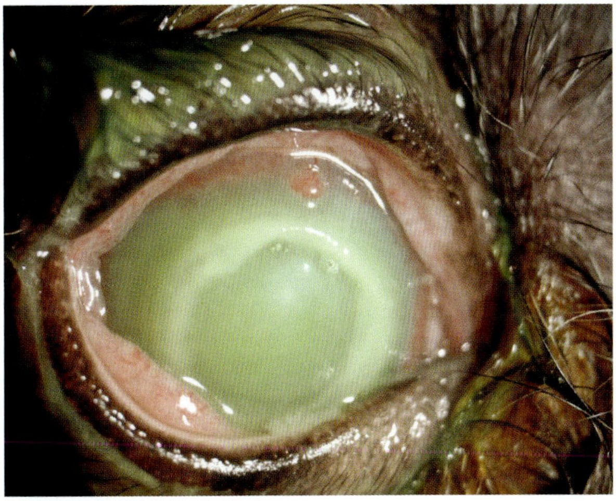

Complicated melting ulcer in a dog who was treated with topical corticosteroids. Generalised corneal degradation.

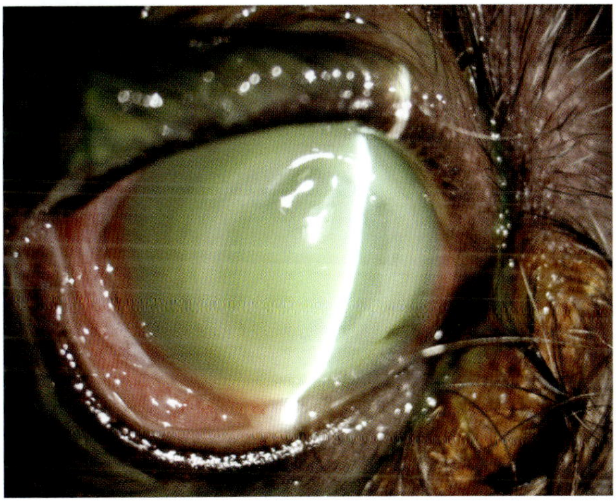

Slit-lamp picture. Close-up showing the depth of the ulcer.

Contraindicated

Use of topical corticosteroids in an ulcerated cornea accelerates degeneration and collagenolysis.

Melting corneal ulcer

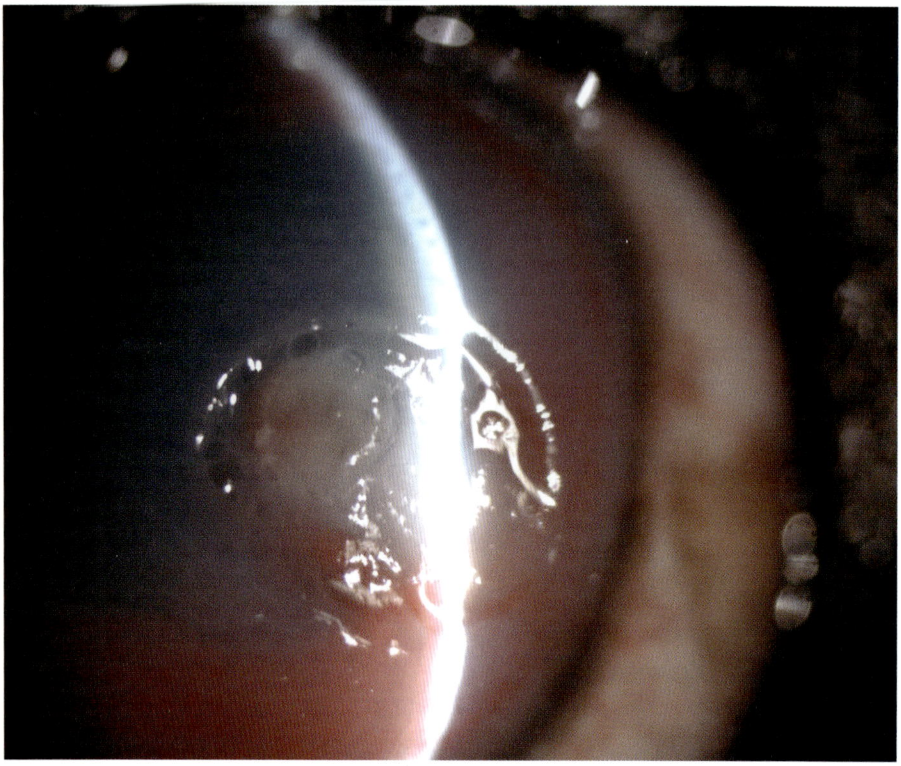

Bullous keratopathy secondary to enzymatic corneal damage caused by proterases and collagenases.
The patient was treated with a local anaesthetic for seven days.

Contraindicated

- Use local anaesthetics only for diagnostic purposes and never for prolonged corneal therapy due to their corneal neurotoxicity.

Treatment

- This type of ulcer requires the addition of anticollagenases such as NAC (N-acetylcysteine) and autologous serum to the topical antibiotic treatment.

Chronic superficial keratitis

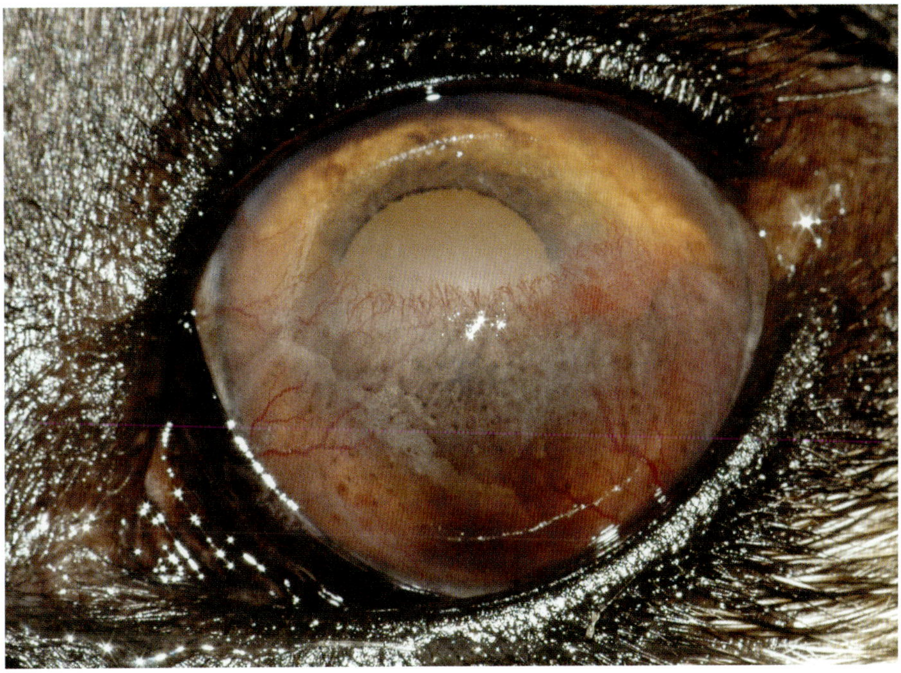

Chronic superficial keratitis (CSK) with neovascularisation, cellular infiltrate, and pigmentation.
Time since onset: three months.
Left eye of the patient pictured below.

Superficial inflammation of the cornea (epithelium, basement membrane, and stroma) characterised by neovascularisation, cellular infiltrate, and/or pigmentary invasion.

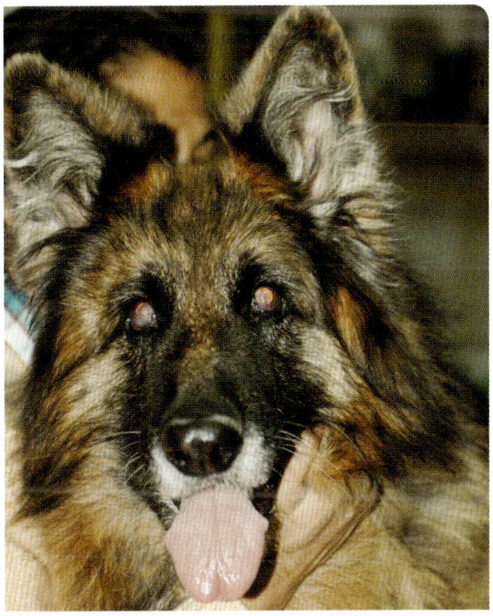

German Shepherd with bilateral CSK.

Chronic superficial keratitis

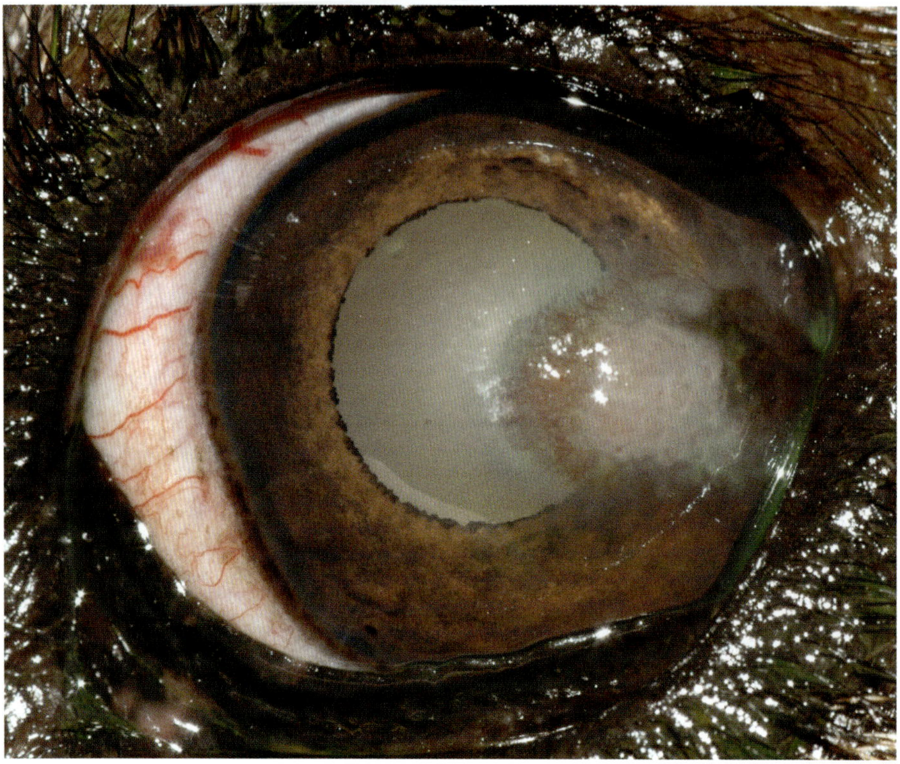

Chronic superficial keratitis in a four-year-old German Shepherd.
Lesion in the temporal area of the cornea.
Close-up of the cellular infiltrate and blood vessels.
Time since onset: 25 days.

Breed predisposition

The German Shepherd is the most commonly affected breed, followed by the Belgian Tervuren. Mixes of these breeds can also suffer from CSK.

Important notes

The younger the patient, the more severe the illness is considered to be.
UV rays of sun exacerbate the inflammatory process.

Chronic superficial keratitis

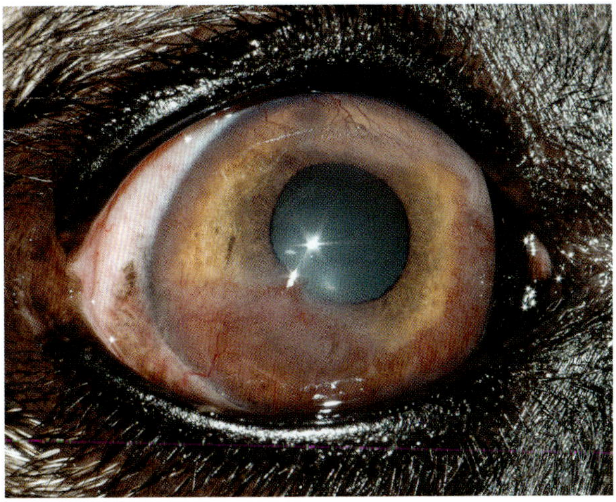

Corneal invasion by blood vessels during the acute phase of CSK.
Seven-year-old German Shepherd.

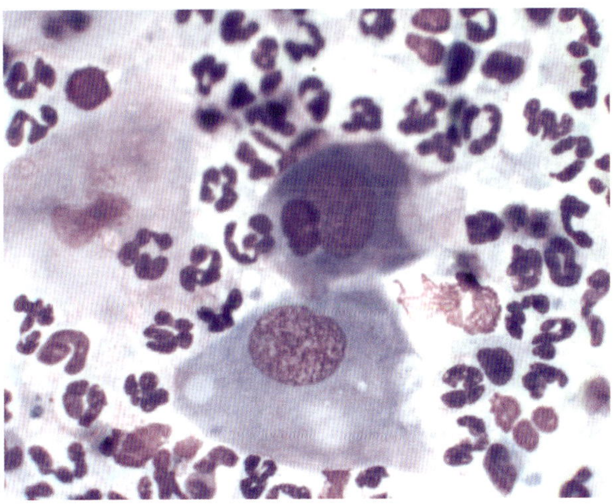

CSK. Primary neutrophilic inflammatory response.
Cytological image courtesy of Cristina Fernández Algarra.

- Corneal invasion by blood vessels (pannus) starts from the temporal region in most cases. The vessels may then extend throughout the cornea.
- They generally affect the superficial stroma.

Chronic superficial keratitis

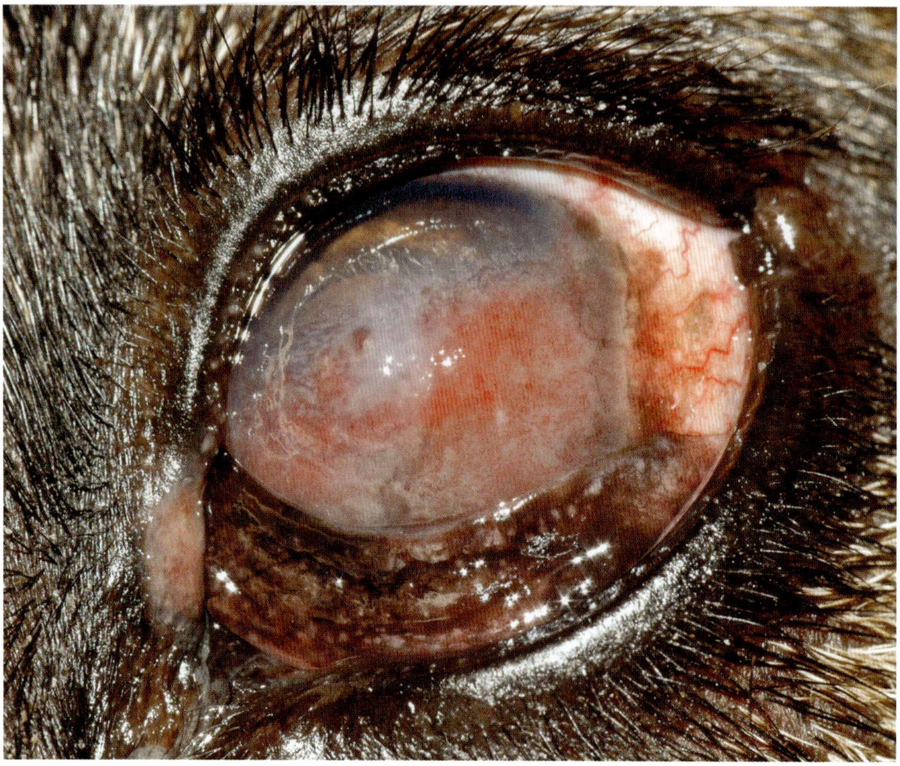

Cellular and vascular infiltration of the cornea of a German Shepherd with very severe CSK. This patient also has a lymphoplasmacytic infiltration of the nictitating membrane.

The most common cells in these phases are fibroblasts, macrophages, and keratocytes. This cellular infiltrate develops in response to the inflammatory process.

Chronic superficial keratitis

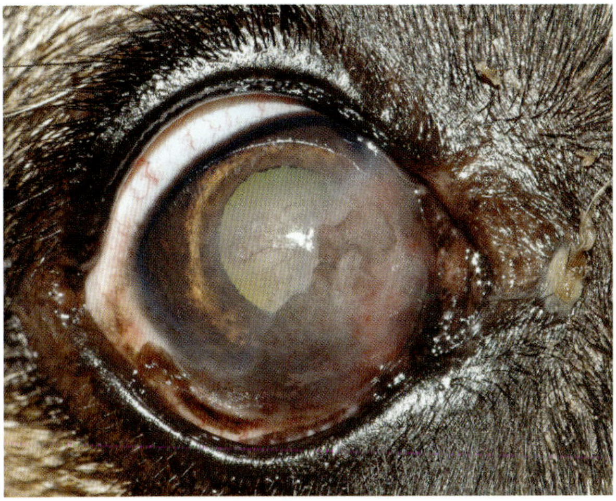

Advanced CSK. Pigmentary invasion in the corneal stroma.
Time since onset: four months, without medical treatment.

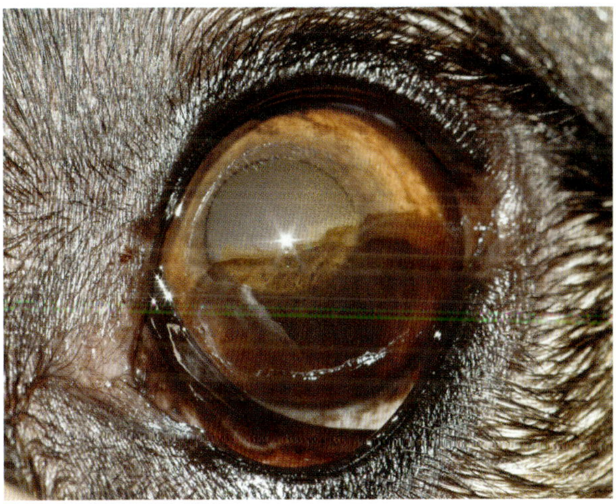

Pigmentation phase in a German Shepherd with CSK. Medical treatment successfully reverses the neovascularisation and cellular infiltration, but it does not fully eliminate the melanotic pigment.

Treatment

- Medical treatment is mainly based on topical immunosuppressants: corticosteroids (dexamethasone), cyclosporine A 0.2 %, or tacrolimus 0.02 %.
- In severe cases, consider subconjunctival and/or systemic routes of drug administration.

Chronic superficial keratitis

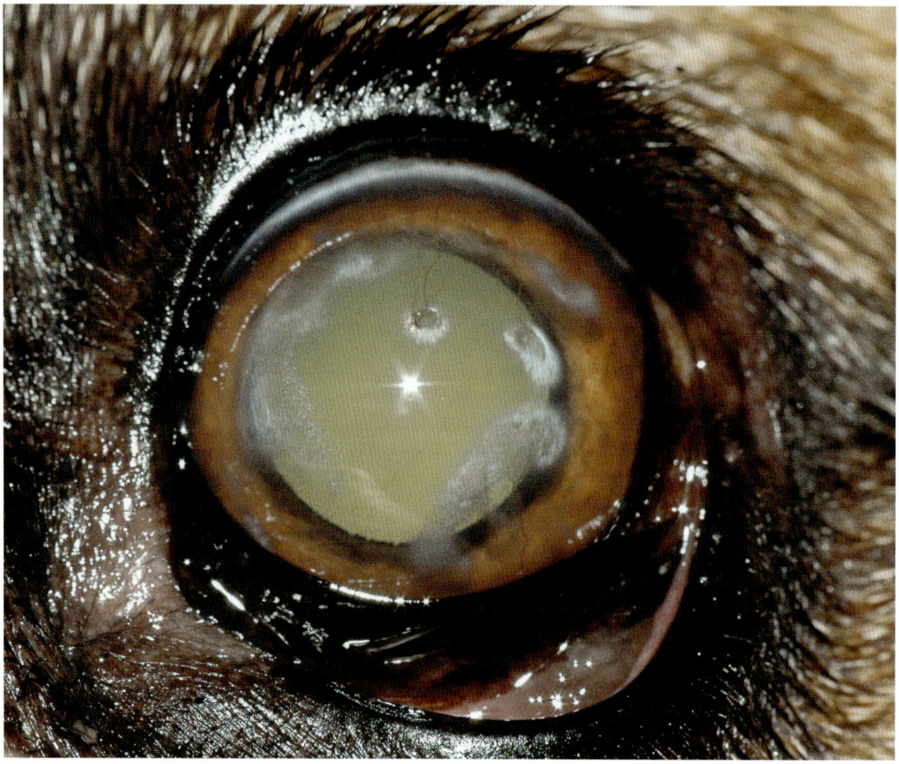

German Shepherd with CSK.

i The appearance of cholesterol deposits in the corneal stroma is rare but occurs in some patients in advanced phases of CSK.

Keratoconjunctivitis sicca

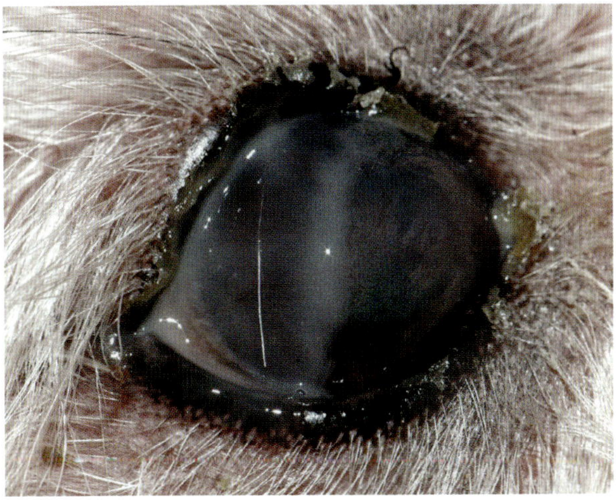

Severe keratoconjunctivitis sicca (KCS) in a six-year-old West Highland White Terrier. Time since onset: two months. Close-up of mucoid secretion, crusts on the palpebral margins, and neovascularisation of the cornea.

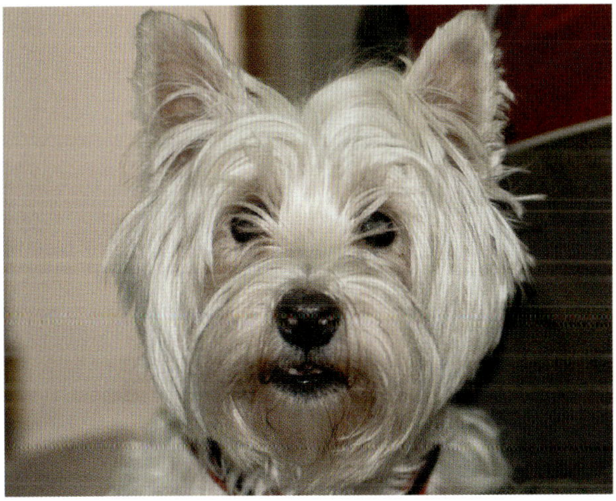

Patient pictured above.

i | Inflammatory disease of the cornea (and the conjunctiva) due to a qualitative and/or quantitative deficiency in the precorneal tear film.

MUCUS on the cornea is pathognomonic for KCS.

Keratoconjunctivitis sicca

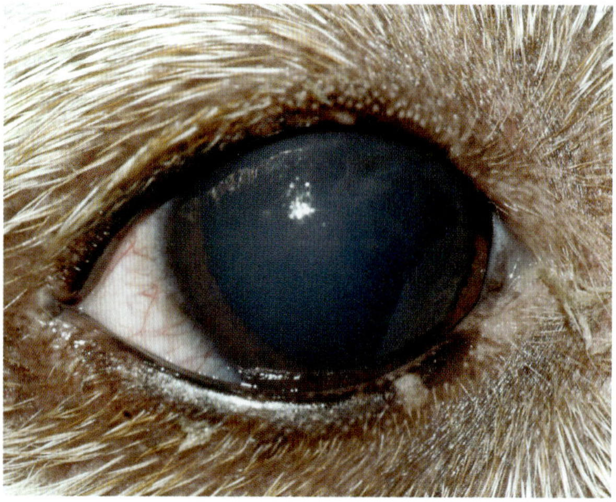

Lack of shine on the cornea is an early sign of KCS. Two-year-old mixed breed dog with mild KCS.

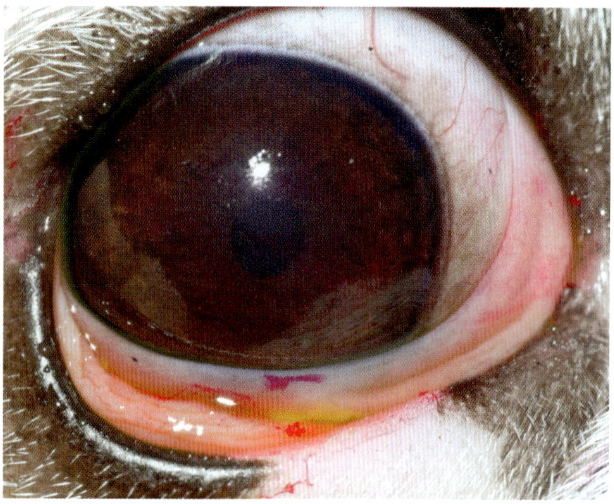

Rose bengal is a vital stain often used for early KCS diagnosis. Close-up of its uptake in the affected areas of the cornea.

i | The normal cornea is transparent, smooth, shiny, and avascular. As KCS progresses, the cornea loses these characteristics.

Keratoconjunctivitis sicca

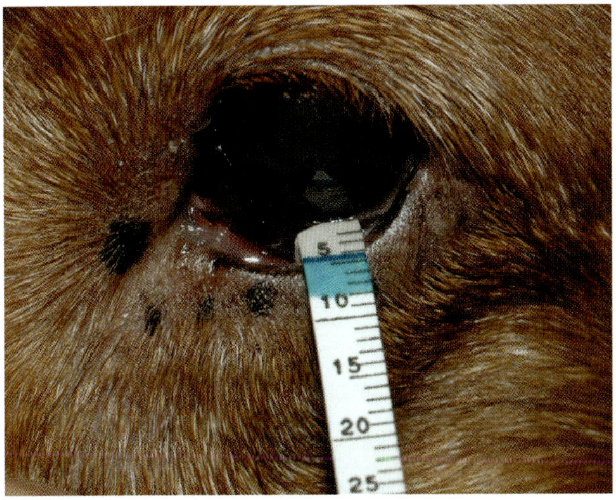

Mild KCS in a Cocker Spaniel.
Schirmer's (simple) test results below 8 mm/min are considered abnormal.

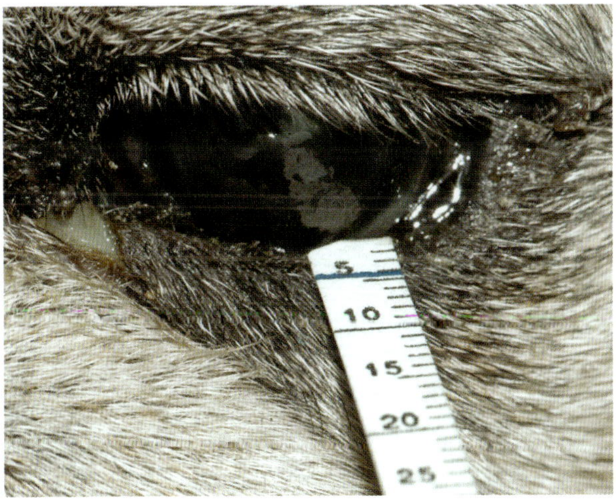

Severe KCS in an English Bulldog.
Very severe hyposecretion.
Schirmer's test 0 mm/min.

Important notes

- The normal Schirmer's test result (in dogs) is 15-20 mm/min.
- Patient with suspected KCS: Schirmer's test result of 8–10 mm/min.
- Patient with KCS: Schirmer's test result of <8 mm/min.

Keratoconjunctivitis sicca

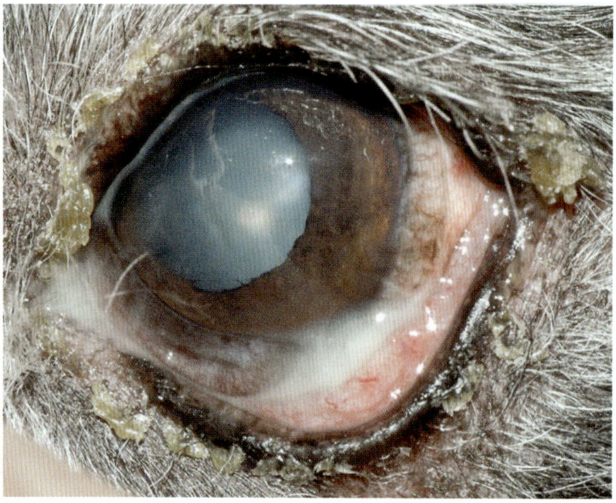

KCS in a West Highland White Terrier. Close-up of the mucoid secretion and conjunctival hypertrophy and hyperaemia. Corneal damage is mild.

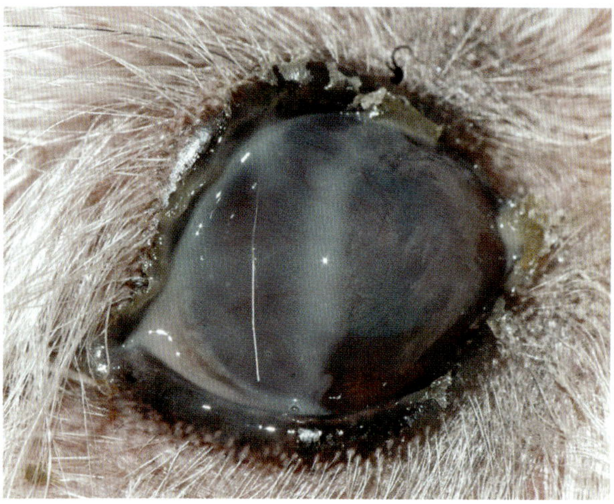

Moderate KCS in another "Westy".
Note the mucus and the corneal neovascularisation.

Breed predisposition

The breeds most predisposed to KCS are the West Highland White Terrier, Yorkshire Terrier, English Bulldog, Cocker Spaniel and Shih-Tzu.

Keratoconjunctivitis sicca

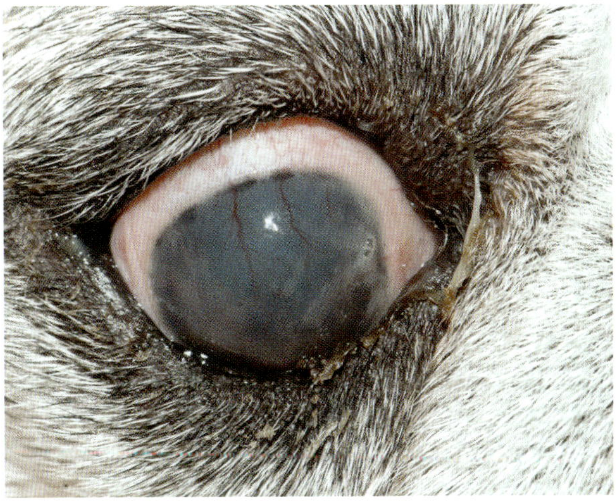

Severe unilateral KCS in a two-year-old English Bulldog. This was due to removal of the nictitating membrane gland (NMG).
Close-up of vascular invasion of the cornea.

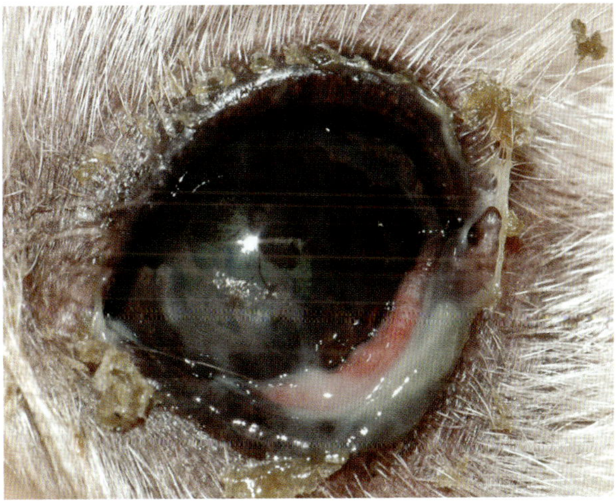

West Highland White Terrier with advanced KCS. Conjunctival hyperaemia and hypertrophy and mucus are present. New vessels and pigment can also be seen on the cornea.

Contraindicated

DO NOT EXCISE THE NMG because this may cause iatrogenic KCS (mainly in predisposed breeds).

Keratoconjunctivitis sicca

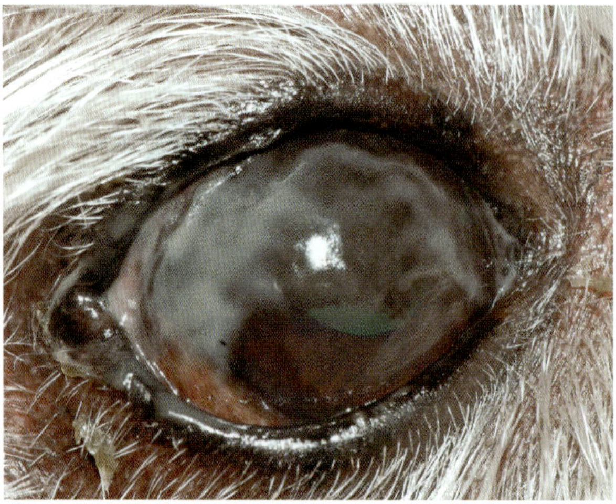

West Highland White Terrier with very severe KCS.
Visual deficit.
Note the large amount of melanotic pigment under the mucus.

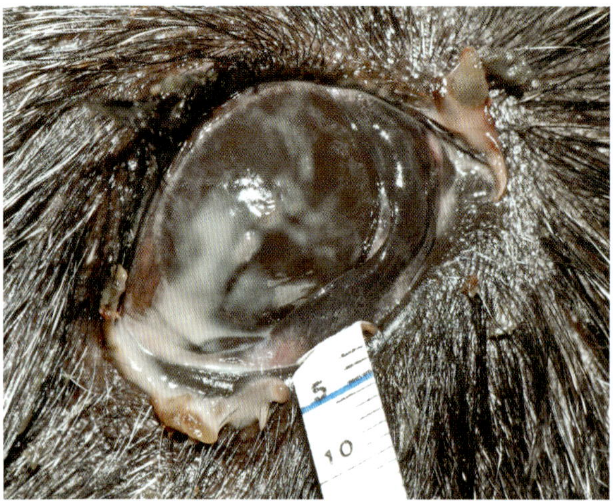

Severe KCS in a Cocker Spaniel.
Total hyposecretion.
Generalised corneal invasion of melanin. Blind eye.

i | In KCS, the patient's vision prognosis is linked to the concentration of pigment in the corneal stroma.

Keratoconjunctivitis sicca

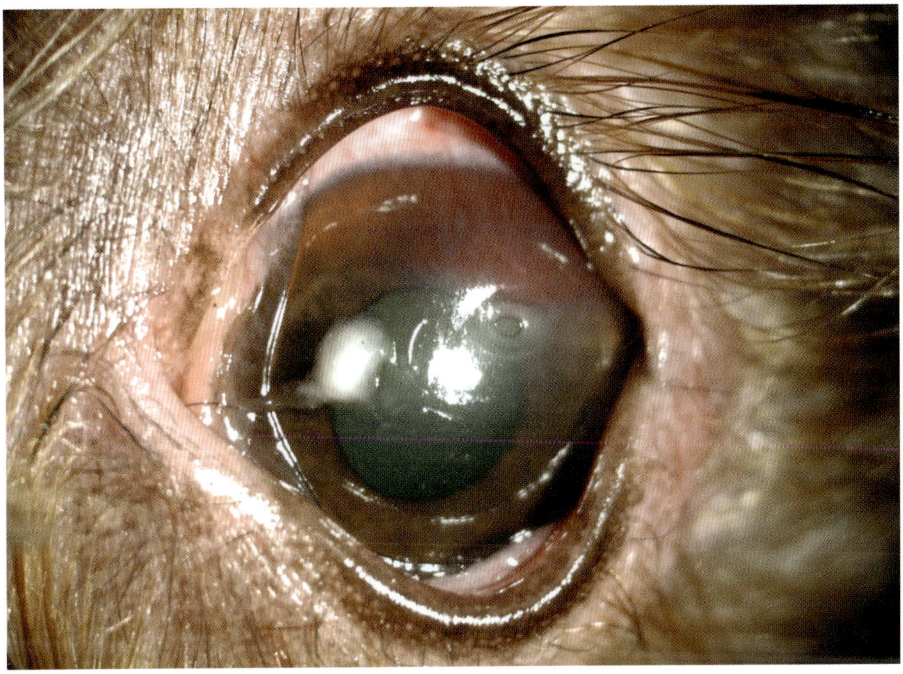

Yorkshire Terrier with a stromal corneal ulcer secondary to severe KCS.

Patients with KCS may present with corneal lesions (stromal ulcers or perforations) or respiratory problems (obstructed nostrils) due to severe tear hyposecretion.

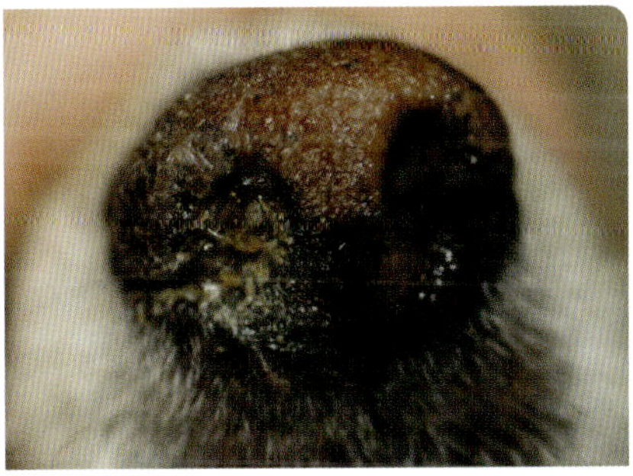

Dry, obstructed nostril in a mixed-breed dog with KCS.

Pigmentary keratitis

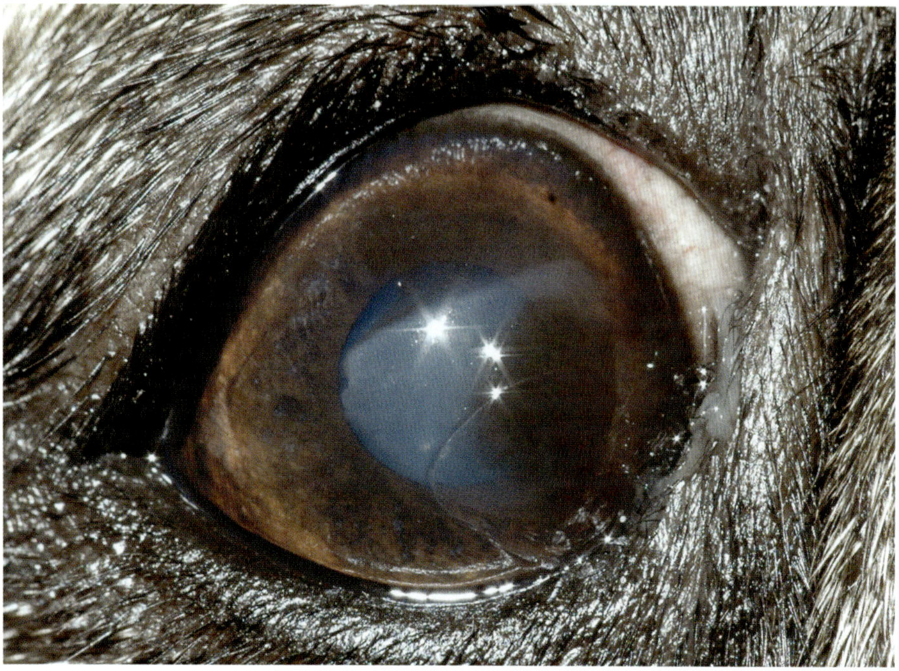

Pigmentary keratitis in a three-year-old Pug. This corneal lesion is characterised by a melanotic pigment invasion from the nasal area of the cornea.

Inflammatory corneal disease related to chronic exposure to irritating stimuli and associated with melanotic pigment, subtle corneal oedema, and neovascularisation.

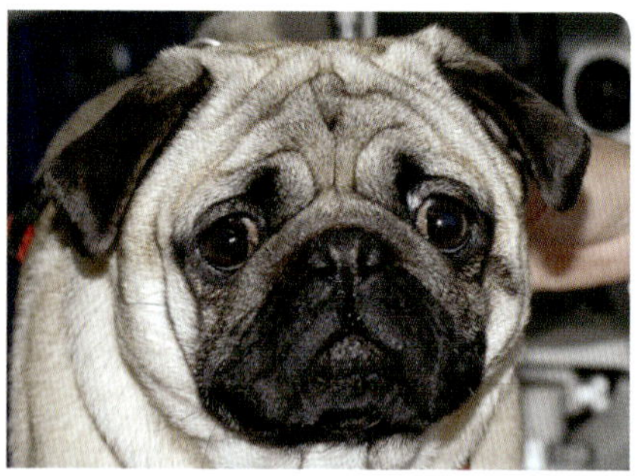

Pug with pigmentary keratitis.

Pigmentary keratitis

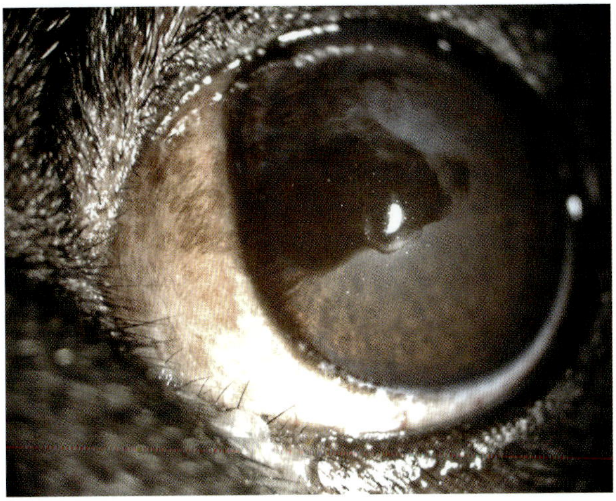

Pigmentary keratitis in a three-year-old Pug. Macropalpebral fissure (euryblepharon), medial entropion, exophthalmos, and lagophthalmos are the risk factors for this corneal disease.

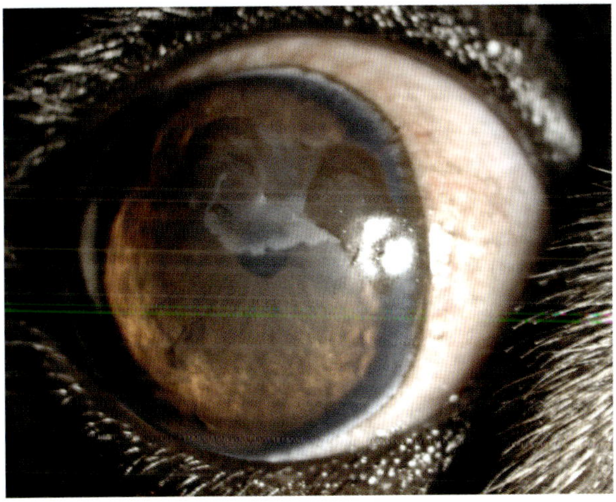

Close-up of the subtle corneal oedema, neovascularisation, and pigmentary invasion in the cornea of a Pug with pigmentary keratitis. Contact with the nasal fold hairs can aggravate the clinical condition.

Pigmentary keratitis

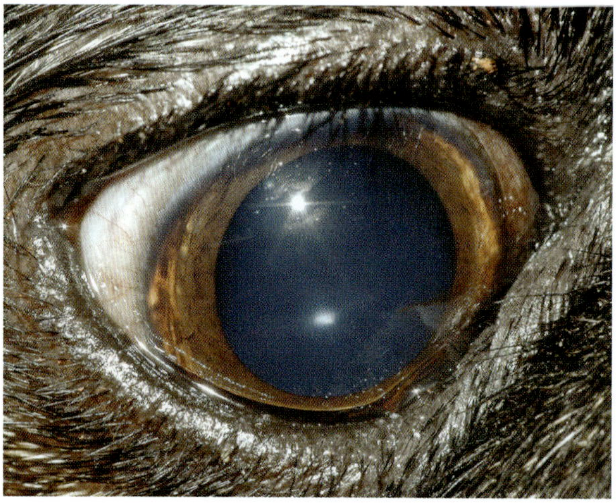

Pigmentary keratitis in a three-year-old Pug. Close-up of the corneal irritation in the nasal area caused by medial entropion and nasal fold trichiasis.

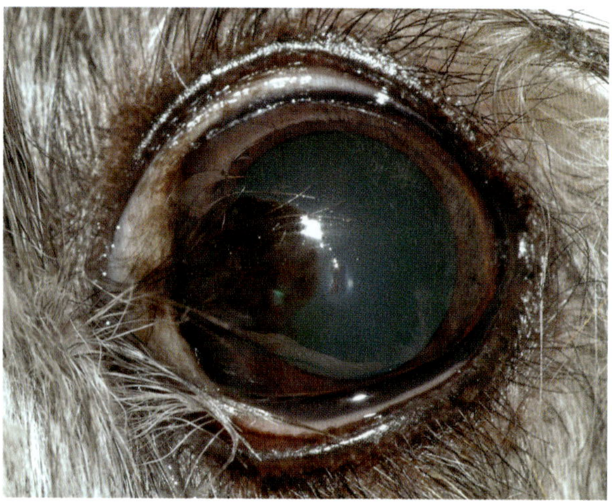

Shih-Tzu with pigmentary keratitis. In addition to exophthalmos and euryblepharon, rubbing of the facial hairs has aggravated the condition in this patient.

Breed predisposition

The breeds at greatest risk for pigmentary keratitis are the Pug, Shih-Tzu, Lhasa Apso and Pekingese.

Pigmentary keratitis

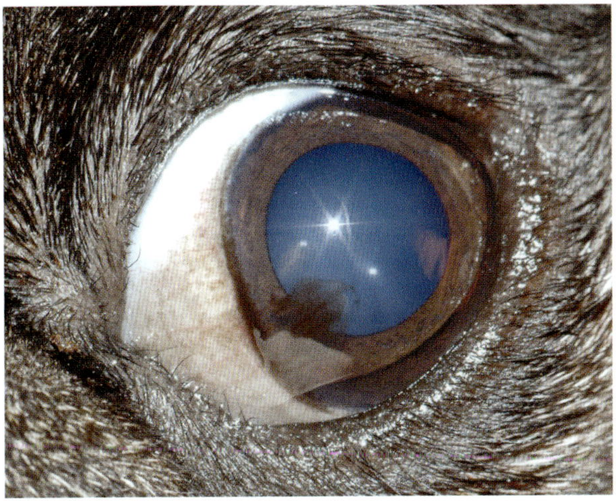

Pigmentary invasion in mild pigmentary keratitis.

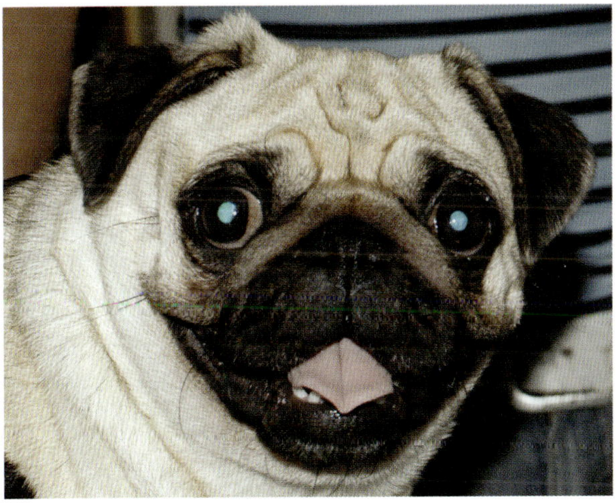

Visual function is unaffected in the early phases of the disease. Note the perfect tapetal reflection in both eyes.

Important notes

Use of cyclosporine A (topical) and artificial tears in the early phases helps minimise melanotic pigment deposition in the cornea.

Pigmentary keratitis

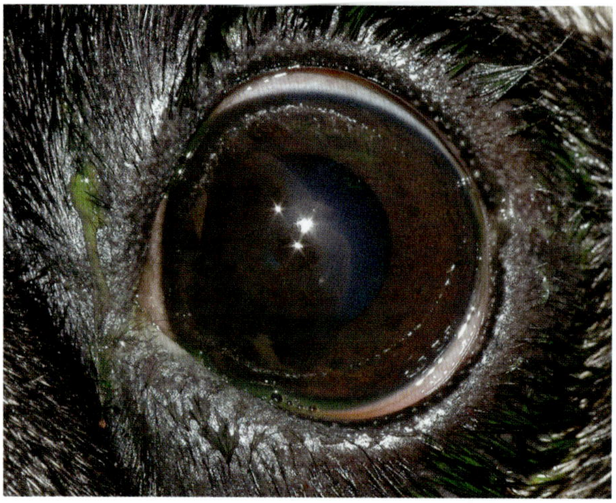

Moderate pigmentary keratitis in a Pug.
As the disease progresses, the pigmentary invasion from the nasal area of the cornea results in a visual deficit.
Time since onset: two years.

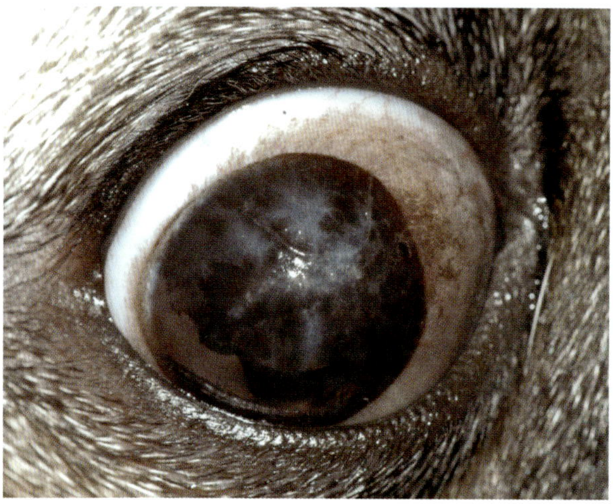

Severe pigmentary keratitis in a Pug. Pigment invades nearly the whole cornea. Close-up of the macropalpebral fissure in this patient.

Pigmentary keratitis

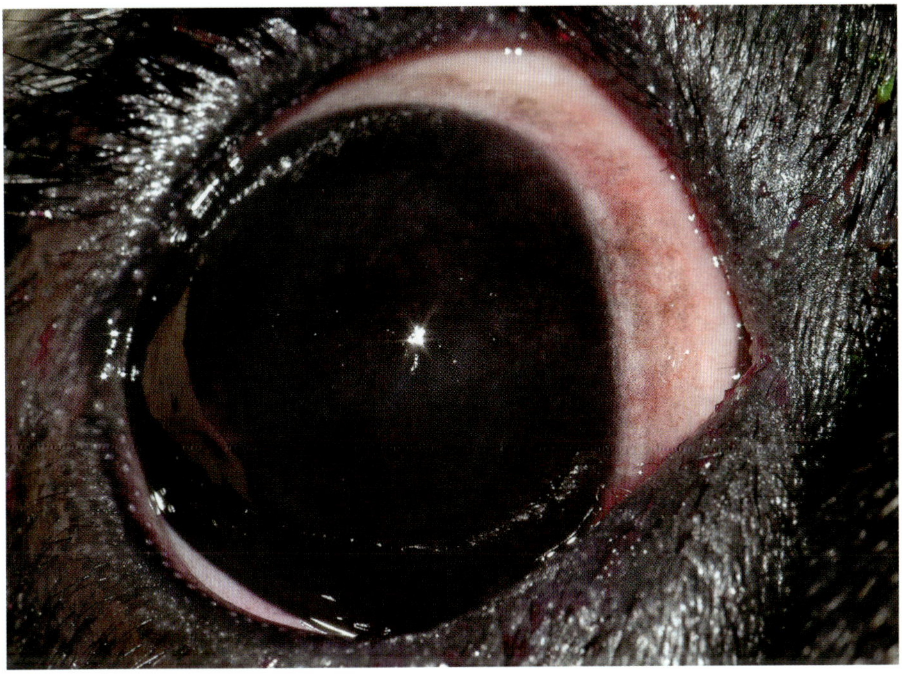

Severe pigmentary keratitis (blind eye). Pigmentary invasion affects the whole cornea. End stage of the disease.

Important notes

- Prompt diagnosis of this disease is key to avoiding blindness.
- All brachycephalic breeds (especially Pugs) should undergo a biomicroscopic examination in the first few months of life to detect melanin deposits in the cornea.

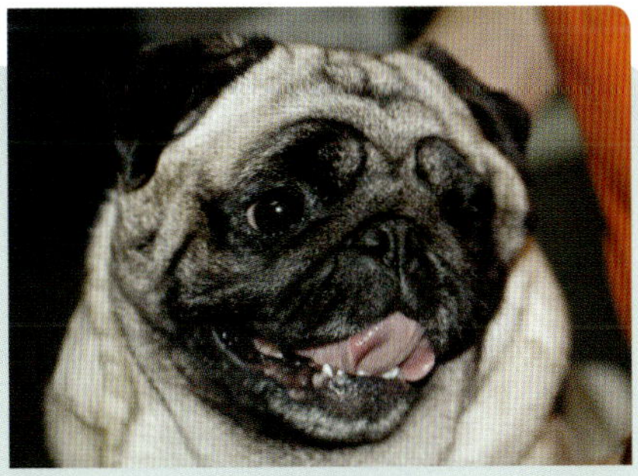

Patient pictured above. Pigmentary invasion blocks the tapetal reflection.

Pigmentary keratitis

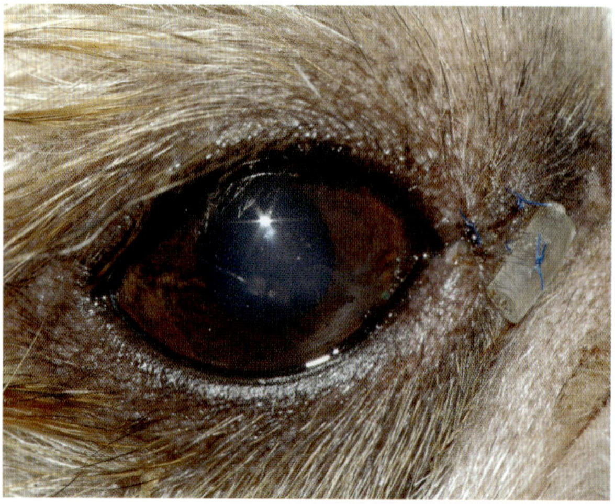

Medial canthoplasty is the surgical technique of choice in patients with pigmentary keratitis.
Shih-Tzu after surgery.

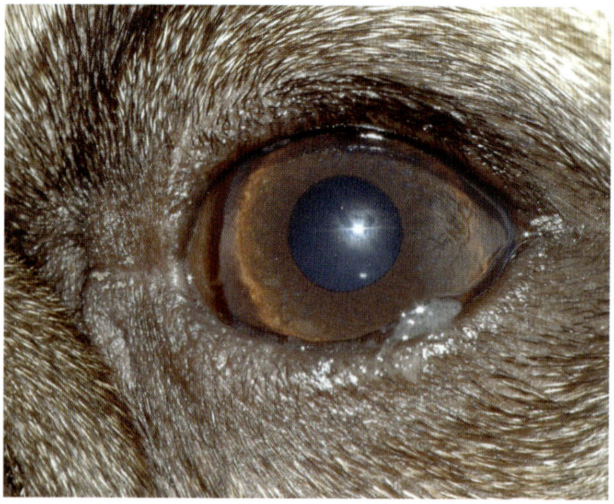

Pug treated surgically. Close-up of the scar on the medial canthus following medial canthoplasty.

Surgical technique

The most common technique is medial canthoplasty, as described by Roberts-Jensen. This surgery reduces the size of the palpebral fissure, corrects medial entropion, protects the cornea from contact with hairs from the face or nasal folds, and improves distribution of the precorneal tear film. The result is elimination of all the factors that chronically irritate the cornea.

Pigmentary keratitis

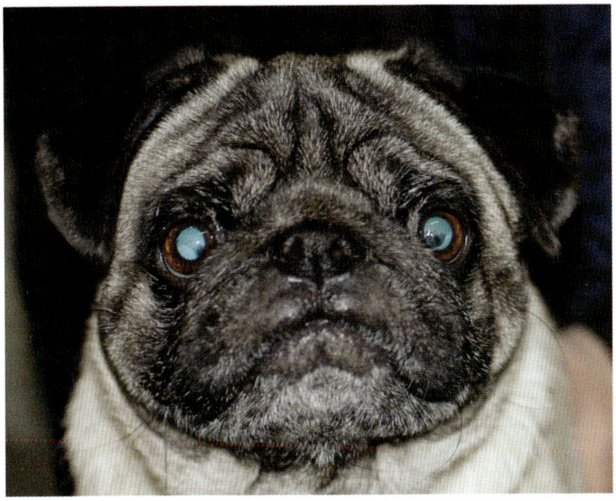

Pug with pigmentary keratitis after medial canthoplasty. Note the smaller palpebral fissure.

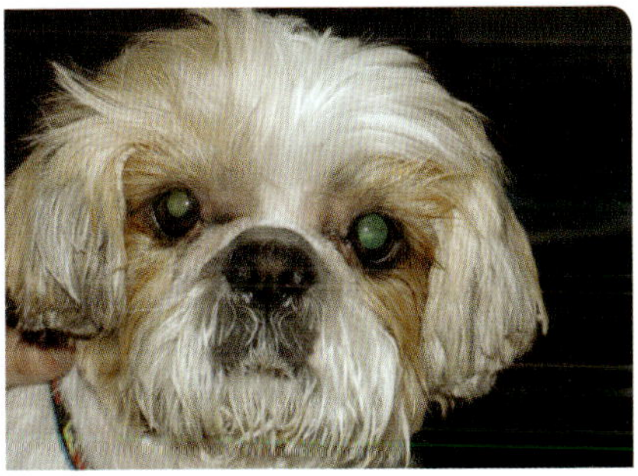

This Shih-Tzu had a medial canthoplasty using the Roberts-Jensen technique.

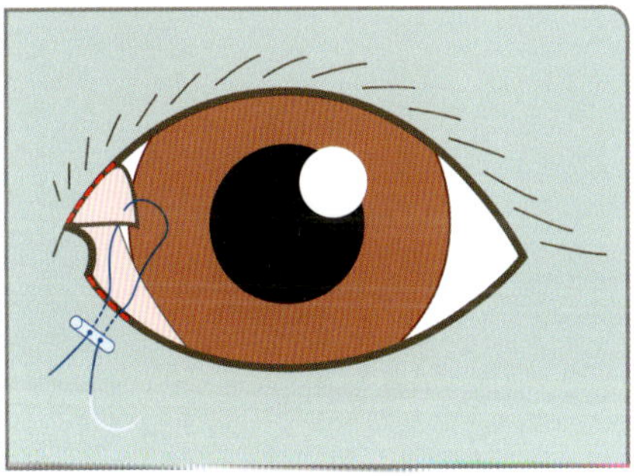

Diagram of the surgical technique.

Surgical technique

- In a medial canthoplasty (Roberts-Jensen), a flap of upper palpebral conjunctiva is created and inserted into a pocket previously created by separating the skin and orbicular muscle from the lower palpebral conjunctiva.
- Be extremely careful not to damage the lower lacrimal punctum or canaliculus.

Feline eosinophilic keratitis

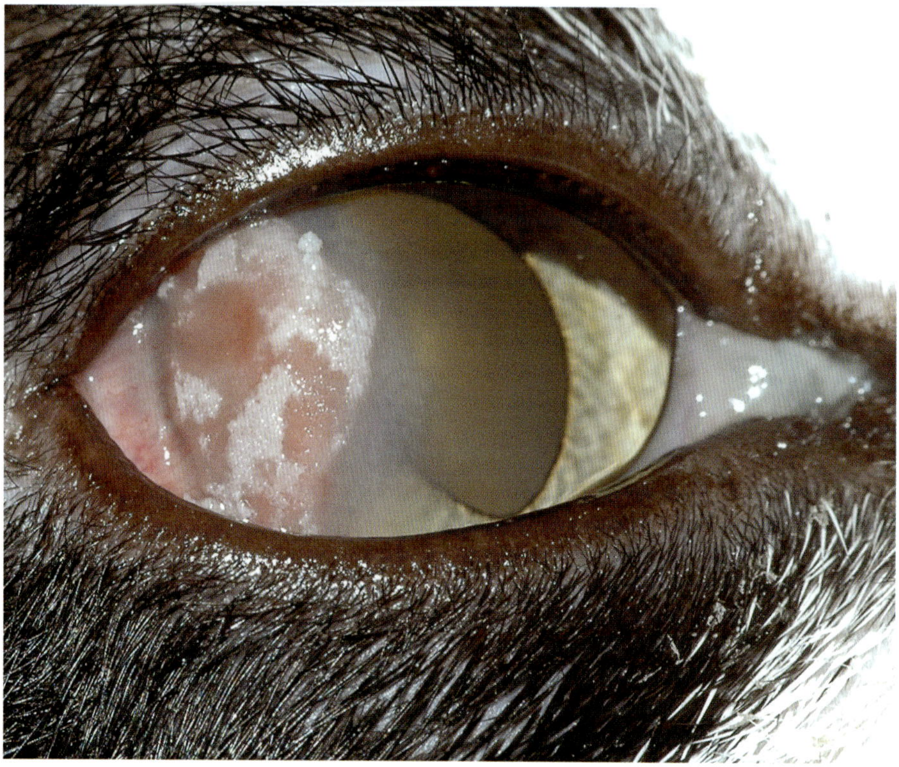

Feline eosinophilic keratitis. Four-year-old domestic shorthair cat. Time since onset: three months with epiphora and blepharospasm.

- The presence of whitish plaques in the outer layers of a cat's cornea, along with neovascularisation, should always suggest feline eosinophilic keratitis.
- It is most commonly located in the dorsotemporal area of the cornea.

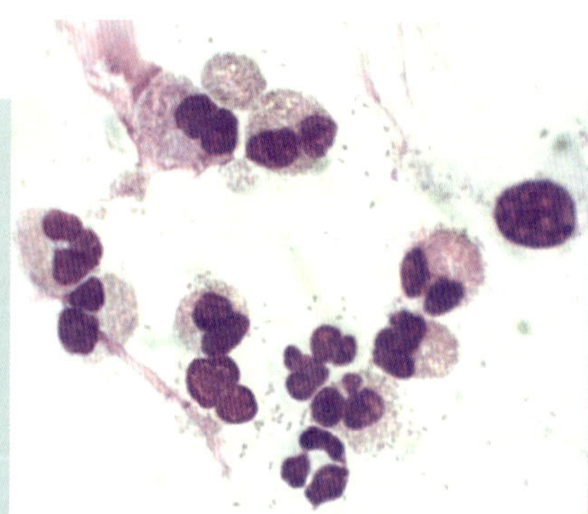

Cytological image of a sample taken from the patient pictured above. Close-up of the eosinophil population.
Image courtesy of Cristina Fernández Algarra (100× immersion).

Feline eosinophilic keratitis

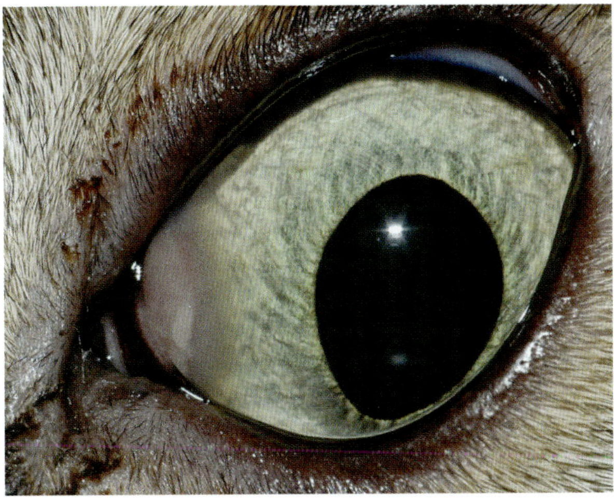

Feline eosinophilic keratitis. Lesions in the nasal area of the cornea are less common than in the temporal area, but the clinical signs are similar (cellular infiltrate and new blood vessels).

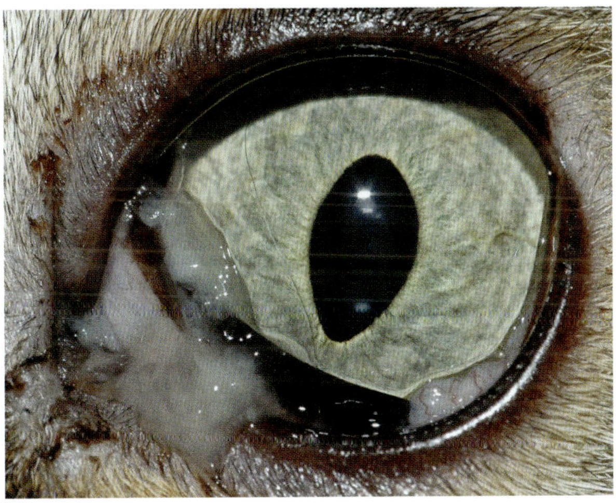

Serous or mucous ocular secretions and blepharospasm are the most common signs.

The definitive diagnosis is based on the results of the corneal cytology.

Eosinophils (including degranulated ones), plasma cells, and mastocytes are the most common cells in these patients.

Feline eosinophilic keratitis

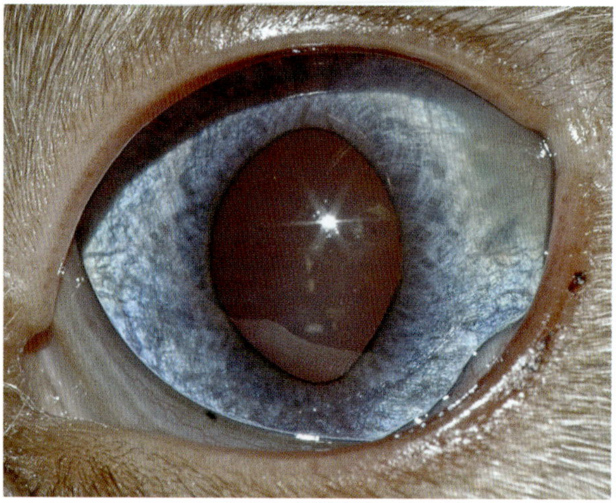

Eosinophilic keratitis, mild, in a Siamese cat. Temporal location. Invasion of blood vessels and cellular infiltrate. Time since onset: 10 days.

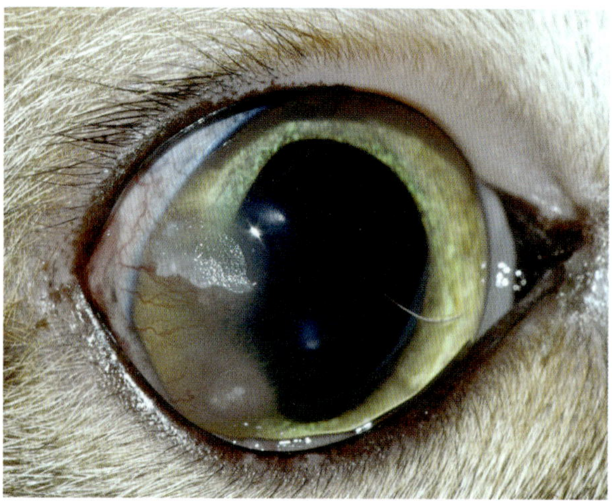

Moderate eosinophilic keratitis. Cellular infiltrate, oedema, and whitish plaques are signs of disease progression. Time since onset: 35 days.

i

The average age of onset of this corneal disease is 4–6 years.

The presentation is generally unilateral but can be bilateral.

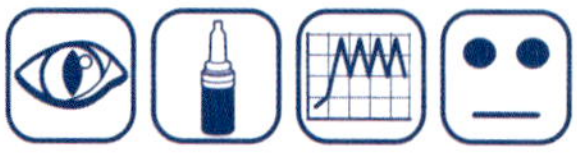

Feline eosinophilic keratitis

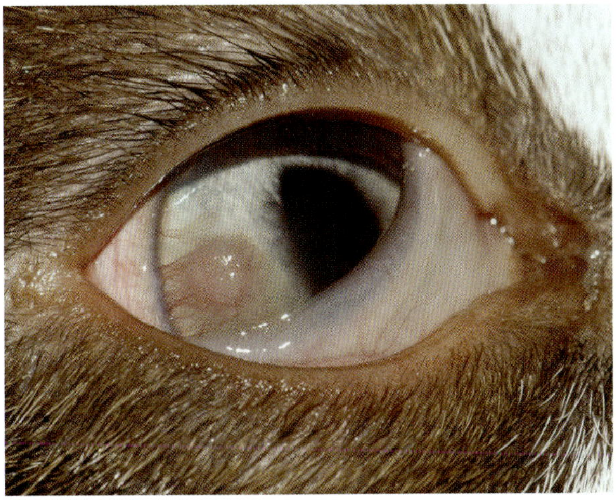

Stromal cellular infiltrate and new blood vessels in a cat with eosinophilic keratitis.

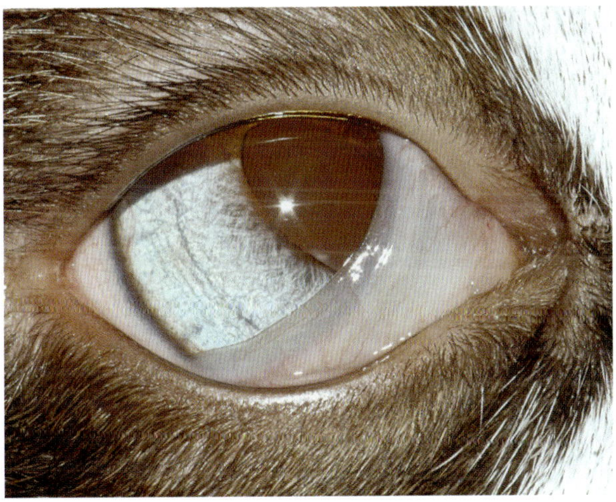

Patient pictured above after 15 days of treatment with dexamethasone eye drops.

- The drugs of choice for feline eosinophilic keratitis are topical corticosteroids (preferably dexamethasone) and topical cyclosporine A, 0.2 % (if tolerated).
- Recurrences are common.

Corneal dystrophy

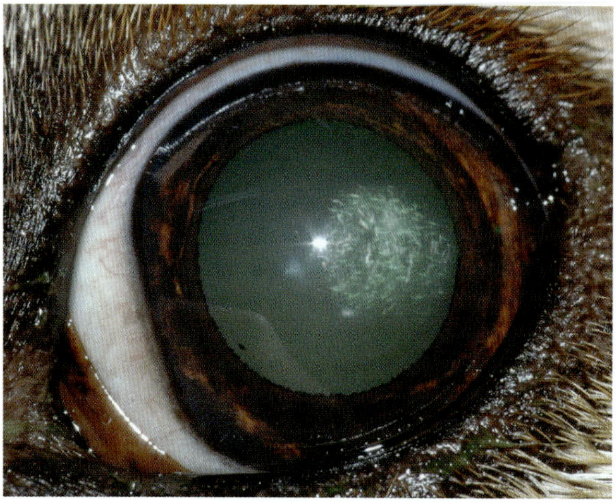

Stromal corneal dystrophy, central, in a four-year-old Beagle.

Presentation: 30 days.

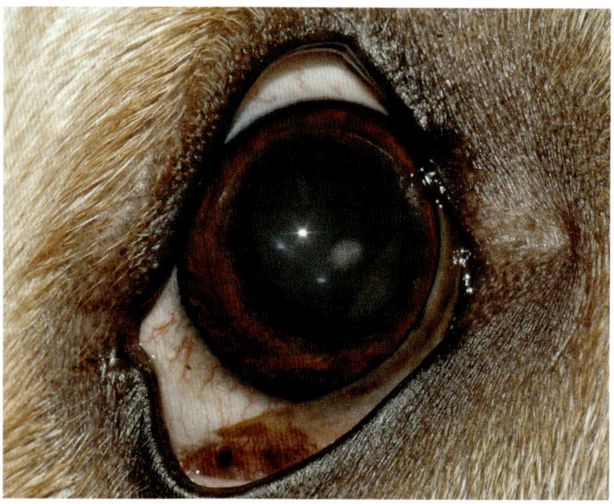

Two-year-old Labrador Retriever with stromal corneal dystrophy. Oval-shaped.

Corneal dystrophy is a noninflammatory corneal disease that is usually bilateral, progressive, and characterised by the presence of whitish deposits (phospholipids or cholesterol).

Corneal dystrophy

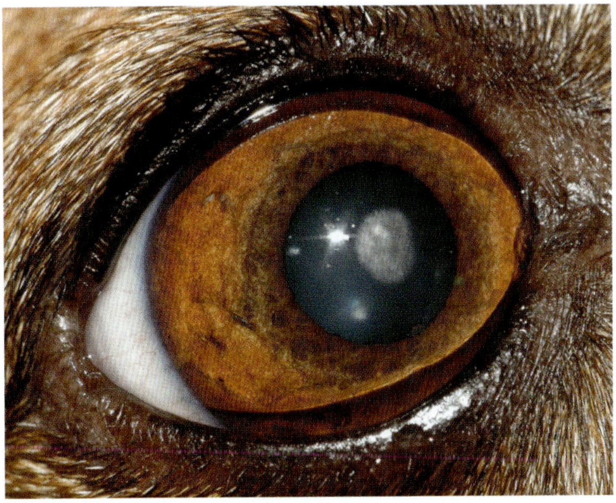

Axial corneal dystrophy in the right eye of a 2.5-year-old Beagle.

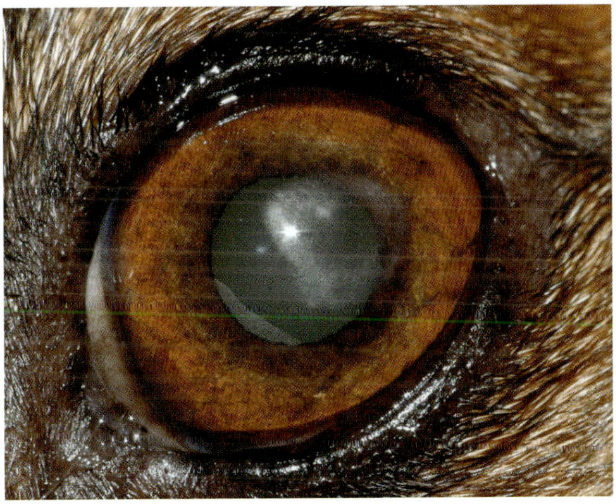

Corneal dystrophy in the left eye of the patient pictured above.

Important notes

- Primary corneal dystrophy generally presents bilaterally and symmetrically. The size of the lesion may vary between the eyes.

Breed predisposition

- Corneal dystrophy has been described in the Beagle, Siberian Husky, Cocker Spaniel, and Airedale Terrier.

Corneal dystrophy

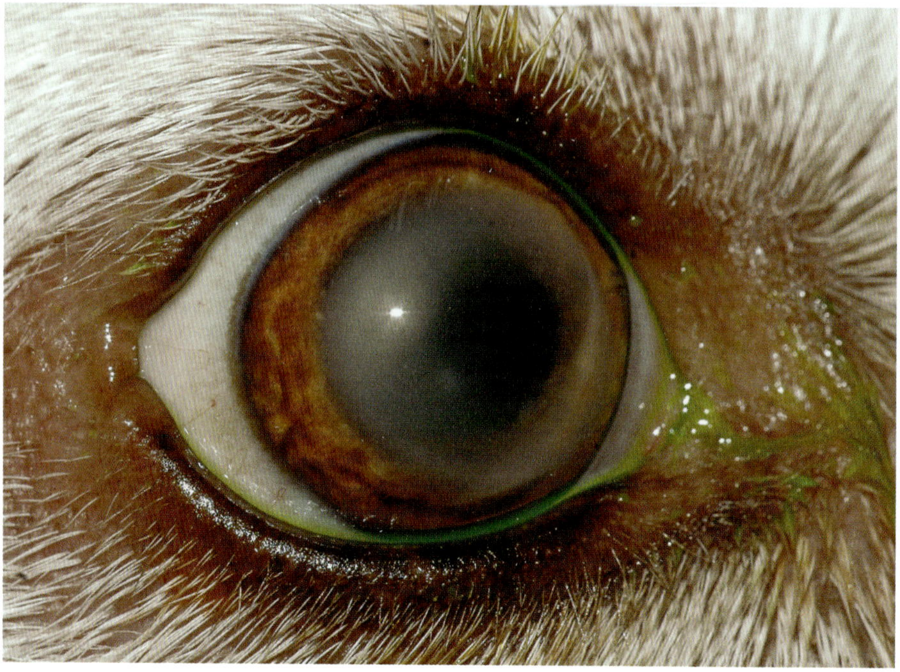

Lipid stromal corneal dystrophy in a five-year-old Husky.
Lesions are often ring-shaped in this breed.

This avascular disease of the cornea has been described as bilateral with a hereditary component in the Husky.

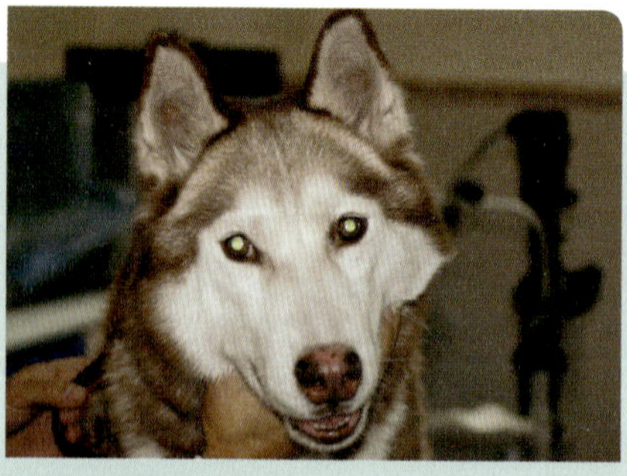

Patient pictured above.
Note the bilateral corneal opacity.

Corneal dystrophy

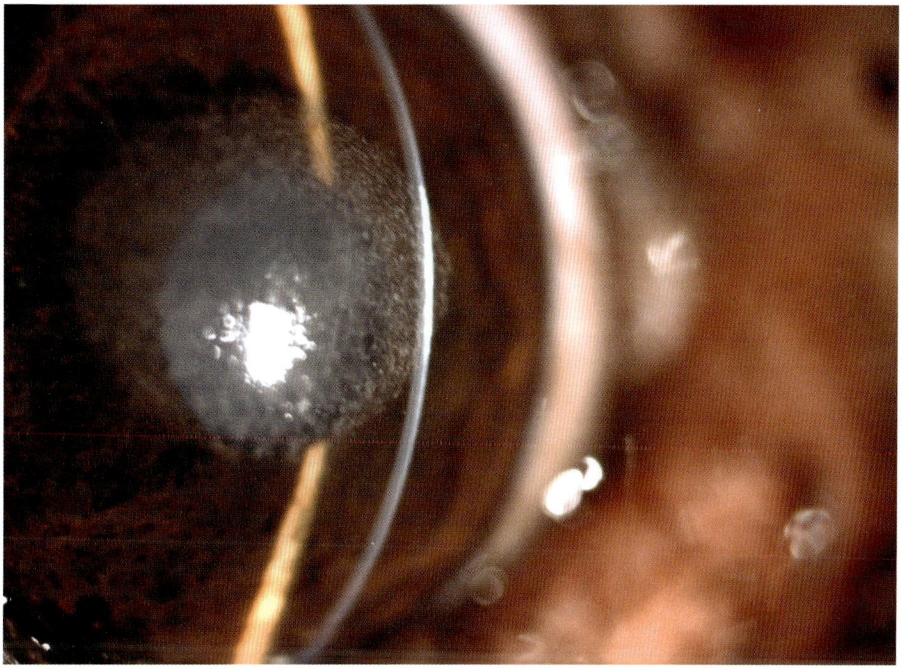

Close-up of the cornea pictured below. Note the stromal location of the dystrophy.
Slit-lamp picture.

Interesting notes

Slit-lamp biomicroscopy is critical for proper location of corneal lesions.

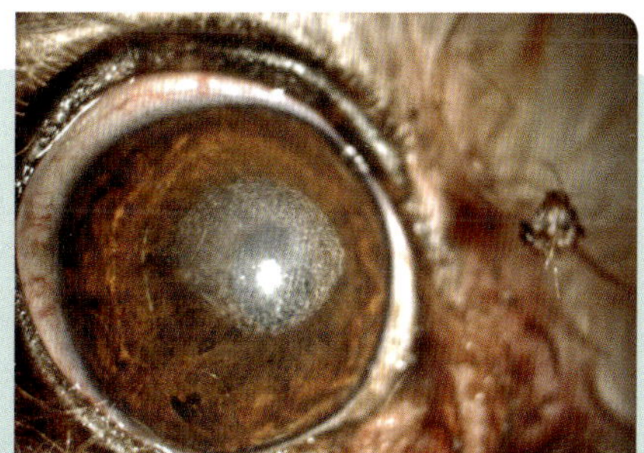

Airedale Terrier with stromal corneal dystrophy.
Axial location and crystalline shape.

Corneal dystrophy

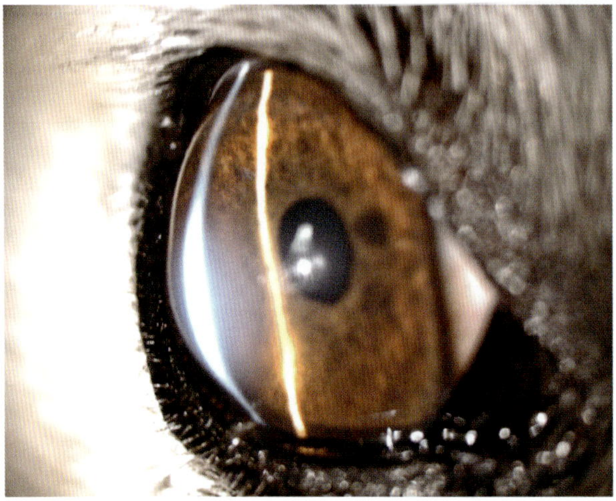

Endothelial corneal dystrophy in a 13-year-old Fox Terrier.

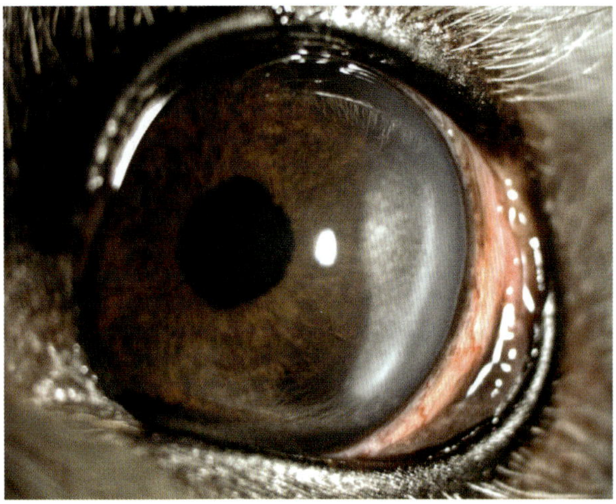

Progressive endothelial corneal dystrophy in the temporal area of the cornea. Fourteen-year-old Fox Terrier. The picture shows age-related iris atrophy.

Breed predisposition

- Endothelial corneal dystrophy has been reported in the Fox Terrier, Boston Terrier, and Dachshund.
- It is a spontaneous progressive disease that tends to start in the temporal area and may affect the entire cornea, causing blindness.

Corneal degeneration

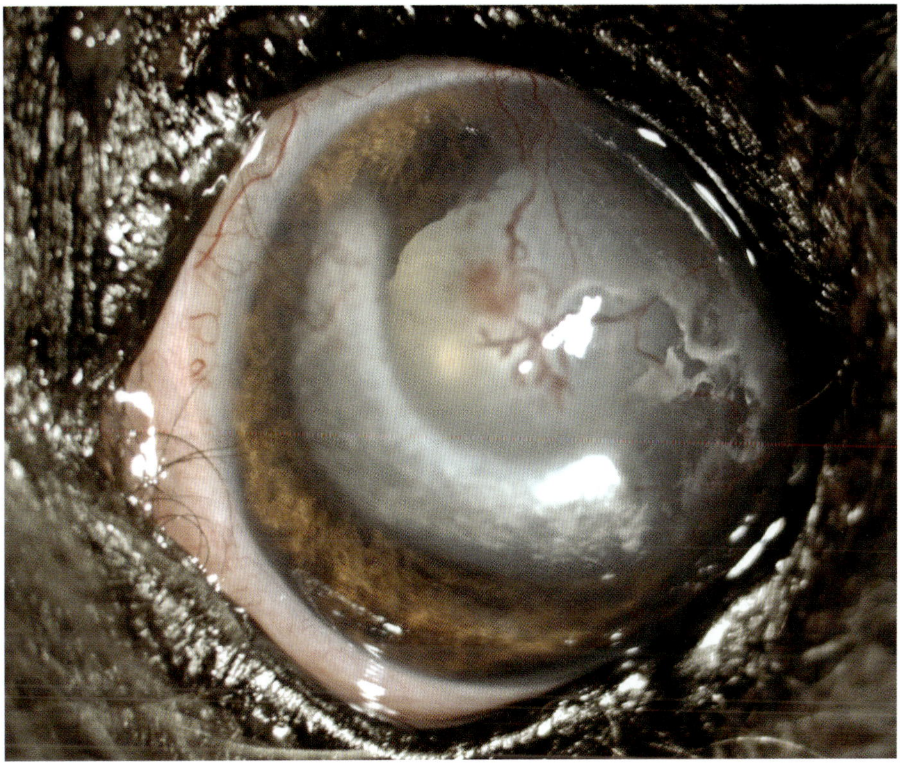

Corneal degeneration in a 14-year-old mixed-breed dog.
Note the new vessels, oedema, and corneal deposits.

Corneal degeneration is an inflammatory corneal disease that is secondary to chronic corneal damage or to a systemic disease.

It may be uni- or bilateral and is generally eccentric.

Corneal degeneration

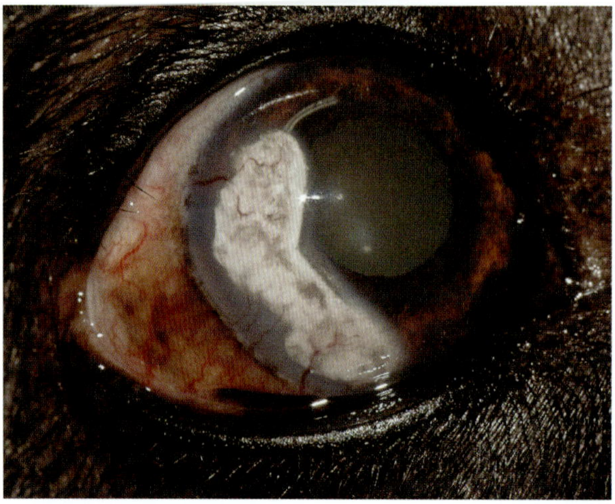

Corneal degeneration in the right eye of a German Shepherd mix with hypothyroidism.

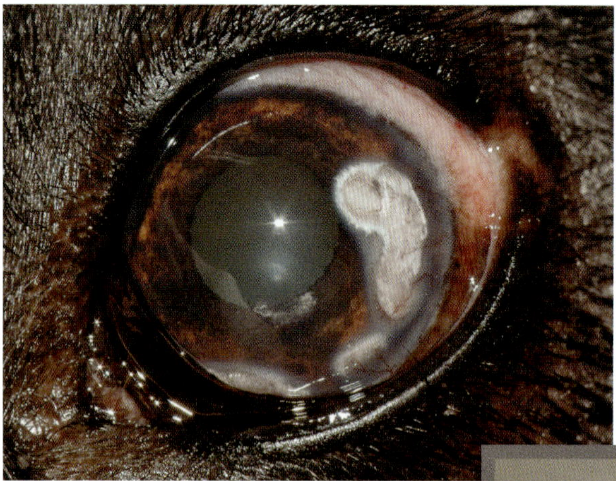

Left eye with the same signs of corneal degeneration (new vessels, deposits, and oedema).

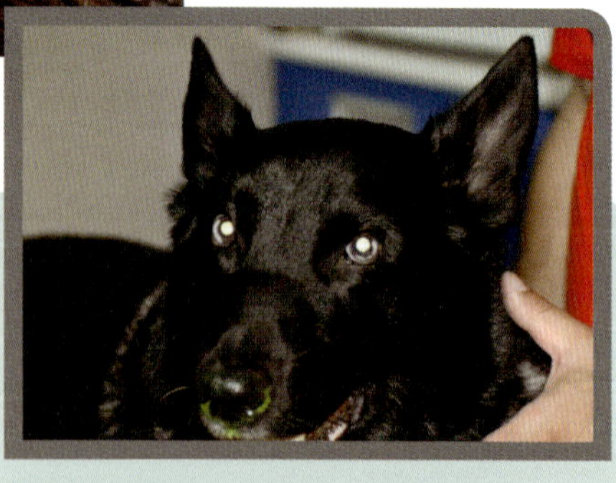

Our patient. Bilateral corneal degeneration.

Important notes

- The systemic diseases most often associated with corneal degeneration are hypothyroidism (described in the Cocker Spaniel and German Shepherd), liver disease, and endocrine diseases (Cushing's syndrome and diabetes).

Corneal degeneration

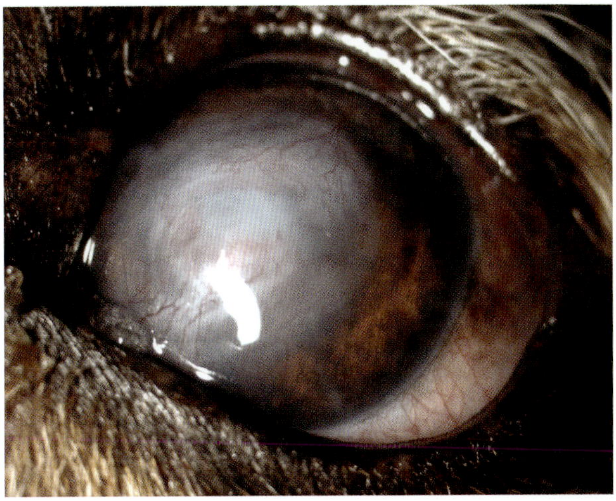

Extensive corneal degeneration secondary to severe ulcerative keratitis in a dog.

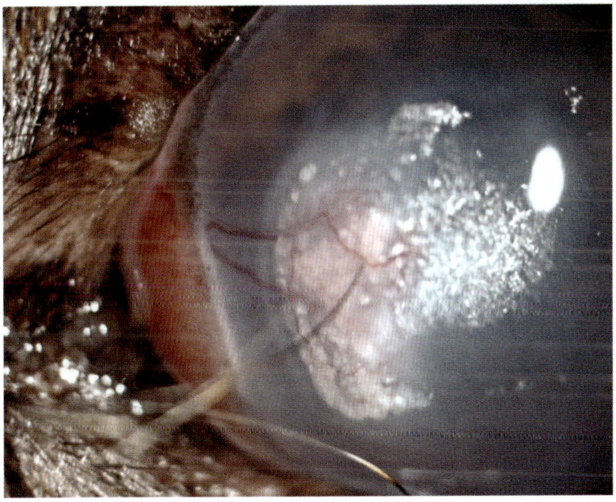

New vessels and calcium deposits in a 15-year-old dog with corneal degeneration.

i

Corneal degeneration may occur in response to a chronic inflammatory process (corneal ulcers, surgeries, episcleritis, etc.).

Calcium or lipid salts may be isolated from these corneal deposits.

Corneal degeneration

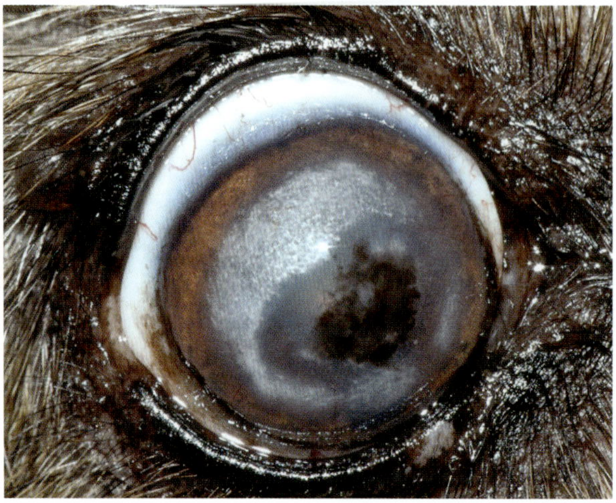

Thirteen-year-old mixed breed dog with chronic corneal degeneration.
Close-up of neovascularisation, pigment deposits, and pigment infiltration.
Time since onset: two years.

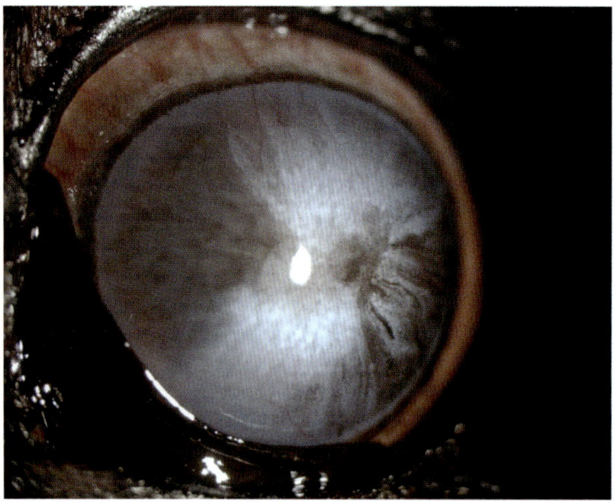

Fifteen-year-old mixed breed dog with very advanced corneal degeneration. Severe visual deficit.

Important notes

- The presence of pigment is a sign of CHRONICITY.
- Medical treatment is designed to minimise neovascularisation and pigment deposition (with cyclosporine A, tacrolimus) and to nourish the cornea (with autologous serum, artificial tears).
- Extreme cases may require surgery (keratoplasty).

Corneal oedema

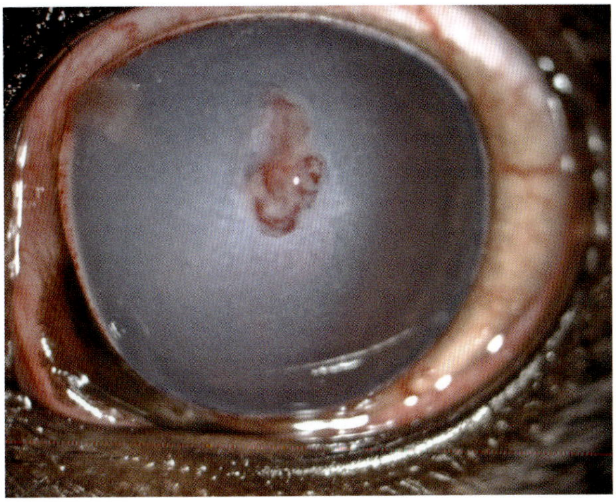

Corneal oedema in a dog that was scratched by a cat. The breach of the epithelial barrier allows fluid to enter the corneal stroma.

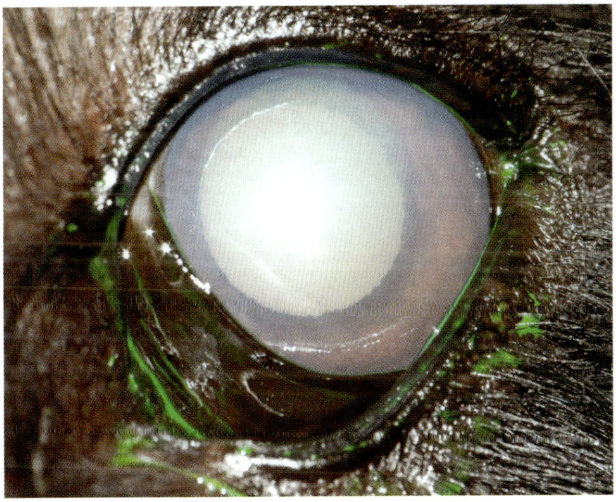

Endothelial damage secondary to uveitis allows aqueous humour into the stroma. Diffuse corneal oedema in a dog with chronic uveitis.

i Any epithelial damage or failure of the endothelial pump can allow fluid to enter the corneal stroma.

Corneal oedema

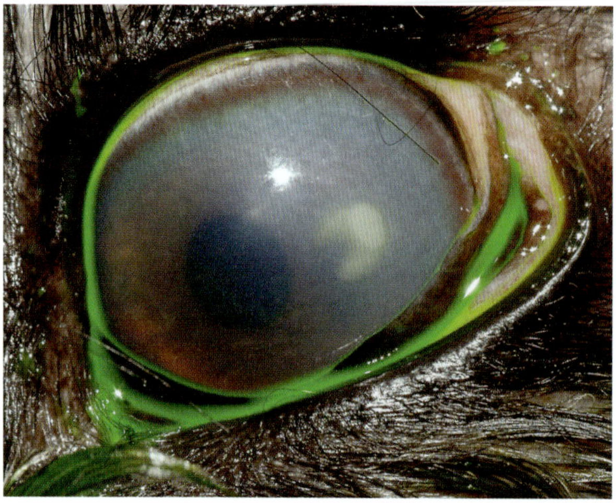

Acute uveitis secondary to corneal contact with a pine processionary caterpillar. Acute corneal oedema.

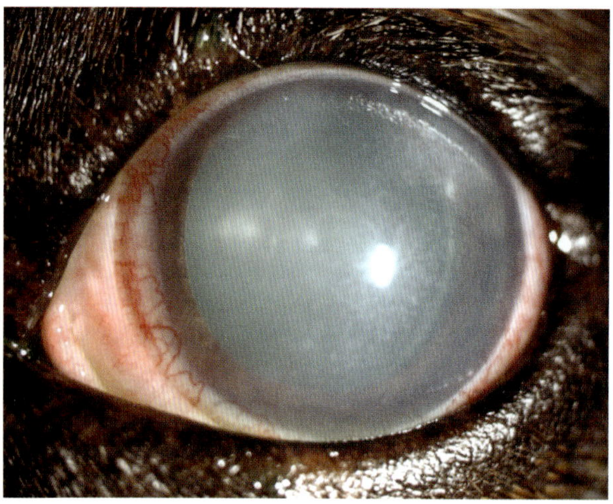

Oedema secondary to endothelial damage caused by acute glaucoma.

i | The most common causes of corneal oedema are ulcers, uveitis, glaucoma, and anterior lens luxation.

Neoplasms

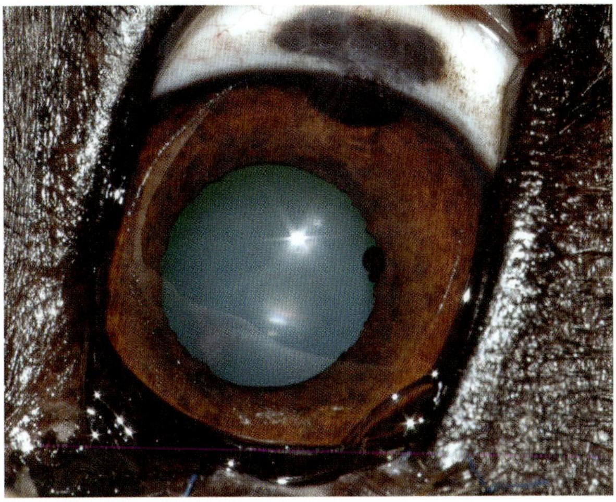

Epibulbar melanoma in a seven-year-old German Shepherd.
Generally benign in behaviour.

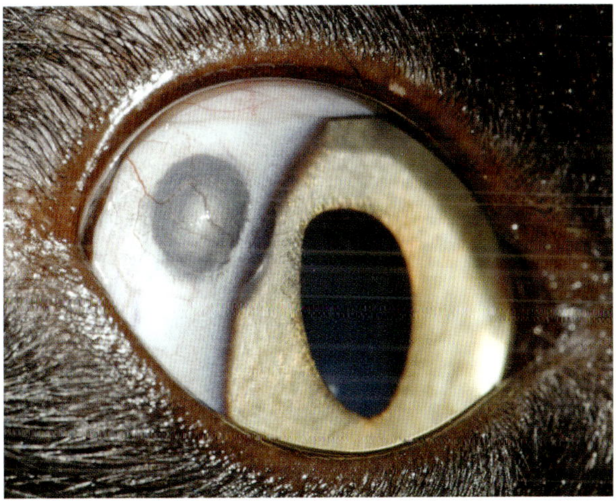

Limbal melanoma with corneal invasion in a six-year-old domestic shorthair cat.

i | Corneal neoplasms are rare. Epibulbar melanoma, squamous cell carcinoma, and fibrous histiocytoma in Collies have been reported.

Foreign bodies

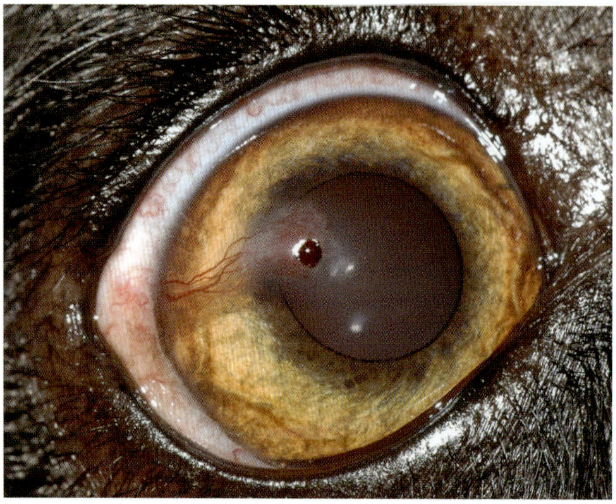

Three-year-old Brittany Spaniel with vascular invasion from the corneoscleral limbus towards the foreign body (from a plant).

Time since onset: 10 days.

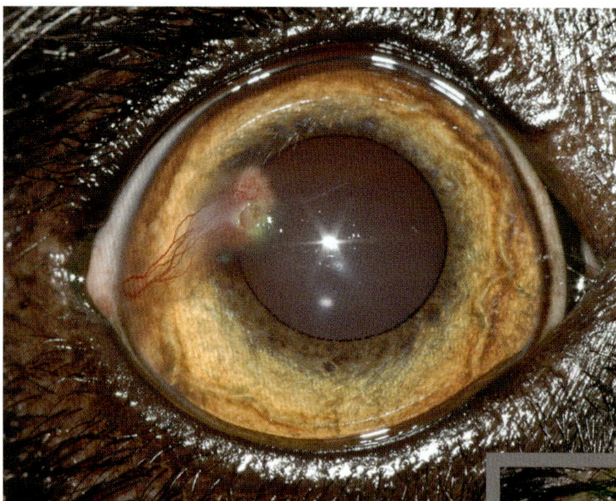

Treatment consists of removing the foreign body (under general anaesthesia).

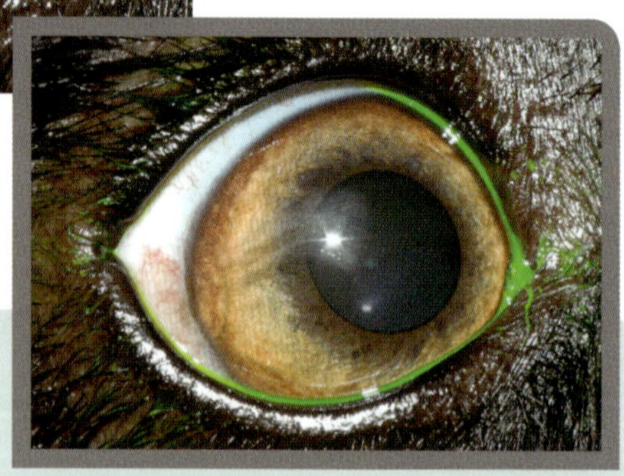

Follow up with medical treatment to induce scarring. Patient 15 days later.

The most common corneal foreign bodies are pieces of leaves, thorns, grass awns, and glass or metal shards.

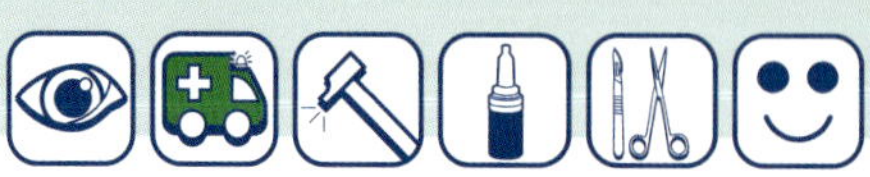

Foreign bodies

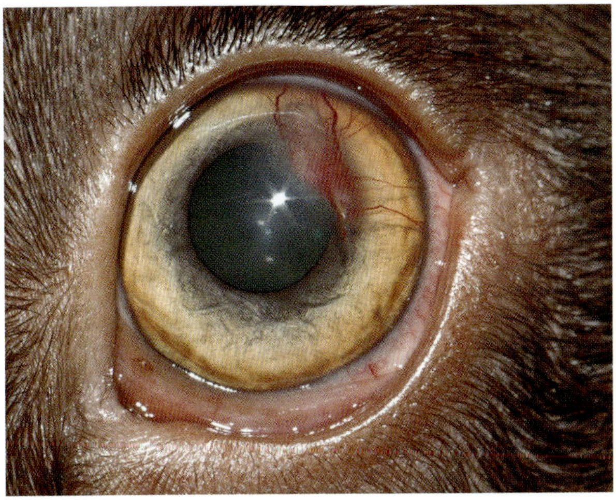

Four-year-old Pointer with a thorn lodged in the dorsotemporal corneal stroma. The end emerges in the para-axial area.
Time since onset: 25 days.

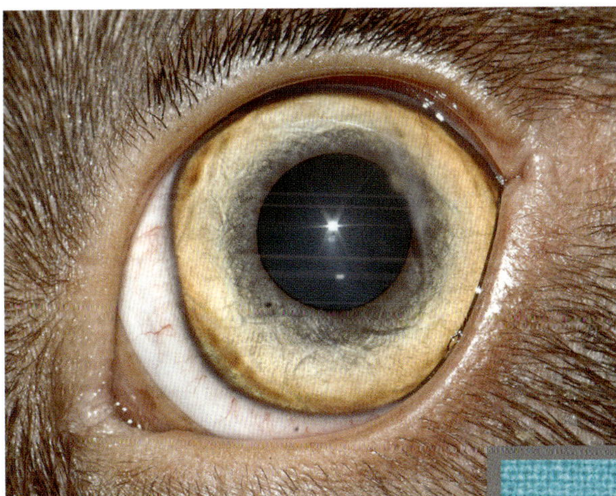

Patient following removal of the foreign body.
Corneal leukoma in the affected area.

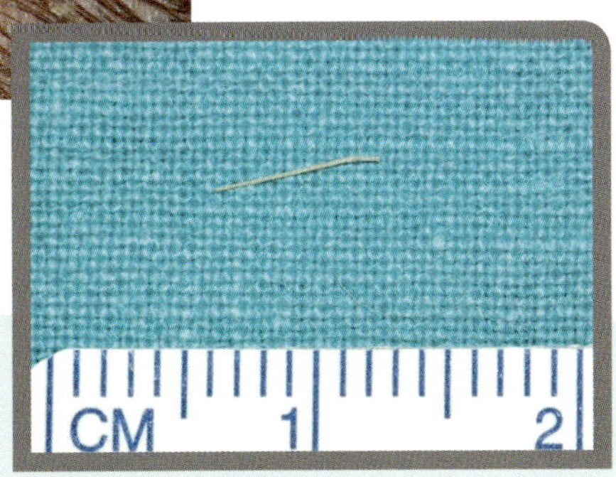

Foreign body. Thorn from a plant.

The main clinical signs in these patients are epiphora and blepharospasm.

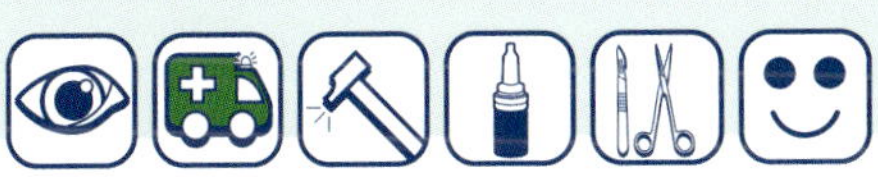

Foreign bodies

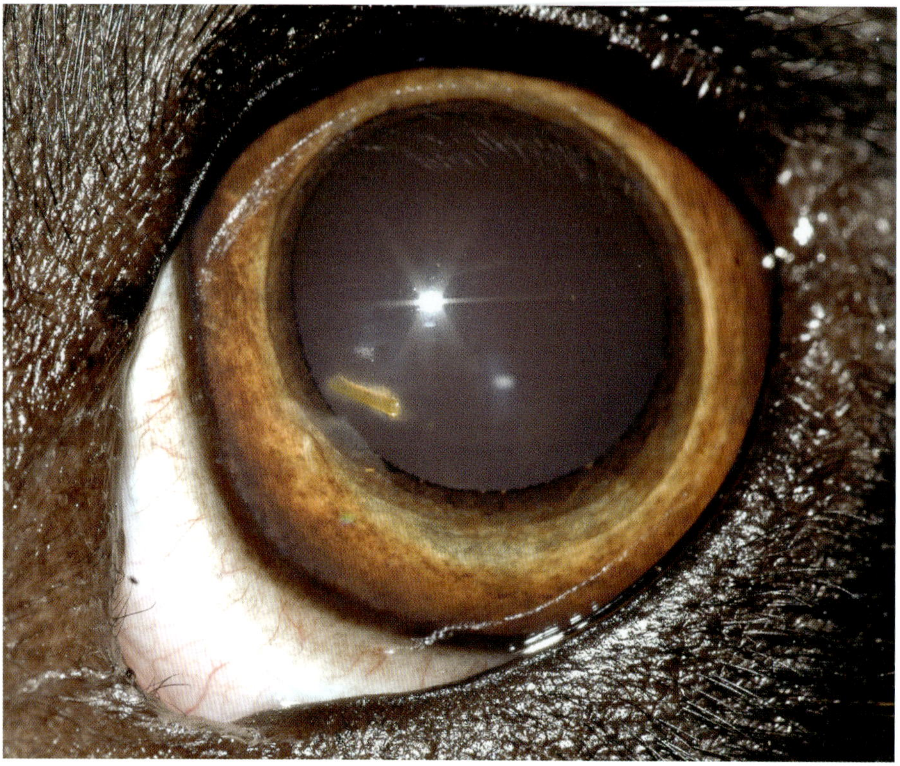

Thorn lodged in the cornea of a hunting dog that put his head in the bushes in search of prey. Time since onset: 12 hours.

Emergency

- Remove the foreign body as promptly as possible to avoid corneal perforation.
- Two insulin needles may be used to remove it.

Foreign bodies

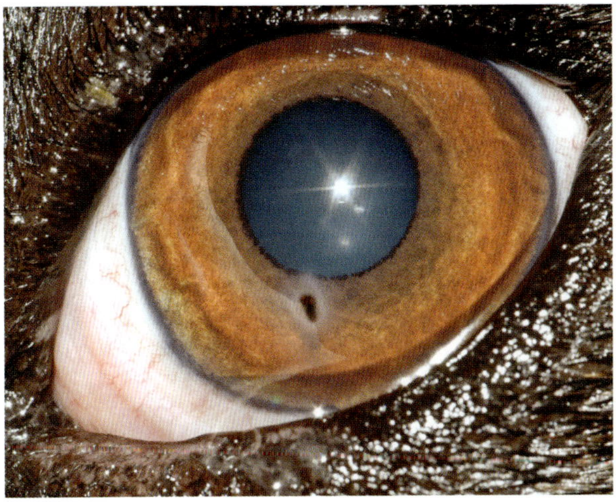

Thorn lodged in the cornea, causing a full-thickness lesion.
Time since onset: six days.

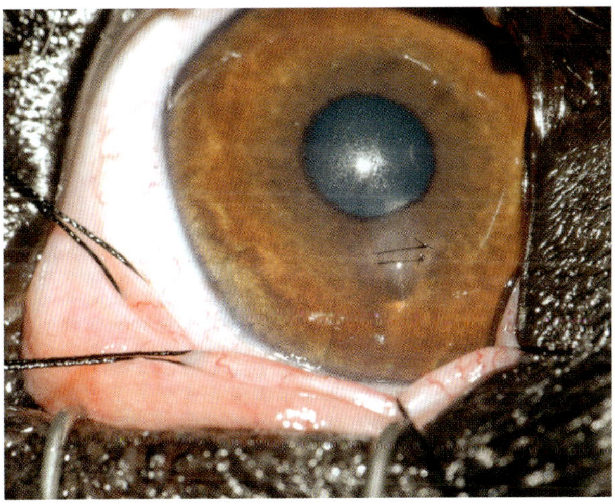

Surgical reconstruction after removal using 9-0 nylon sutures.
Include only $^{2}/_{3}$ of the corneal thickness.

Important notes

- Always use general anaesthesia when extracting foreign bodies that affect the deeper layers of the cornea.

Contraindicated

- When removing the foreign body, ensure that no other material enters the eye.
- DO NOT USE FORCEPS. 25-gauge needles are recommended.

Feline corneal sequestrum

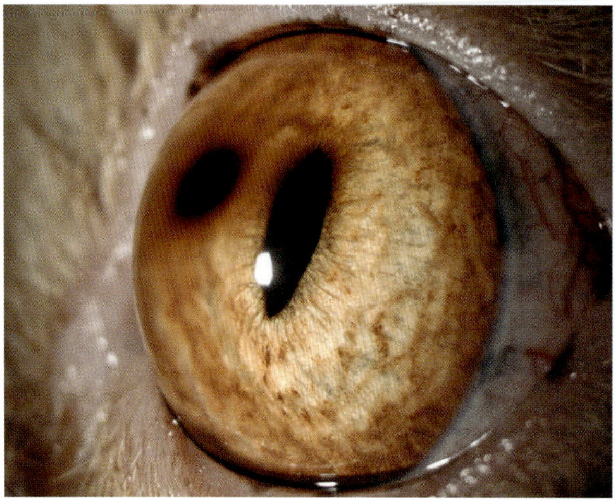

Corneal sequestrum in a two-year-old Persian cat. Close-up of the dark corneal lesion. Do not confuse with a foreign body.

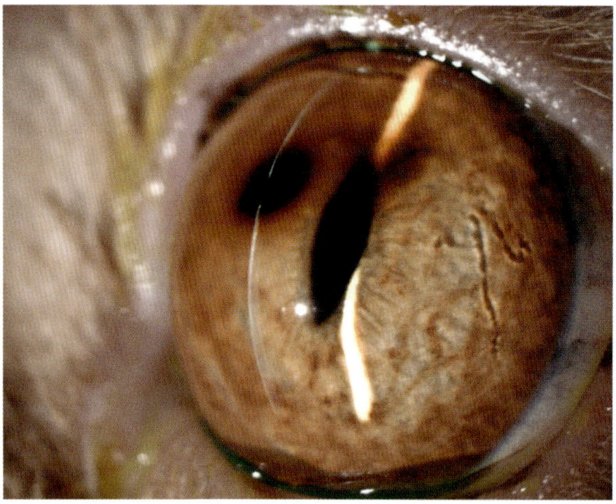

Patient pictured above. Use a slit lamp to examine the condition of the stroma.

i

Feline corneal degeneration (corneal sequestrum) is characterised by focal degeneration of collagen fibres and the presence of brown pigment (in advanced stages) in the corneal stroma.

The most likely cause of this lesion is chronic irritation of the cornea, though other aetiologies such as stromal dystrophy and feline herpesvirus type 1 have been described.

Feline corneal sequestrum

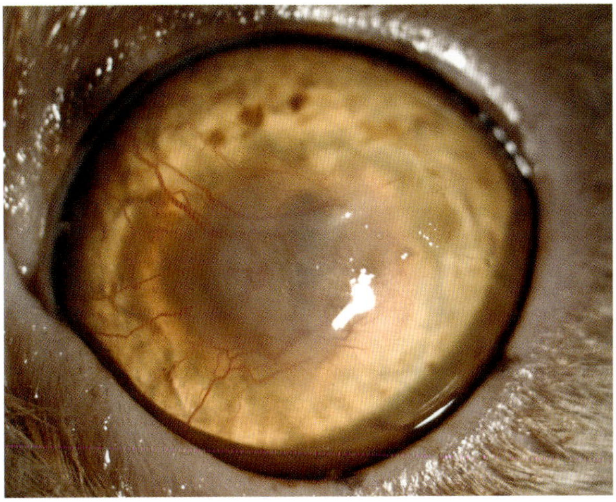

Feline corneal degeneration with prolific neovascularisation.
Time since onset: 35 days.

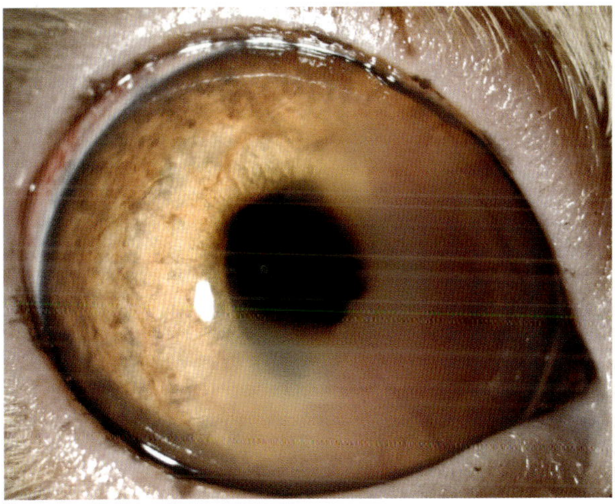

In the most advanced stages, new blood vessels appear along with a blackish, brown plaque.

Breed predisposition

The breeds most predisposed to develop a corneal sequestrum are Persians, Himalayans, and Exotic Shorthairs, but it can occur in any cat.

Feline corneal sequestrum

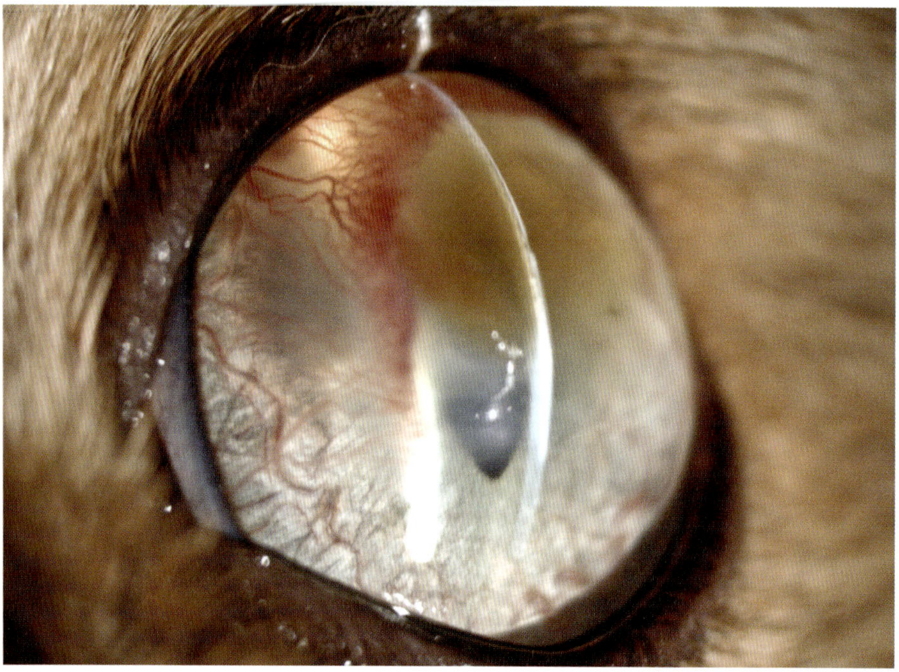

As the disease progresses, the corneal sequestrum induces a loss of stromal structure. The degeneration of collagen fibres can be appreciated using a slit lamp.

Interesting notes

A corneal sequestrum is histologically characterised by the presence of dry, degenerate collagen fibres. It may be considered a form of stromal necrosis.

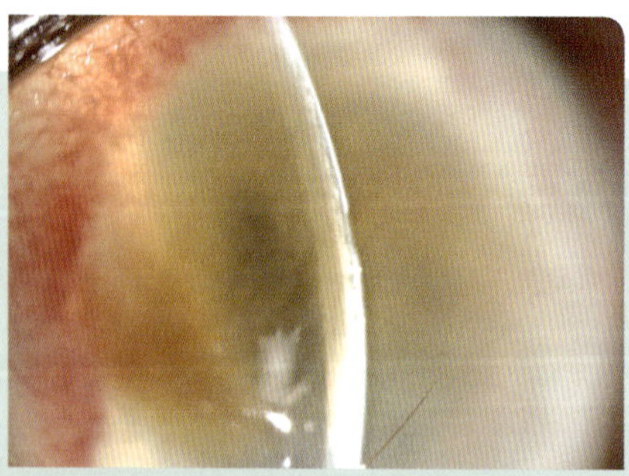

Close-up of the loss of corneal structure in the patient.

Feline corneal sequestrum

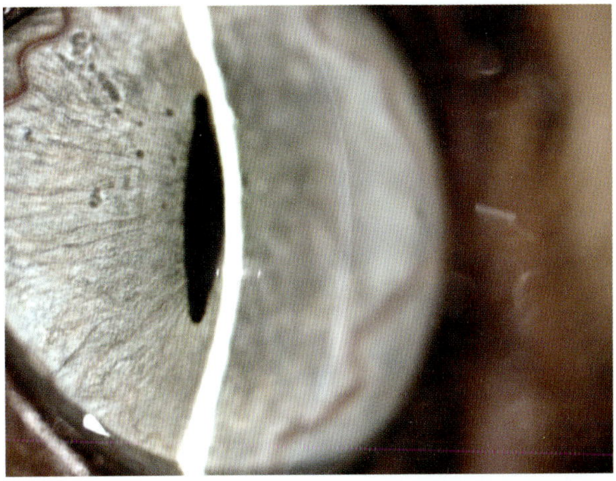

Normal contralateral eye of the patient pictured previously. Slit-lamp picture.

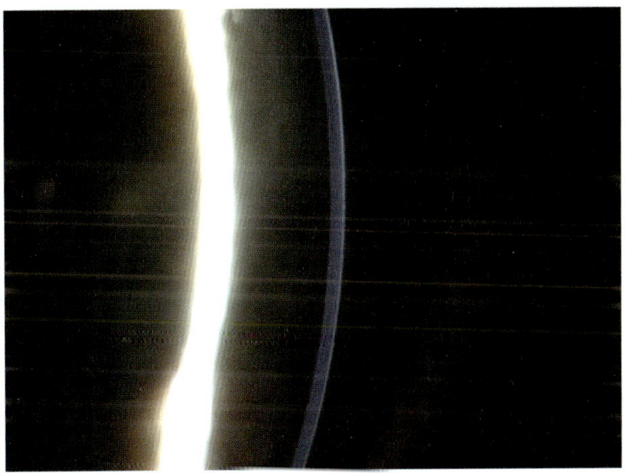

Optical close-up of the normal corneal structure.

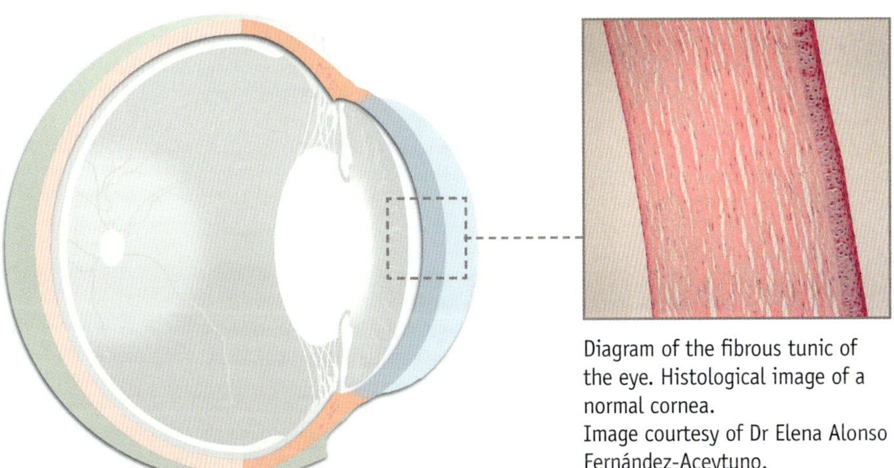

Diagram of the fibrous tunic of the eye. Histological image of a normal cornea.
Image courtesy of Dr Elena Alonso Fernández-Aceytuno.

Feline corneal sequestrum

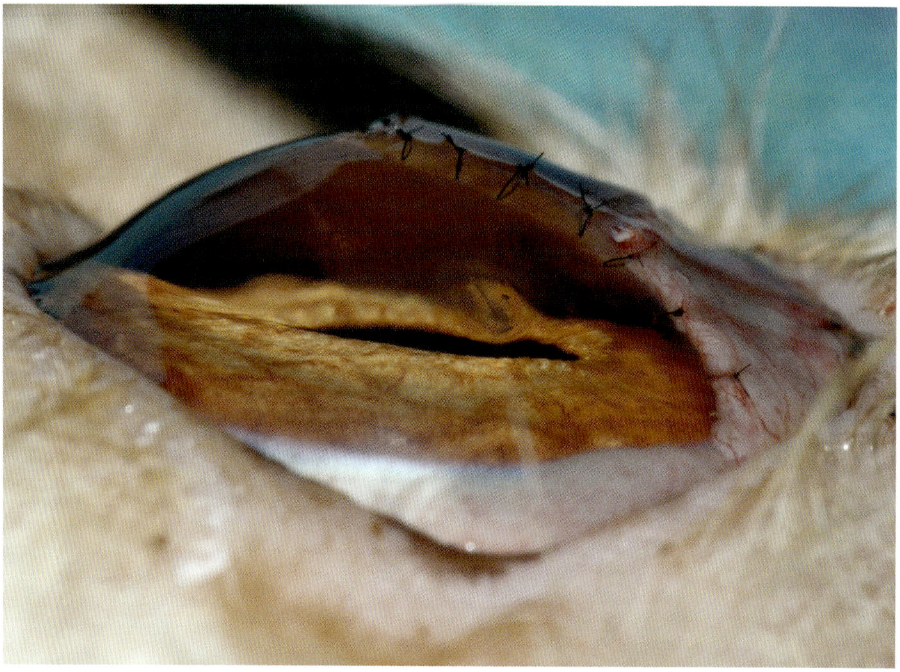

Corneal scleral conjunctival transposition in the patient from page 212 (a two-year-old Persian cat), to surgically treat a corneal sequestrum.

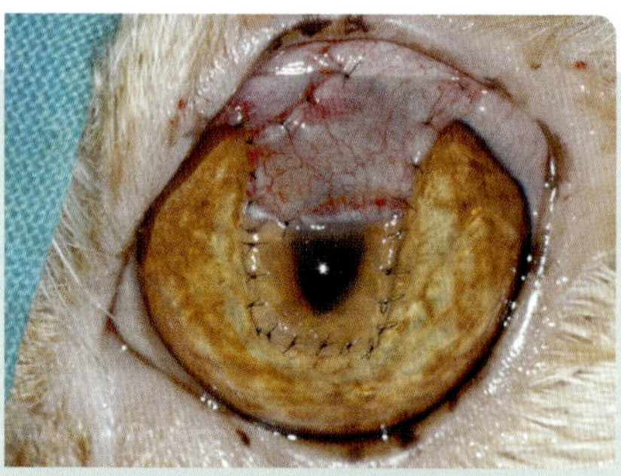

Front view of the flap.

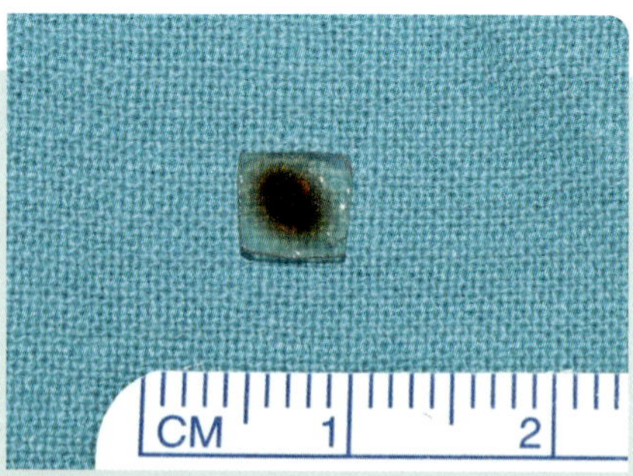

Close-up of the excised corneal sequestrum.

Surgical technique

Corneal scleral conjunctival transposition is the surgical technique of choice for feline corneal sequestrum. It involves an autologous sliding lamellar keratoplasty, which barely distorts the corneal curvature.

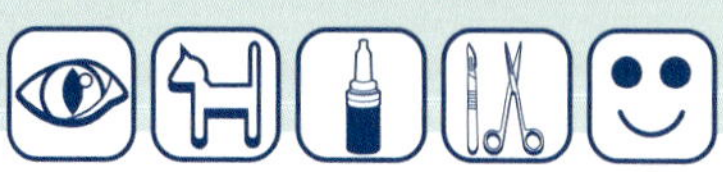

Feline corneal sequestrum

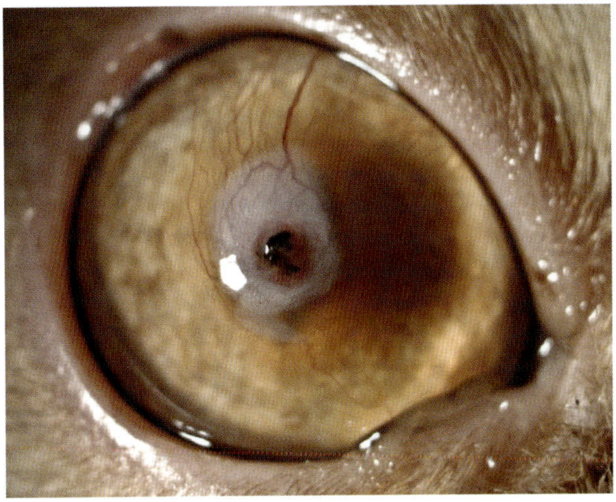

Feline corneal sequestrum in the central (axial) area of the cornea in a Persian cat. Corneal scleral conjunctival transpositions involve the transposition of healthy peripheral corneal tissue to the axial area after removal of the lesion (sequestrum).

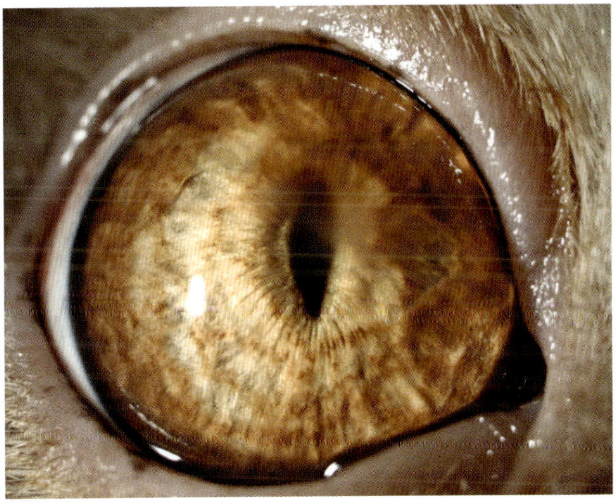

The patient's cornea two months after treatment.

Interesting notes

- The postoperative use of topical corticosteroids (dexamethasone) and cyclosporine A improves corneal transparency.
- An alternative to a corneal scleral conjunctival transposition is the use of porcine intestinal submucosa or cornea (fresh or frozen) following a keratectomy.

Feline corneal sequestrum

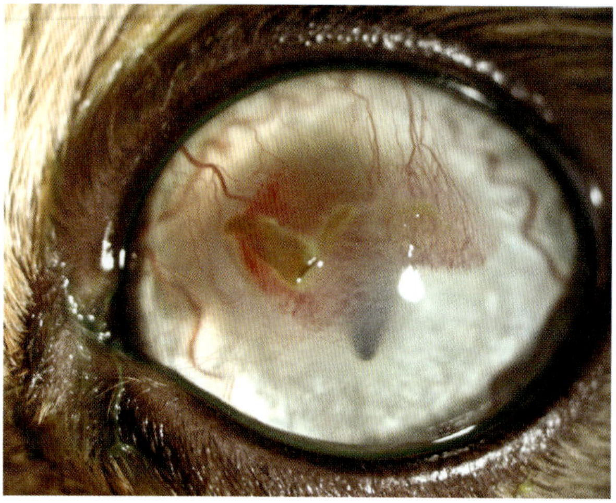

Corneal sequestrum in the process of extrusion in a cat.

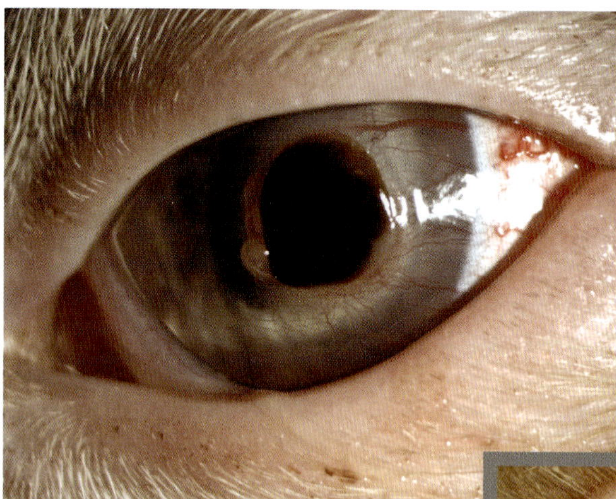

Spontaneous extrusion of a degenerate plaque in a Persian cat.

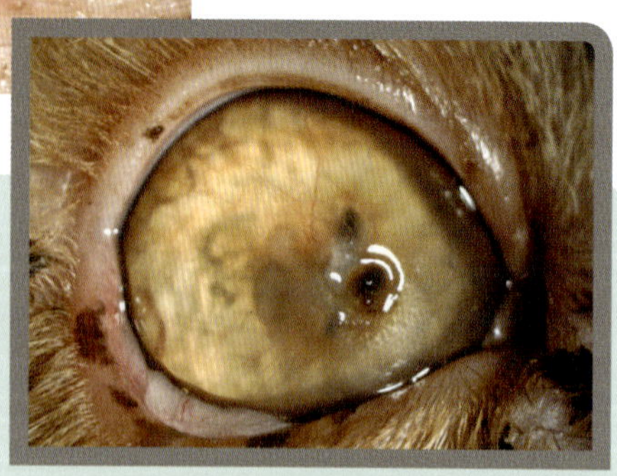

Deep corneal sequestrum. Note the corneal depression in the reflection of the flash.

Important notes

- Corneal sequestra may spontaneously be extruded in some cases. However, do not wait for this to occur because the disease may progress (even lead to perforation) and recurrence is common.

Dermoid cyst

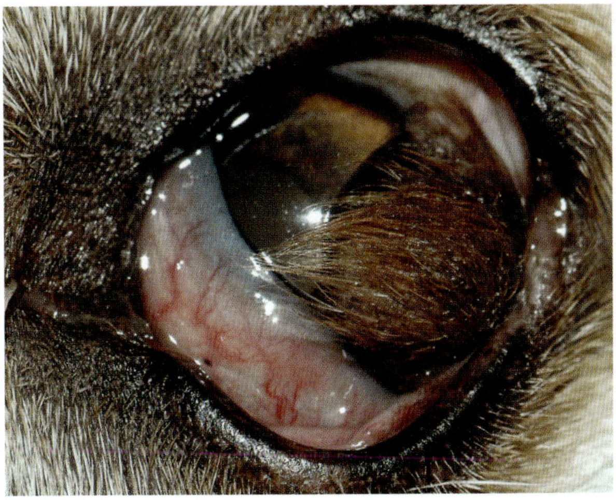

Congenital corneal dermoid cyst in a two-year-old mixed-breed dog.
Patients with dermoids generally present with epiphora and blepharospasm due to hairs rubbing on the cornea and/or conjunctiva.

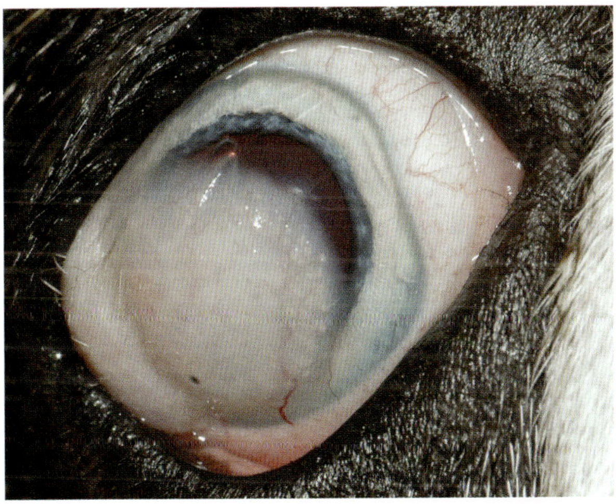

Dermoid cyst in a French Bulldog puppy; it involves more than 3/4 of the full corneal surface. This patient has a visual deficit in the affected eye.

Treatment

The treatment of choice for corneal or corneal conjunctival dermoid cysts is surgical excision through superficial keratectomy.

Corneal abscess

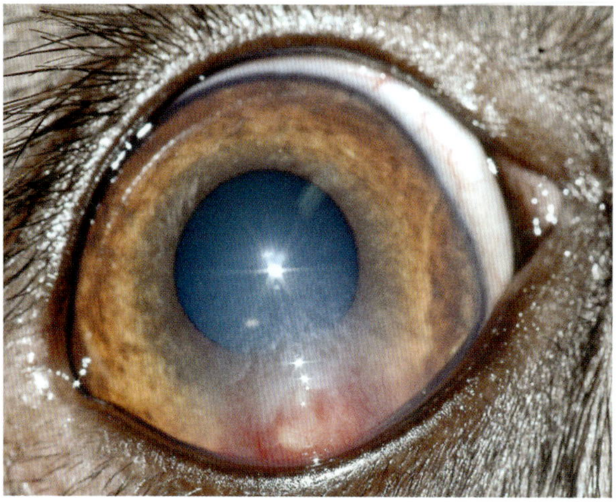

Corneal abscess in a seven-year-old mixed-breed dog. Patient who often goes into the fields.
Time since onset: 25 days.

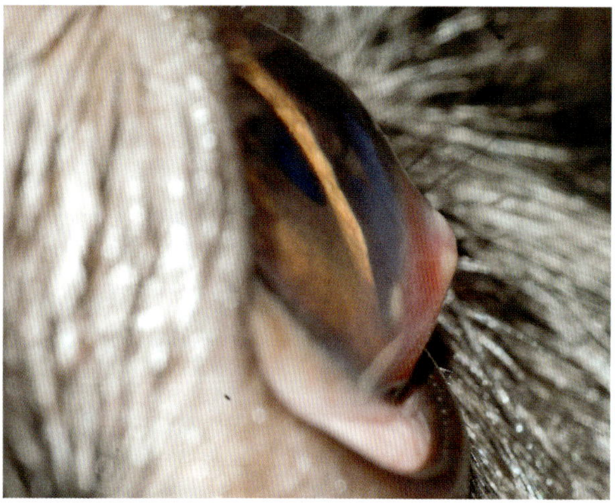

Lateral view of the eye. Close-up of the size and site of the abscess.

Treatment

- Long-term medical treatment with culture and sensitivity testing may be sufficient to resolve the infection as long as the causal agent (often a stromal foreign body) is eliminated.
- Surgical treatment (drainage of the abscess and/or keratectomy) should be considered in cases where medical treatment is not curative.

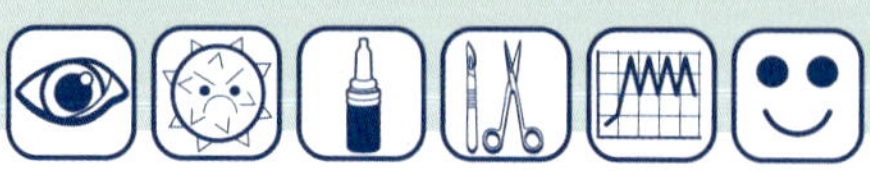

Episcleritis

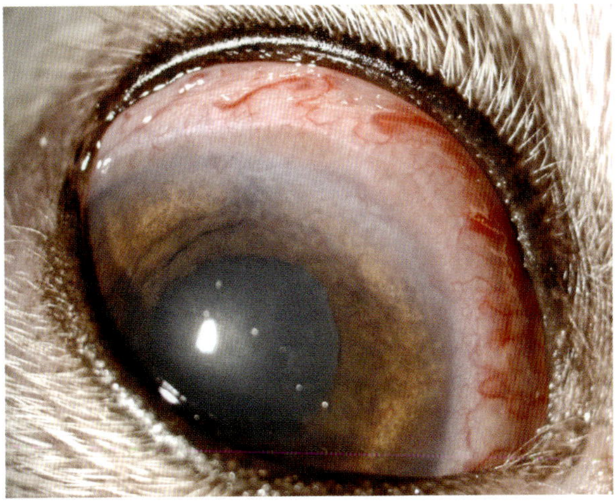

Moderate episcleritis in a seven-year-old mixed-breed dog. Conjunctival hyperaemia and marked episcleral injection. Time since onset: 20 days. Mild blepharospasm is present.
Corneal oedema and neovascularisation in the area closest to the episcleral inflammatory reaction are common.

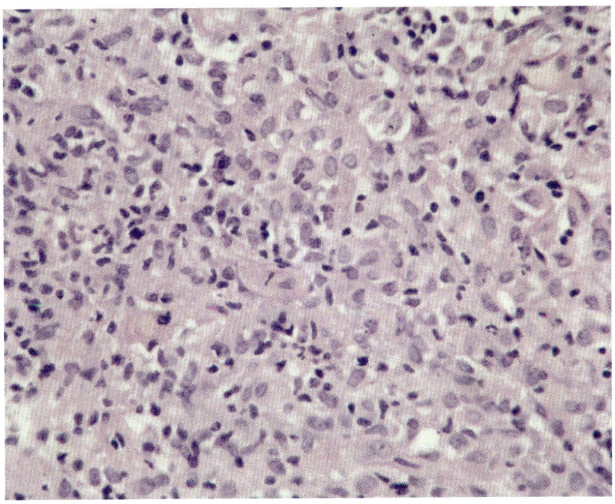

Dense cellular infiltrate that is predominantly lymphocytic, plasmacytic, and neutrophilic. Chronic granulomatous episcleritis in the patient pictured above. Image courtesy of Histovet.

i | Episcleritis is a proliferative inflammatory disease that may be nodular or diffuse. It affects the episcleral tissue and is generally chronic. It tends to be benign in behaviour and of immune origin.

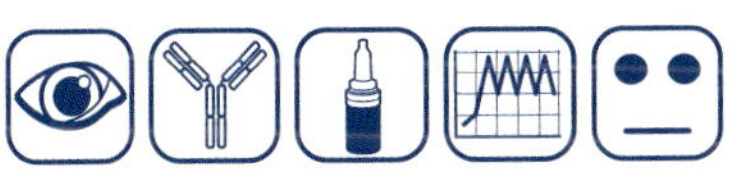

Episcleritis

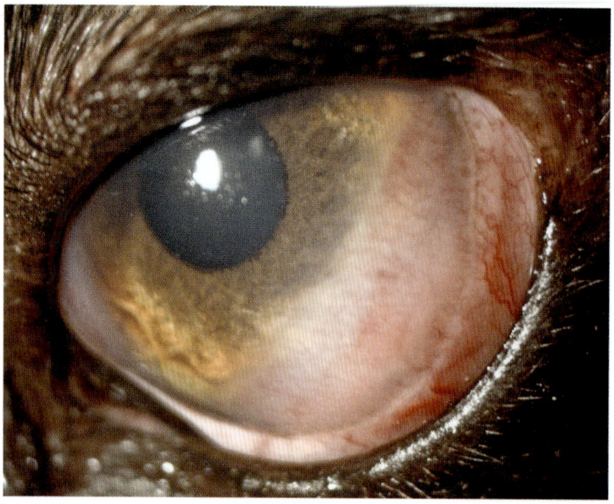

Nodular diffuse episcleritis in a dog with leishmaniasis. Diagnosis confirmed using immunohistochemistry.

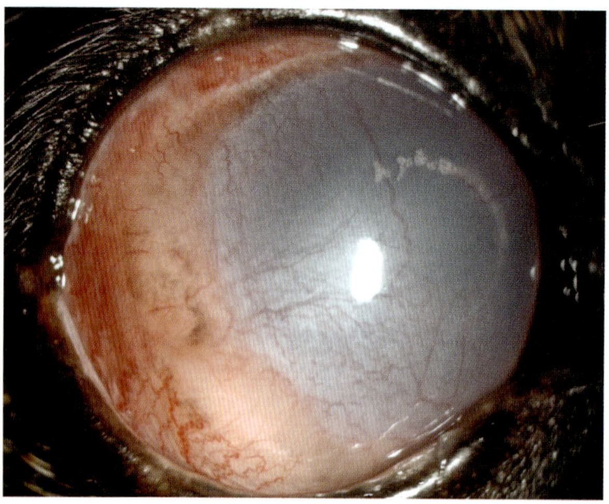

Severe inflammatory episcleral reaction with generalised corneal compromise. Canine leishmaniasis.

Interesting notes

- Certain infectious processes (*Leishmania*) or trauma can result in episcleritis in dogs.
- There is a definitive breed predisposition: Cocker Spaniel, Shetland Sheepdog, Collie and Rottweiler are the breeds most predisposed to this inflammatory disease.

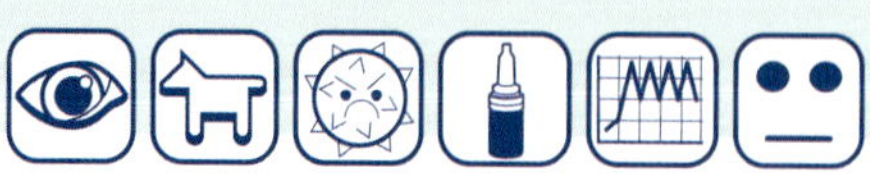

Episcleritis

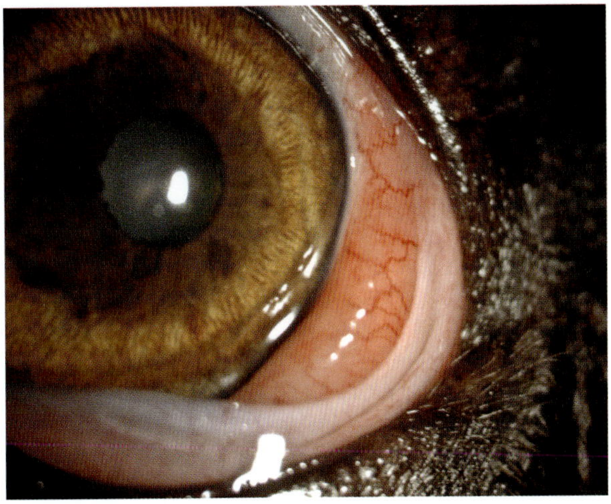

Nodular episcleritis in a five-year-old Rottweiler mix. Episcleral neovascularisation in the ventronasal area.

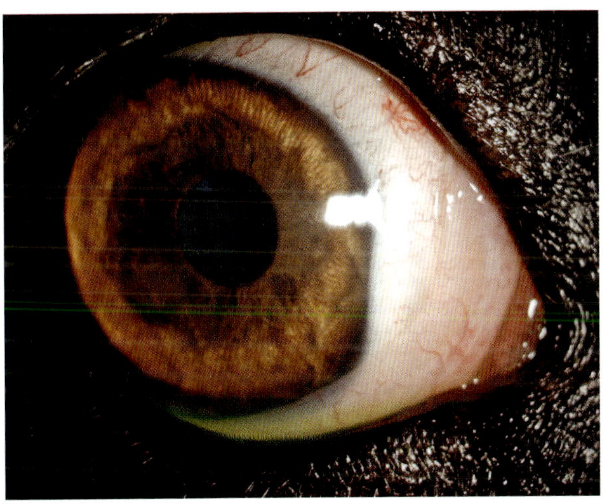

Patient three months after treatment.

Treatment

- Medical treatment involves topical and/or subconjunctival corticosteroids. The drugs of choice are topical dexamethasone and methylprednisolone acetate or subconjunctival triamcinolone. Very severe cases may require the limited use of systemic azathioprine (orally).
- An excisional biopsy is considered diagnostic and is an element of the surgical treatment.

Uvea

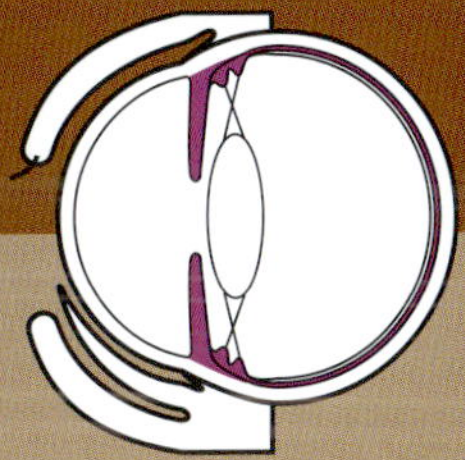

Iris hypoplasia

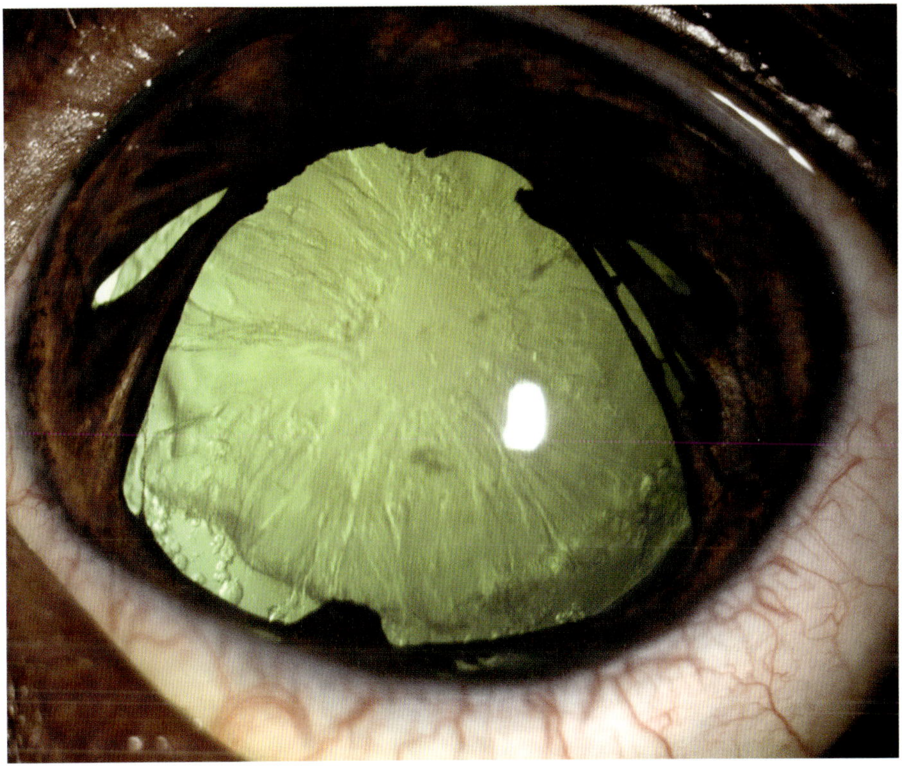

Severe uveal hypoplasia in an eight-month-old Shih-Tzu.

The iris underdevelopment prevents the normal entry of light. There is no normal pupillary aperture. In this case, the hypoplasia is accompanied by a persistent pupillary membrane and congenital cataracts.

i

This is a congenital disorder of uveal development that is manifested by a partial lack of iridal tissue. A complete lack of iris is also called aniridia.

The presentation is often bilateral, though each eye may be affected to a different degree.

Iris hypoplasia

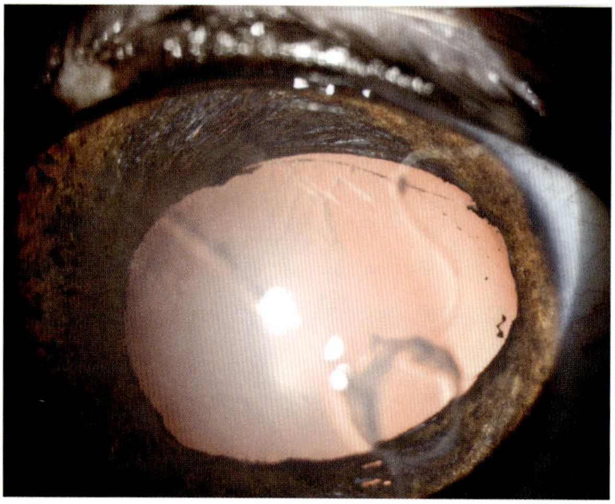

Moderate iridal hypoplasia in a one-year-old Shih-Tzu. The owner noted a brighter shine from one eye than the other and stated that light bothered his pet. Since the patient lacked a normal pupillary aperture, photophobia was a logical consequence.

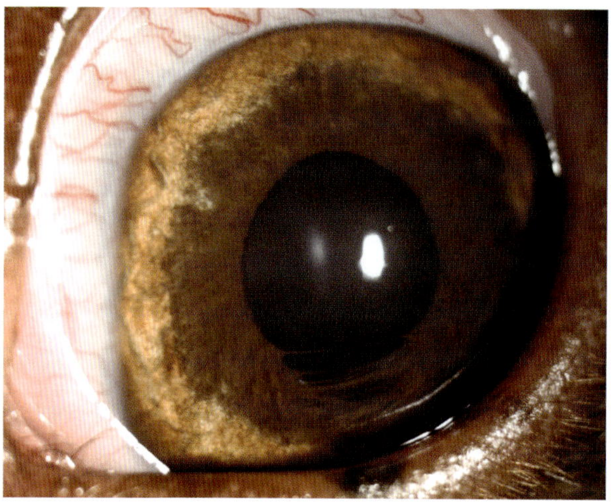

Two-year-old mixed breed dog with mild uveal hypoplasia.

Breed predisposition

- This condition has been described in the Catalan Sheepdog (Villagrasa, 1994), Shih-Tzu, and Rottweiler.
- THERE IS NO TREATMENT.

Iris heterochromia

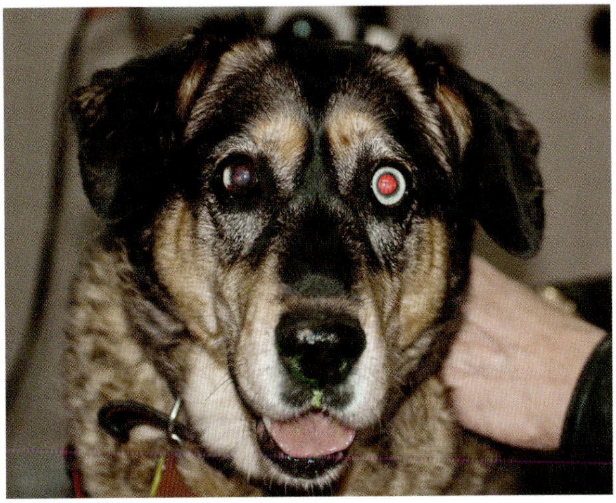

Iris heterochromia in a seven-year-old dog.

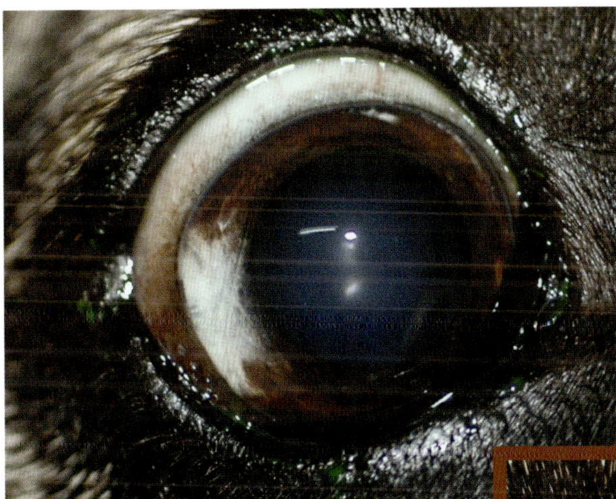

Patient's right eye.

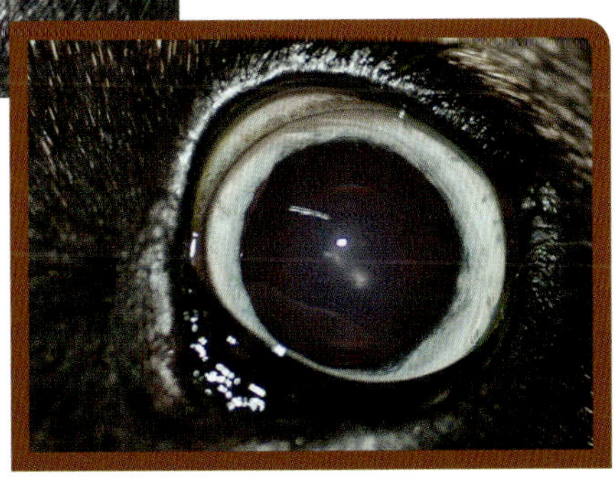

Patient's left eye.

This involves varying pigment concentrations in the iris. Differences in iris colouring may affect one or both eyes.

Heterochromia iridum indicates colour variation of one eye relative to the contralateral one, and heterochromia iridis is colour variation within one eye.

Iris heterochromia

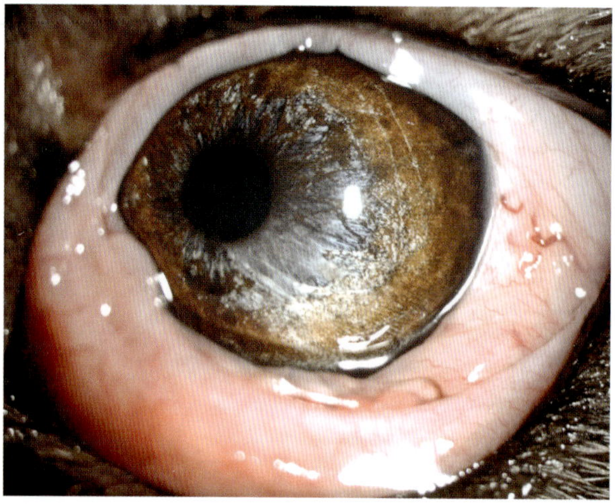

Heterochromia iridis (colour variation in the same iris), in the left eye of an English Bulldog.

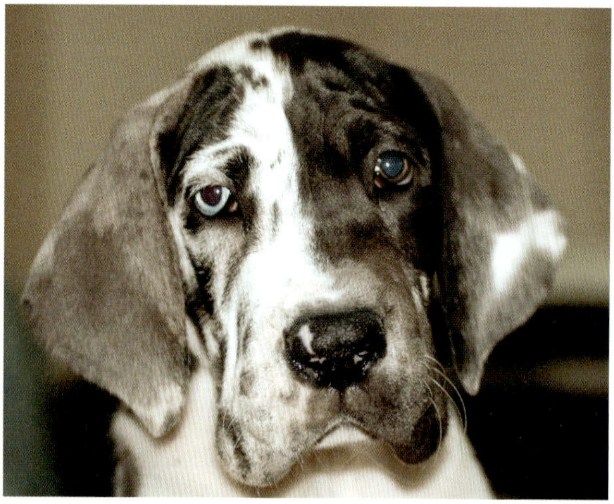

Heterochromia iridum (two irises of different colours) in a Great Dane puppy.

Breed predisposition

- This congenital disease is due to a deficit in the maturation of melanin pigment.
- It has been described in the Siberian Husky, Alaskan Malamute, and Dalmatian.
- Waardenburg syndrome (deafness, white coat, and iris heterochromia) has been noted in cats and Great Danes.

Persistent pupillary membrane

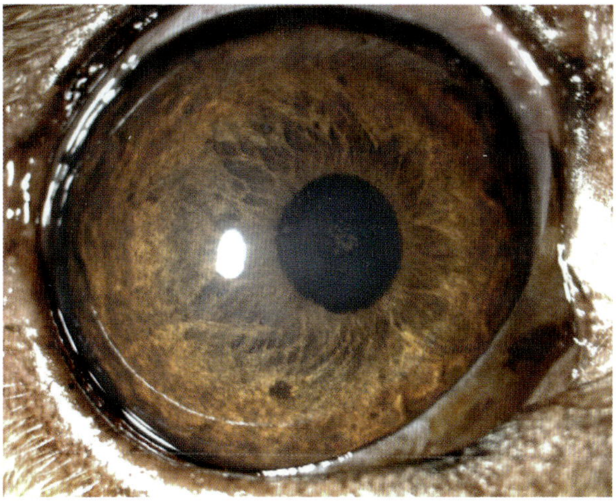

First-degree persistent pupillary membrane (PPM). Pupillary membrane remnants are located on the anterior lens capsule.

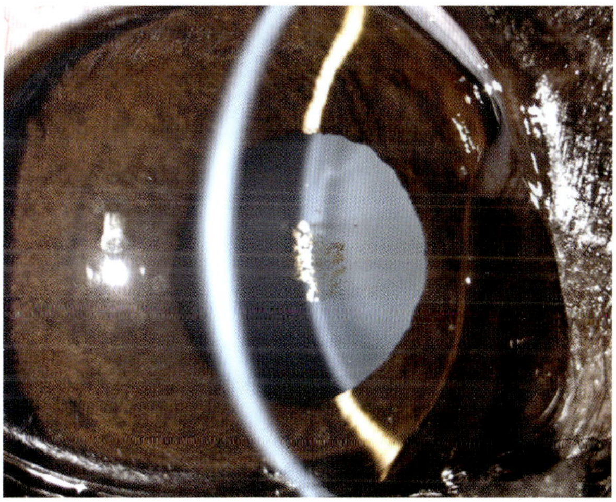

A slit lamp helps us precisely locate the PPM.
Picture from the patient shown above.

i | Defect in the resorption of the mesoderm that keeps the pupillary orifice open during embryonic development and normally disappears following birth.

Persistent pupillary membrane

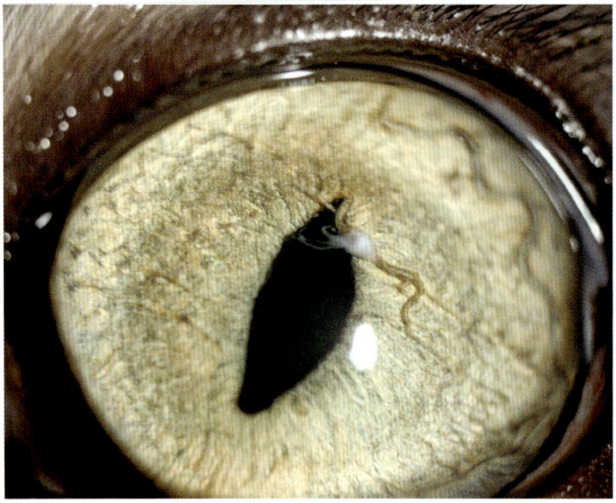

Second-degree PPM in a cat. The fibres of the pupillary membrane cross the pupillary aperture from one side of the iris to the other.

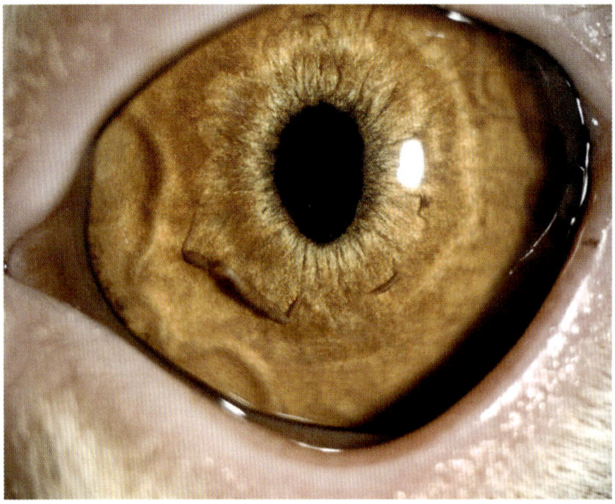

In second-degree PPM, the pupillary membrane strands do not attach to neighbouring structures (cornea or lens). Feline patient.

Breed predisposition

- The most predisposed dog breeds are the Cocker Spaniel, Mastiff, Rottweiler and Dachshund.
- This occurs less often in cats.

Persistent pupillary membrane

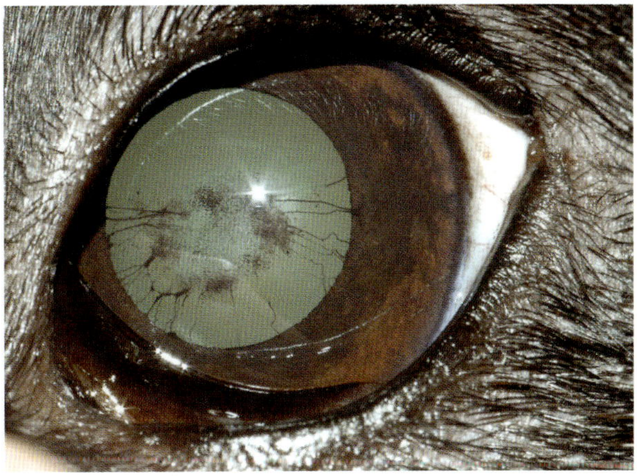

Third-degree PPM in a dog. In these cases, fibres of the persistent pupillary membrane run from the iris collarette to the anterior lens capsule.

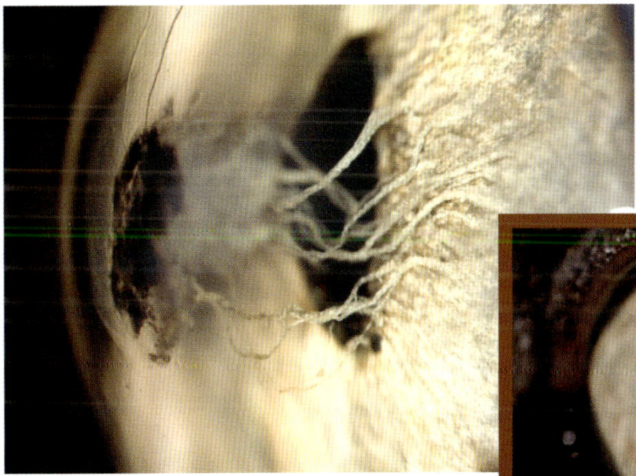

Fourth-degree PPM in a cat. This phase is characterised by adhesion between the pupillary membrane fibres and the corneal endothelium, with the ensuing inflammatory reaction. Feline patient.

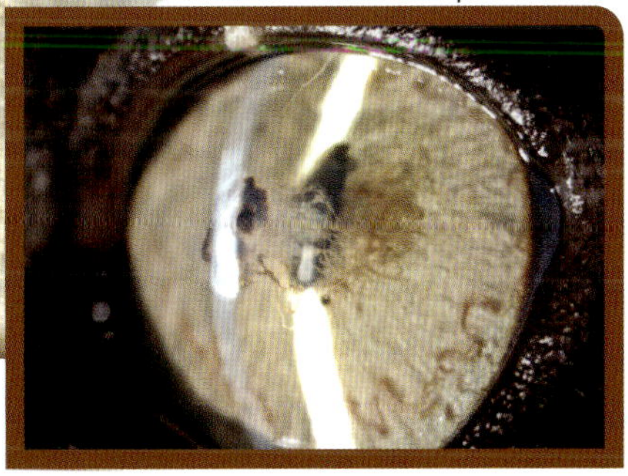

Location of the lesion above with a slit lamp. Adhesion to the endothelium.

Important notes

- It is critical to examine PPM with a slit lamp to assess the intraocular condition.
- PPM always originates from the iris collarette (border between the pupillary zone and ciliary zone).

Uvea

Uveitis

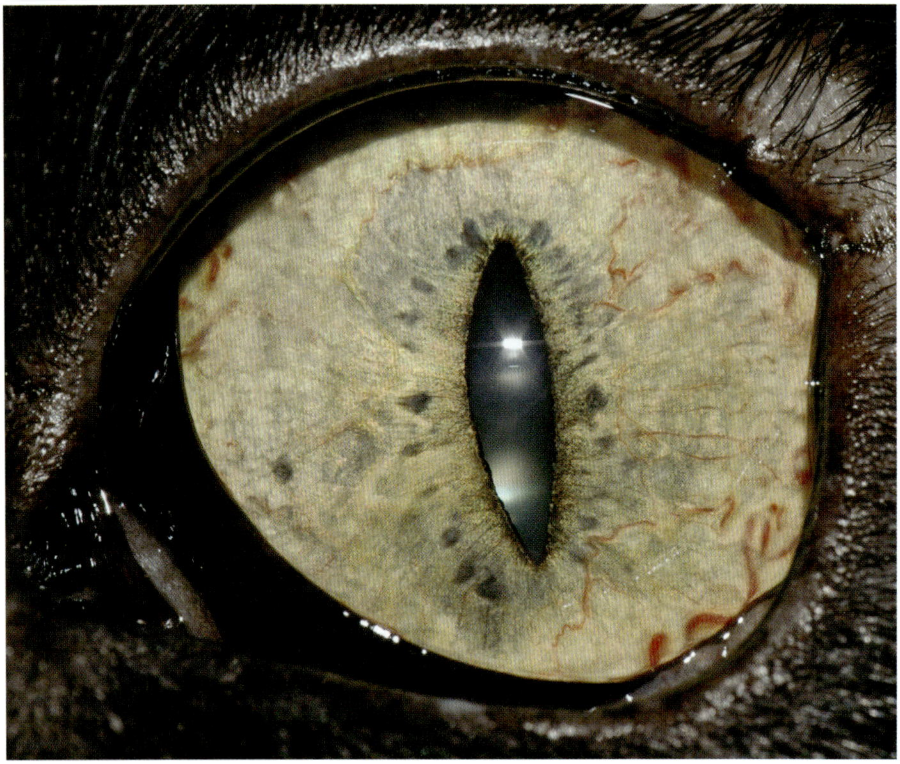

Chronic granulomatous uveitis in a cat with toxoplasmosis.
Close-up of rubeosis (neovascularisation) of the iris and peripupillary granulomas.
Time since onset: two months.

- Uveitis (inflammation of vascular eye tissue) can occur in the following areas:
  - Anterior uvea (iritis and/or cyclitis).
  - Posterior uvea (choroiditis).
- Inflammation of the area between the iris and the choroid is known as pars planitis.
- If it affects the whole uvea, it is called panuveitis.

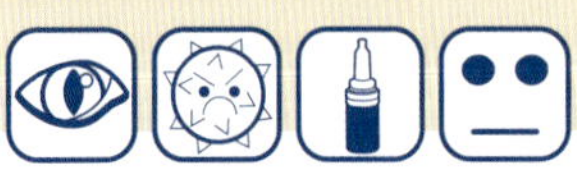

Uveitis

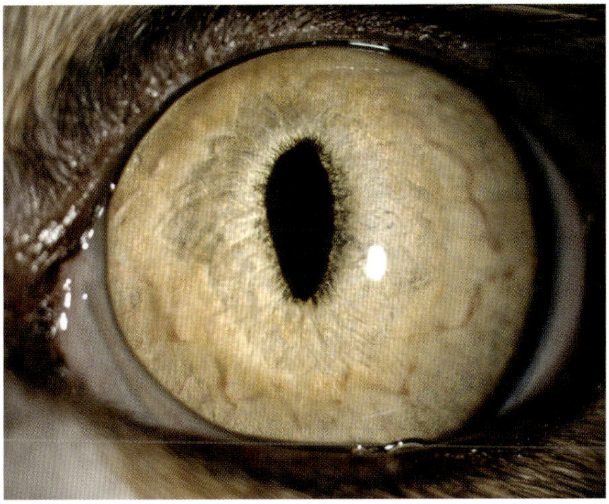

Mild iris oedema and congestion in a cat with uveitis.
Note the blurry, turbid appearance of the iris.
Early clinical sign.
Time since onset: 24 hours.

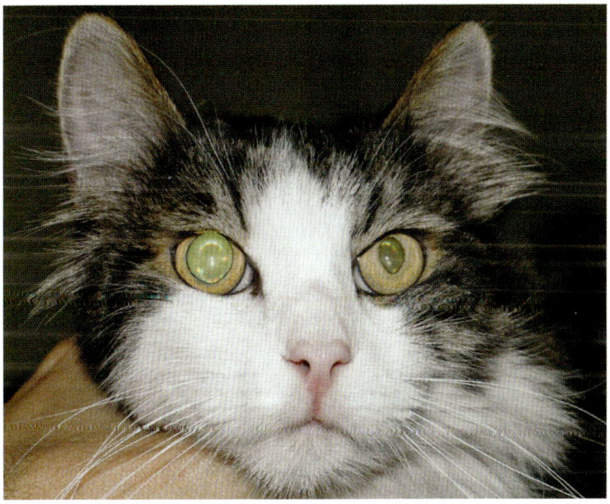

Miosis caused by inflammatory constriction of the iris is pathognomonic for uveitis. Anisocoria in the patient pictured above.

The initial clinical signs of uveitis are:

- MIOSIS.
- UVEAL CONGESTION.
- TYNDALL EFFECT.

Uveitis

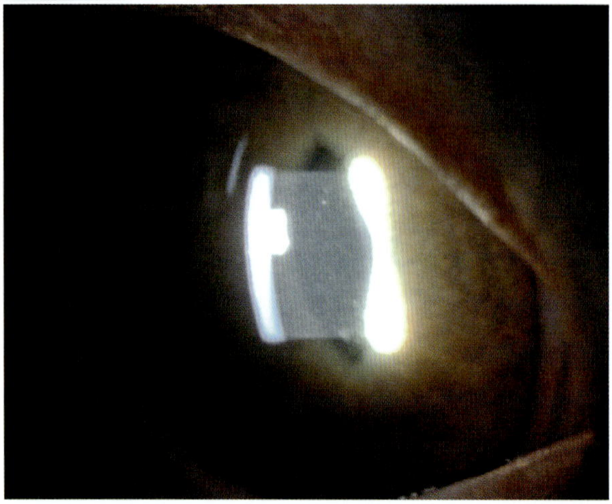

Tyndall effect in a cat with uveitis. Slit-lamp picture. The turbidity of the aqueous humour is caused by the concentration of inflammatory cells.

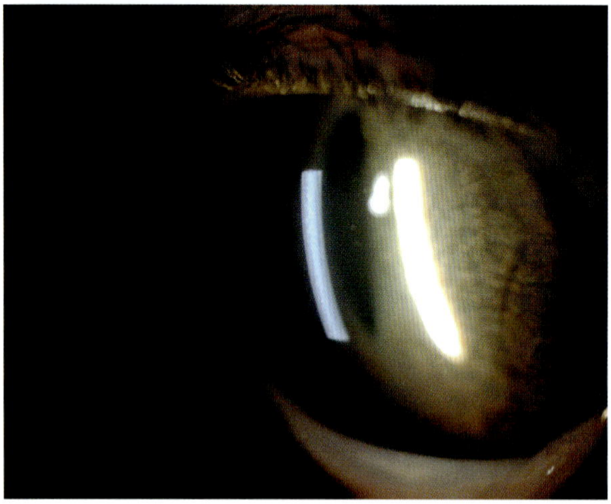

Normal eye. Close-up of the anterior chamber with no inflammatory material. The Tyndall effect is not present.

Interesting notes

Use a narrow slit to identify the Tyndall effect.

Tyndall effect: lack of transparency of the anterior chamber due to the concentration of inflammatory cells that are extravasated from blood vessels. The effect is similar to a ray of sunlight permeating a dust cloud inside a dark room. Slit-lamp biomicroscopy is used to demonstrate this.

Uveitis

Infectious

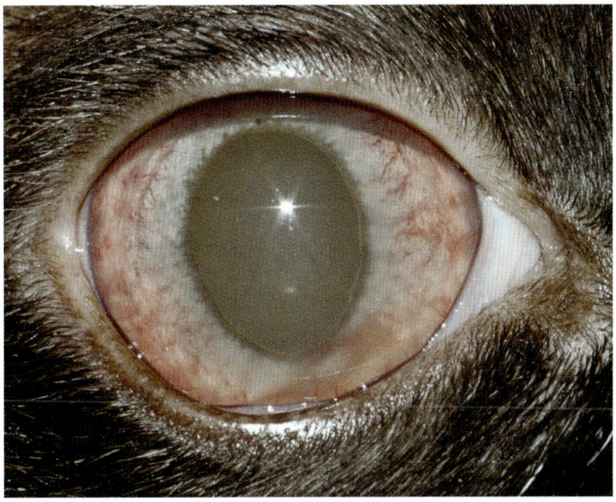

Iridal rubeosis (neovascularisation) in acute uveitis in a cat.
Acute presentation (48 hours since onset).
Feline immunodeficiency.

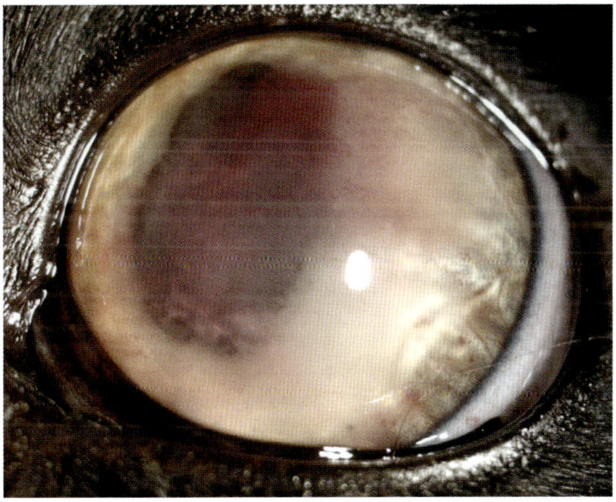

Domestic shorthair cat with acute uveitis due to feline immunodeficiency virus (FIV). Fibrin in the anterior chamber.

The infectious diseases that often induce uveitis in cats are as follows:

- FELINE LEUKAEMIA (FELV).
- FELINE IMMUNODEFICIENCY (FIV).
- TOXOPLASMOSIS.
- FELINE INFECTIOUS PERITONITIS (FIP).

Uveitis

Infectious

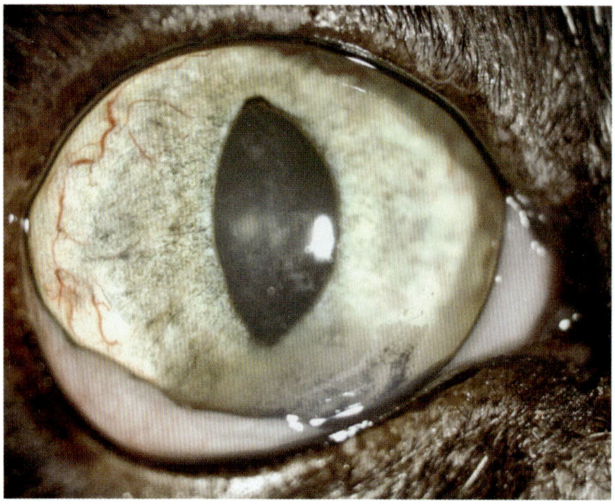

Hypopyon (cells and fibrin in the anterior chamber) in a cat with uveitis.
Another sign of uveitis is visible: iridal rubeosis.
Cause: feline immunodeficiency.

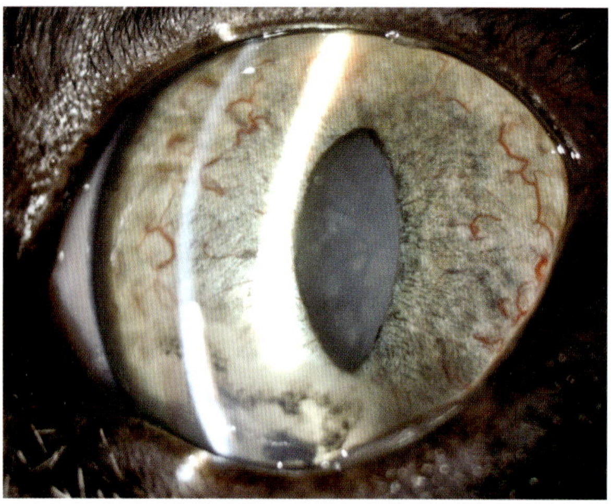

Left eye of the patient pictured above. The uveitis signs are similar to those in the right eye (hypopyon and rubeosis).
Cataracts are secondary to uveitis and signify chronicity.
Slit-lamp picture.

Interesting notes

- Feline uveitis tends to occur with conjunctival chemosis (see upper picture). This does not occur with canine uveitis.

Uveitis

Infectious

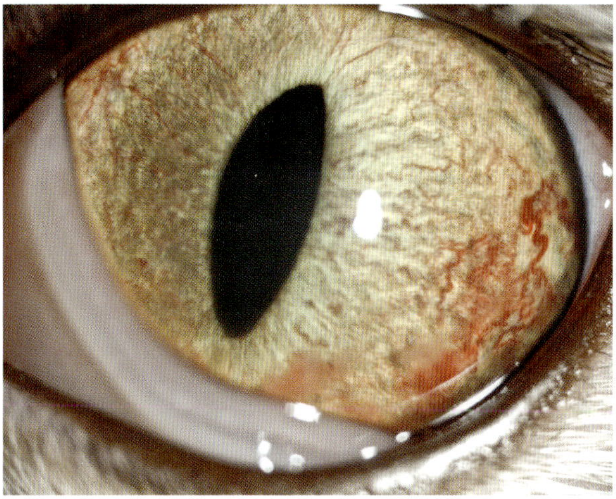

Hypopyon (cells and fibrin in the anterior chamber) in a cat with uveitis.
The ocular discomfort causes protrusion of the nictitating membrane.
Cause: feline leukaemia.

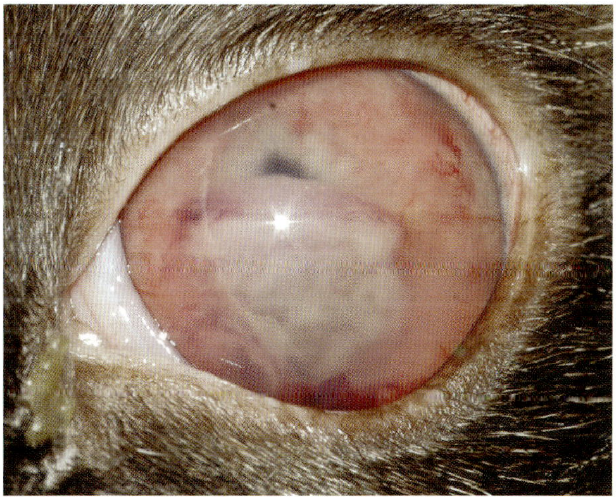

Very severe uveitis secondary to FIP.
Hypopyon.

i | Feline uveitis associated with infectious diseases often presents bilaterally. In some cases, it affects one eye at first and the contralateral eye a few days later.

Uveitis

Infectious

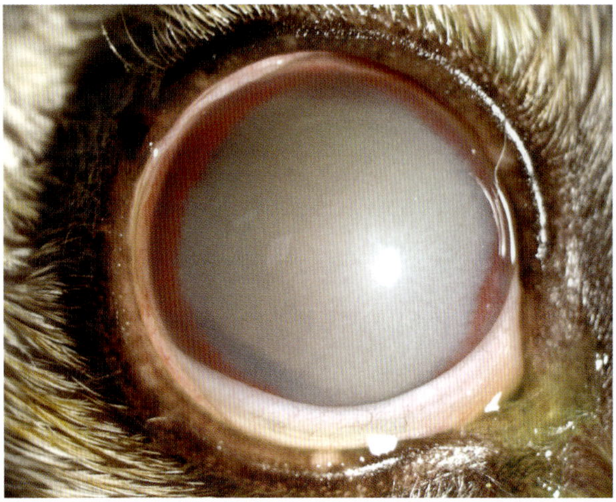

Acute uveitis in a dog. Pericorneal ring and generalised corneal oedema. Time since onset: 48 hours. Intraocular pressure: 7 mmHg.

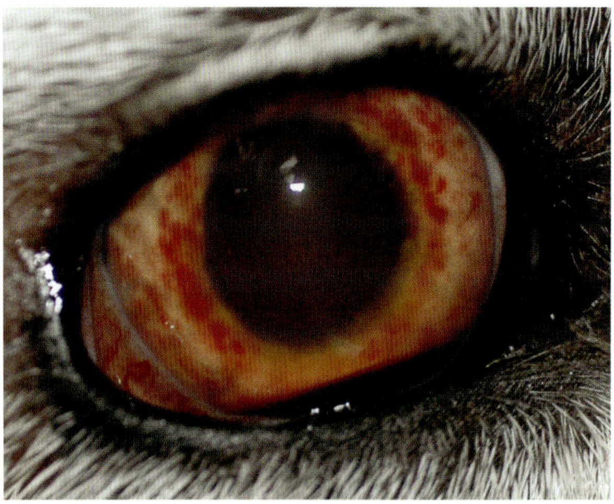

Siberian Husky with acute uveitis (iridal rubeosis and hyphaema). Patient with ehrlichiosis.

Corneal oedema and a pericorneal ring are characteristic of canine uveitis, in contrast to feline uveitis.

Important notes

- In uveitis, the vessels that invade the cornea are THIN, SHORT, PARALLEL, AND NONBRANCHING.

Uveitis

Infectious

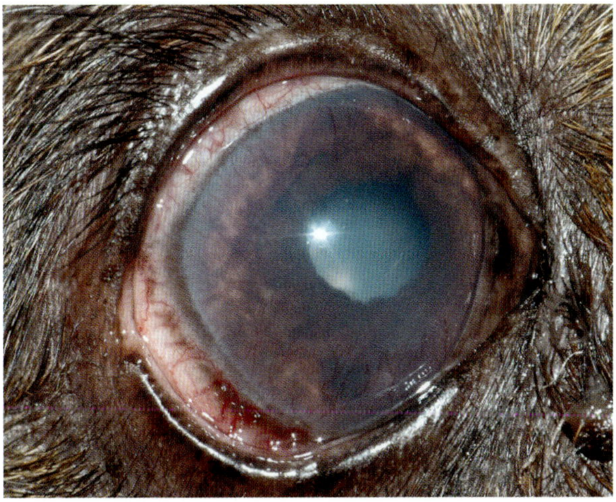

Leishmania-induced uveitis. This type of uveitis is often associated with keratitis (keratouveitis).

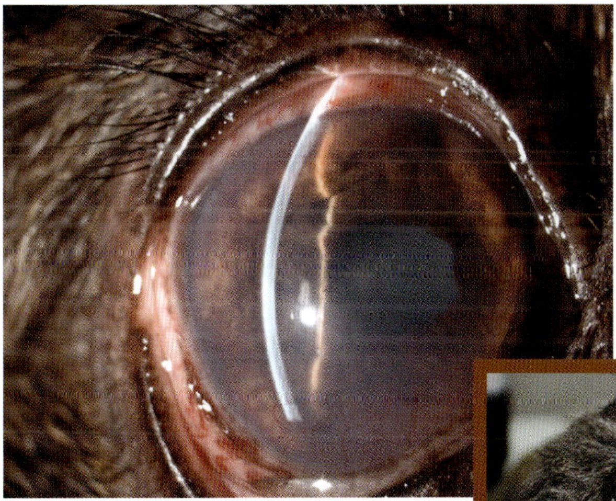

Slit-lamp picture of the right eye of the patient pictured above. Close-up of the corneal oedema and iris inflammation.

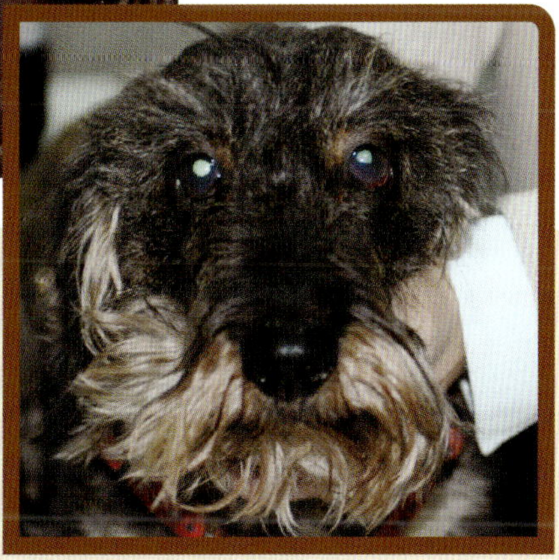

Our patient. Bilateral lesion.

The infectious diseases that most commonly cause uveitis in dogs are as follows:

- LEISHMANIOSIS.
- EHRLICHIOSIS.
- LEPTOSPIROSIS.
- BACTERIAL INFECTIONS (pyometra, prostatitis, periodontal disease).

Uveitis

Lens-induced

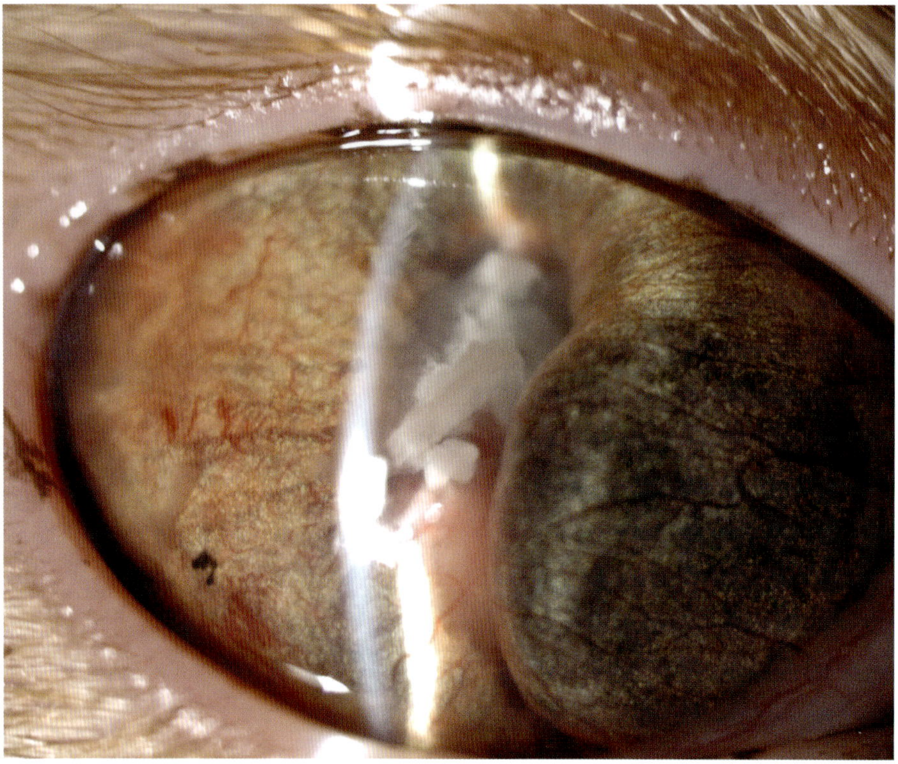

Lens-induced uveitis in a cat.
This patient was scratched by another cat, which perforated the cornea and lens.
The release of lenticular material, specifically the lens proteins, caused severe uveitis.
Close-up of cortical material leaking out of the lens and the uveal reaction (rubeosis).

Interesting notes

The embryonic development of the lens is distinct from that of other intraocular structures. When lens proteins are released from the capsule, they trigger a severe immune response inside the eye.

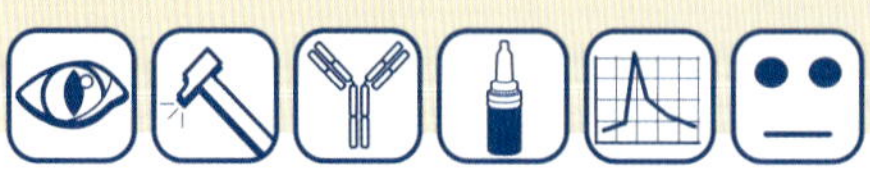

Uveitis

Lens-induced

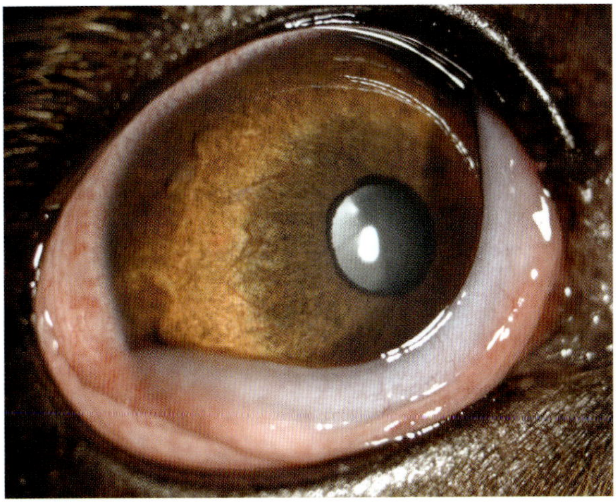

Lens-induced uveitis in a three-year old Beagle with a mature cataract.
Time since onset: 24 hours.

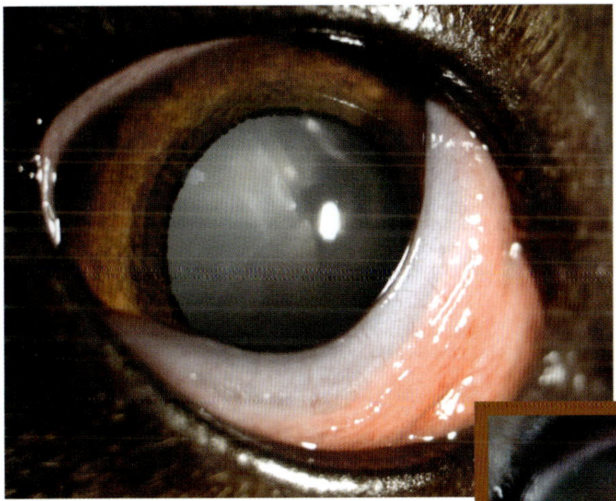

Pupil of the eye pictured above, three hours after topical administration of tropicamide.
Resistance to mydriasis is a characteristic sign of uveitis.

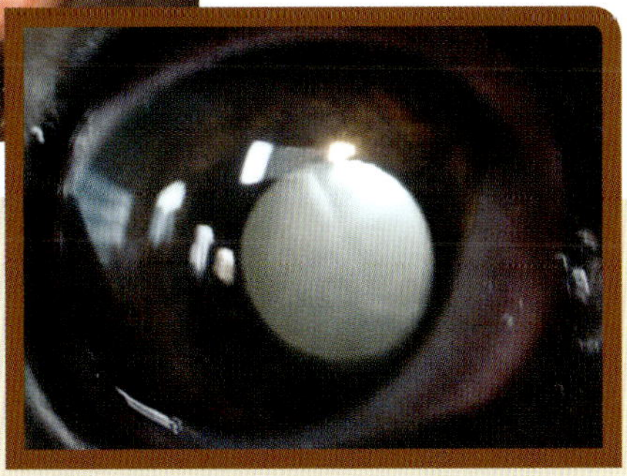

Tyndall effect in the patient's right eye.

Important notes

Lens-induced uveitis is highly inflammatory, and patients (especially dogs) present with severe blepharospasm. MIOSIS, RUBEOSIS OF THE IRIS, THE TYNDALL EFFECT, and PROTRUSION of the nictitating membrane are common signs.

Uveitis

Traumatic

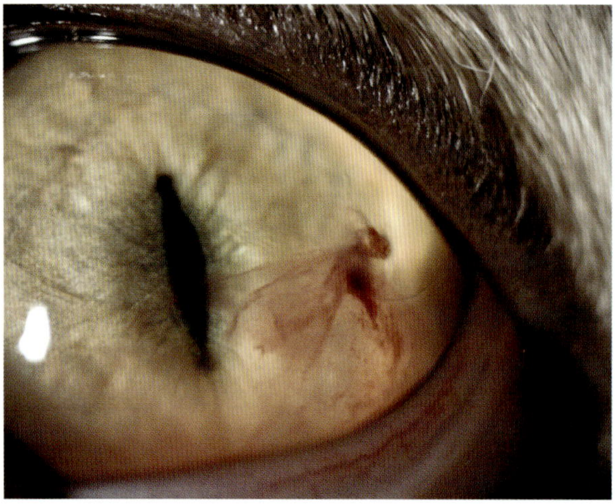

Traumatic uveitis in a cat. A glass shard perforated the cornea and reached the iris. Time since onset: 36 hours. Close-up of the miosis and fibrin in the anterior chamber and of the corneal injury.

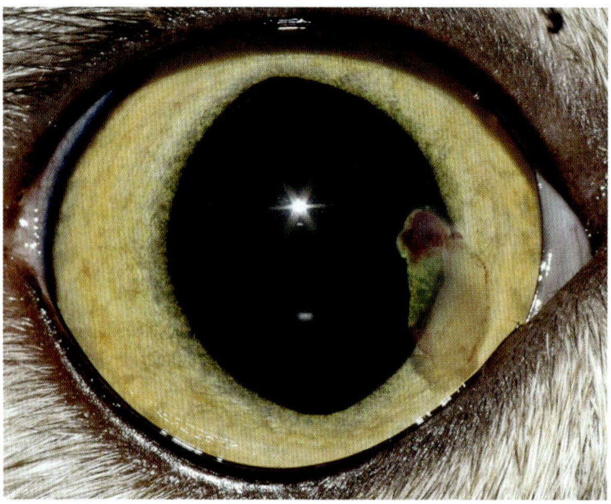

Twenty-four hours after treatment with anti-inflammatories and cycloplegics, the pupil is dilated and the fibrin concentration has decreased.

Interesting notes

- Traumatic uveitis may be perforating (corneal perforation with direct uveal damage), contusion-related (strong direct impacts to the eye) or postoperative (cataract surgery).

Uveitis

Traumatic

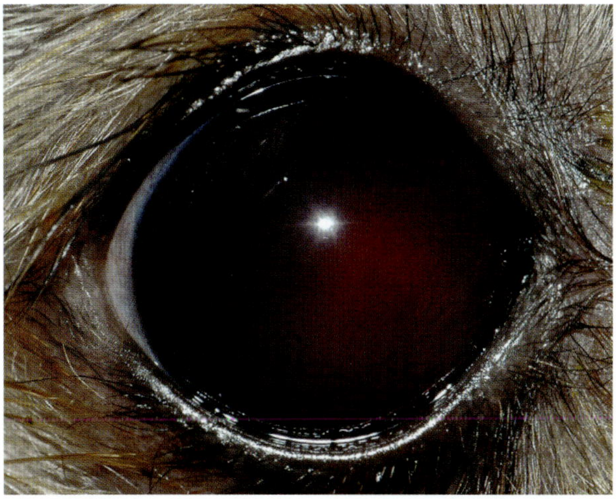

Hyperacute traumatic uveitis in a Yorkshire Terrier with an ocular contusion. Hyphaema after 12 hours.

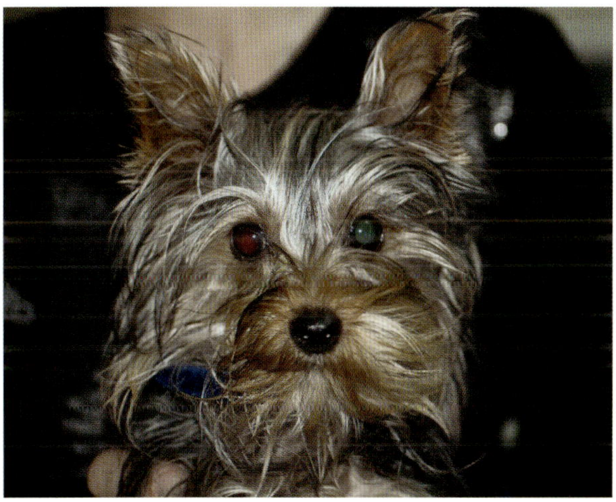

Intraocular haemorrhage, secondary to uveal damage, obscures the tapetal reflection in the patient's right eye.

Emergency

Uveitis with severe intraocular haemorrhage requires prompt, frequent, and long-term medical treatment to minimise sequelae.

Uveitis

Traumatic

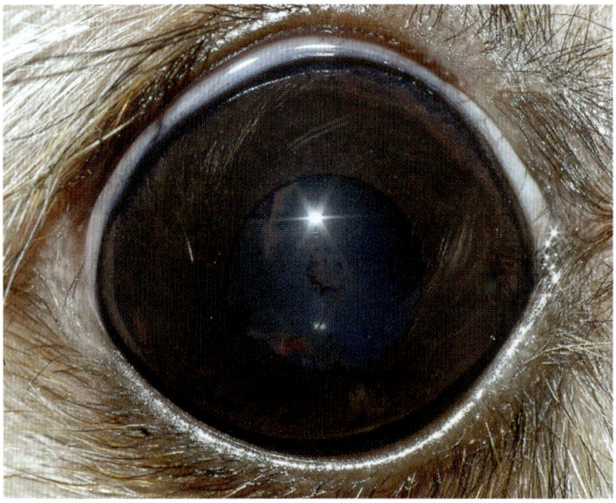

Eye of the patient from the previous case after five days of medical treatment.

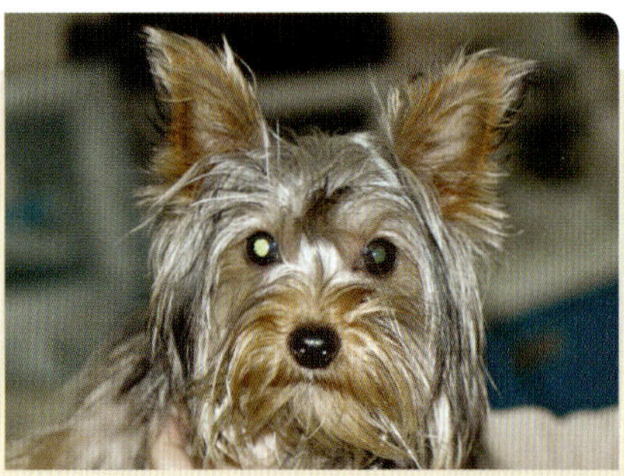

Note the tapetal reflection in the affected eye.

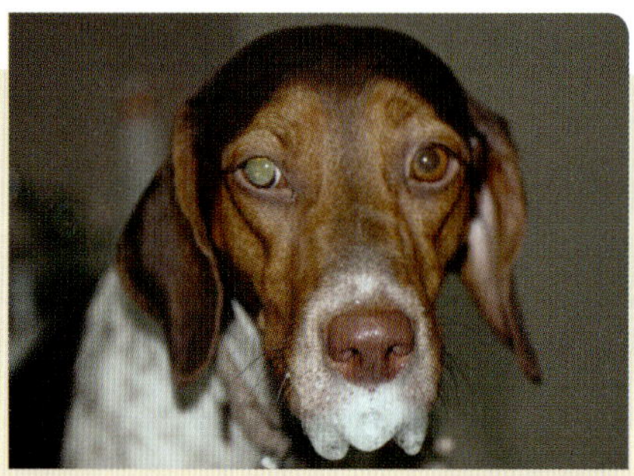

Atropine eye drops can cause hypersalivation (DO NOT USE IN CATS).

Treatment

- ANTI-INFLAMMATORIES
  - Topical: corticosteroids in acetate form have good penetration of the anterior chamber (prednisolone acetate, six times daily).
  - Subconjunctival: prednisolone acetate or triamcinolone.
  - Systemic corticosteroids or NSAIDs.
- CYCLOPLEGICS
  - Atropine or tropicamide (in case of a risk of glaucoma, or in KCS).

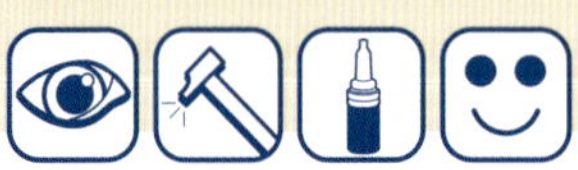

Uveitis

Reflex

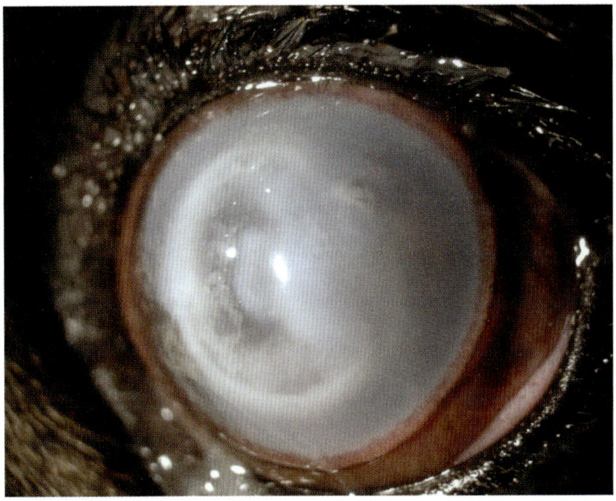

Reflex uveitis secondary to severe corneal damage (deep complicated melting corneal ulcer).
Note the pericorneal ring and corneal oedema characteristic of uveitis.

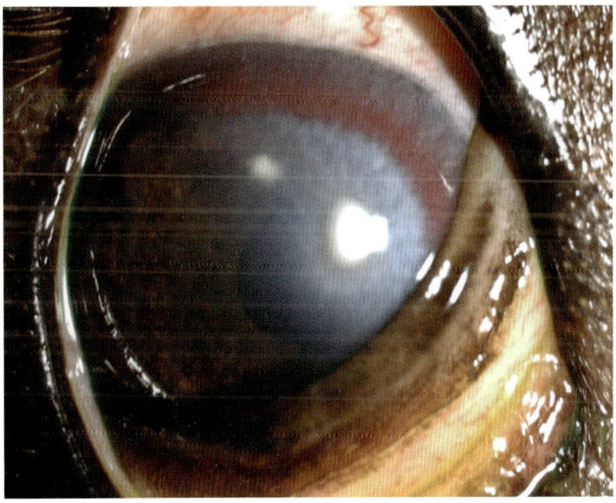

Uveal inflammatory reaction secondary to corneal damage caused by a pine processionary caterpillar. Miosis and corneal oedema are present.

Important notes

- Reflex uveitis results from the response of the trigeminal nerve endings to a severe corneal injury.

Uveitis

Idiopathic

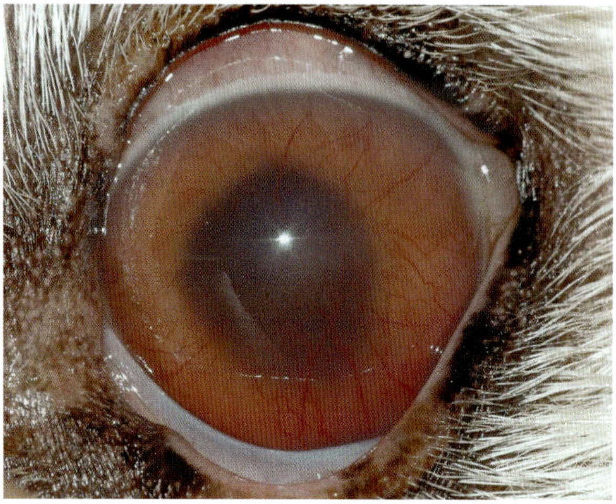

Chronic uveitis with inflammatory compromise of the cornea (keratitis) in the right eye of a seven-year-old Samoyed.
Time since onset: three months.
No cause of uveitis was detected in haematological, biochemical, serological, or endocrine tests.

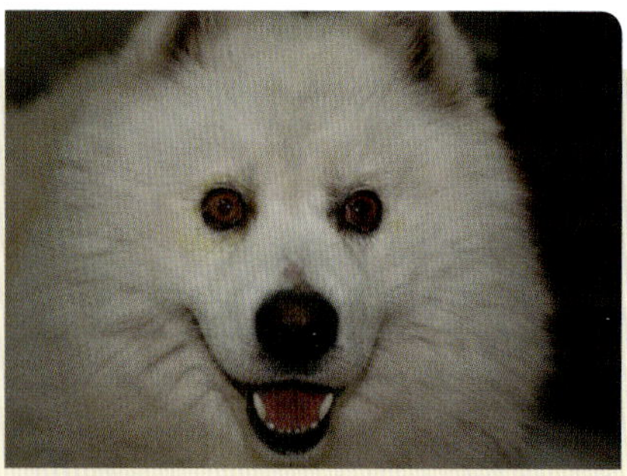

Our patient.

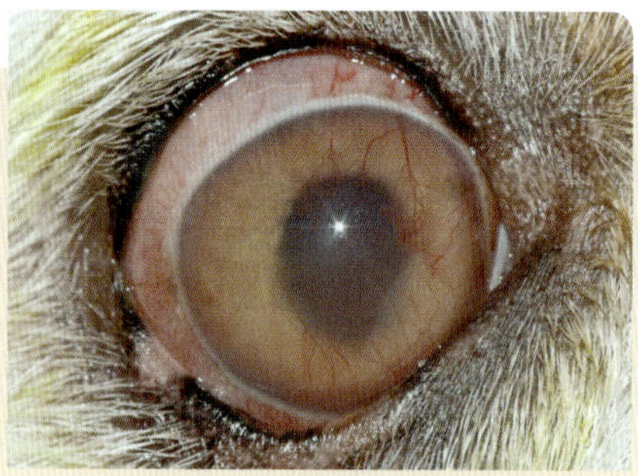

Patient's left eye. Severe keratouveitis. Rubeosis of the iris and oedema.

Interesting notes

- Many cases of uveitis are of unknown aetiology, mainly in cats.
- In histopathological studies (postmortem), many of these uveal inflammatory reactions appear to be predominantly mononuclear.

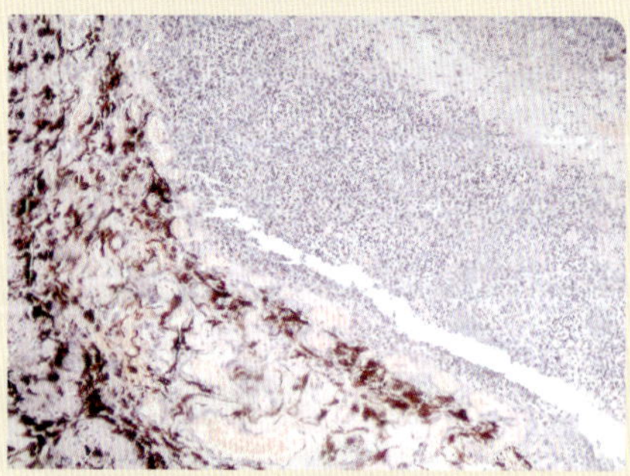

Chronic diffuse pyogranulomatous uveitis. Image courtesy of Histovet.

Uveitis

Sequelae

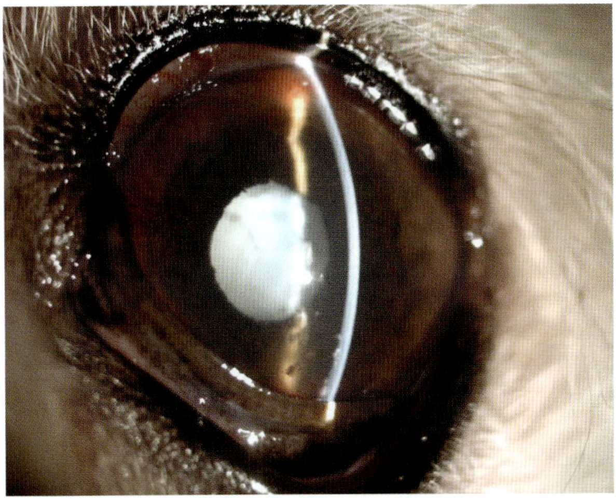

Cataract secondary to canine exudative uveitis.
Mature cataract and keratic precipitates (clinical sign characteristic of uveitis).

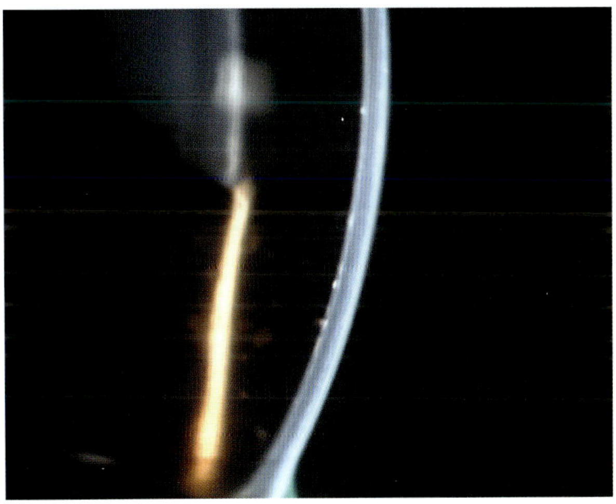

Close-up of the keratic precipitates (inflammatory cells adhered to the corneal endothelium) of the patient pictured above.

Important notes

- Changes in the composition of the aqueous and vitreous humour associated with uveitis may cause cataract formation.

Uveitis

Sequelae

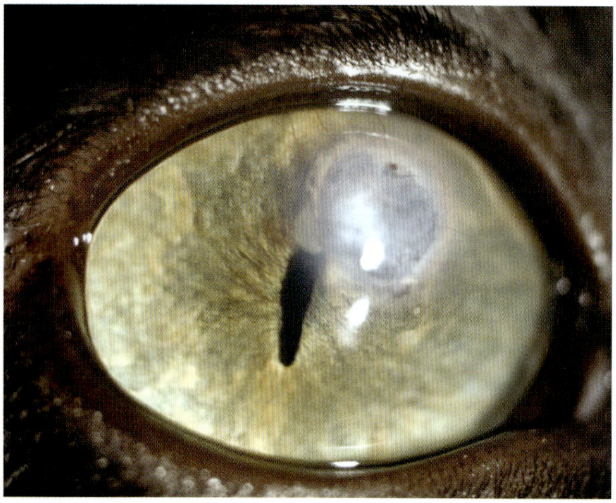

Anterior synechia in a cat resulting from a perforated cornea.
Time since onset: five months.
Close-up of the corneal scar (leukoma) and neovascularisation towards the lesion.

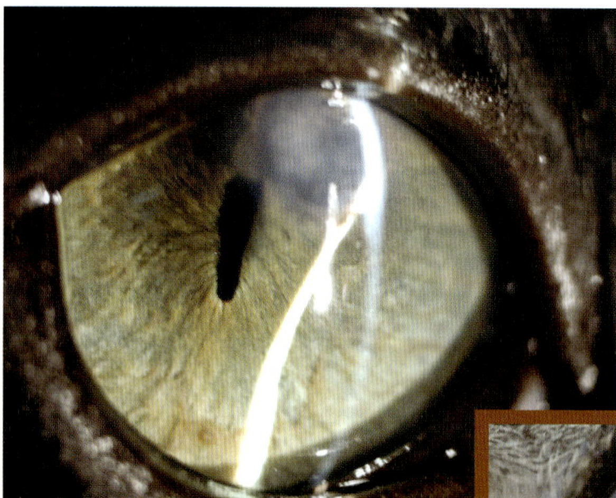

Close-up of the anterior synechia (adhesion of the iris to the corneal endothelium). A cross-sectional view using a slit lamp helps locate the lesion.

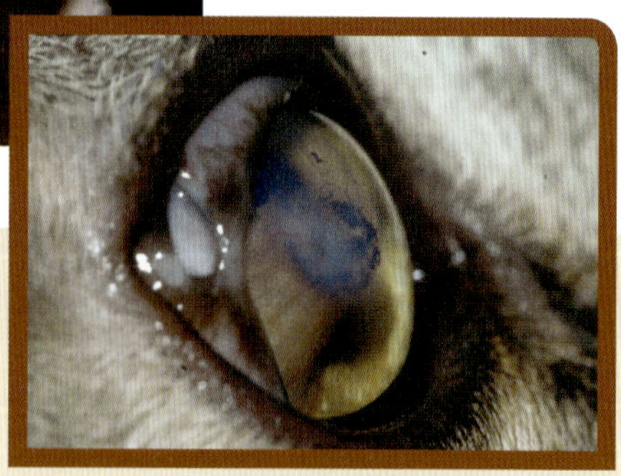

Anterior synechia in a cat resulting from severe uveitis.

- SYNECHIAE (adhesions of the iris) can be:
  - ANTERIOR: adhesion between the iris and the corneal endothelium.
  - POSTERIOR: adhesion between the iris and the anterior lens capsule.

Uveitis

Sequelae

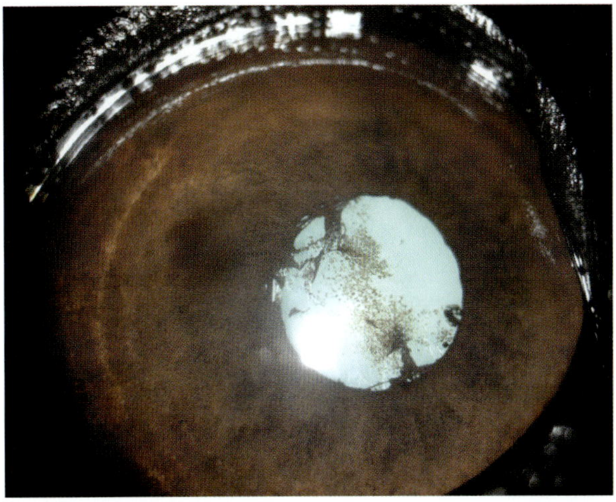

Posterior synechia in a dog resulting severe post-traumatic uveitis.
Close-up of the iris adhesions to the lens, as well as inflammatory material.

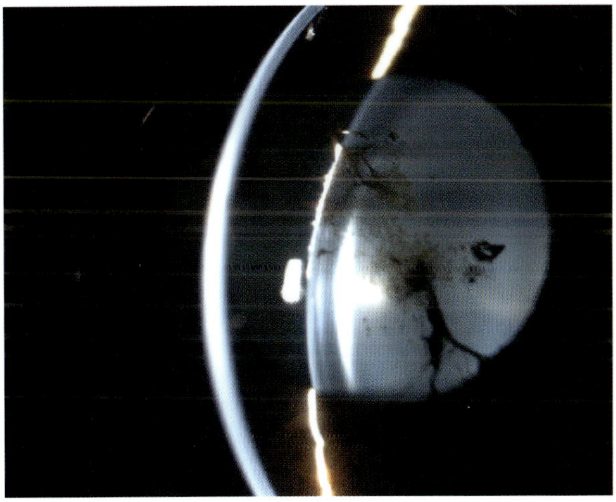

The slit lamp reveals the adhesion of the iris to the anterior lens capsule.

Important notes

Do NOT confuse SYNECHIAE with PPM (persistent pupillary membrane). Synechiae always start at the edge of the pupil, while PPMs originate from the iris collarette.

Uveitis

Sequelae

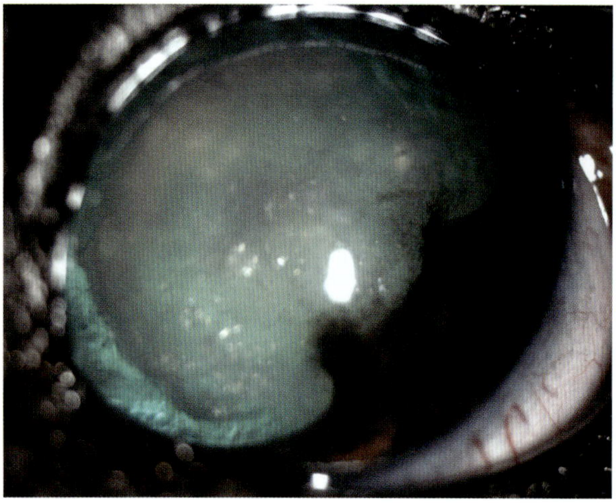

Posterior synechia and immature cataract (in progress), in a dog.

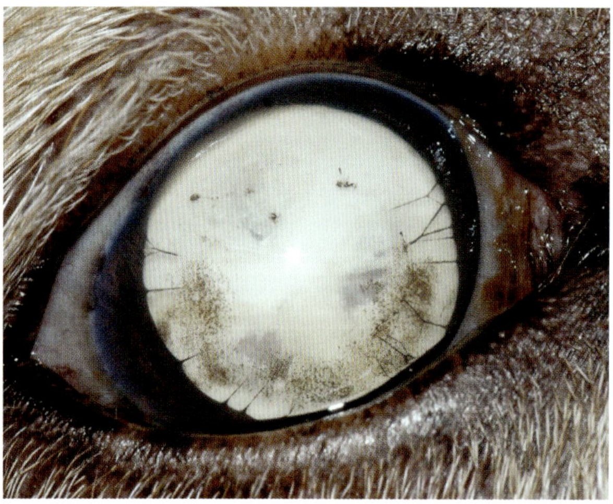

Posterior synechiae, inflammatory remnants, and mature cataract in a dog, seven months after a uveitis episode.

Interesting notes

- The more severe the uveal inflammation, and the later the uveitis is treated, the more synechiae form and the higher the risk of other sequelae (cataracts, retinal detachment, etc.).

Uveitis

Sequelae

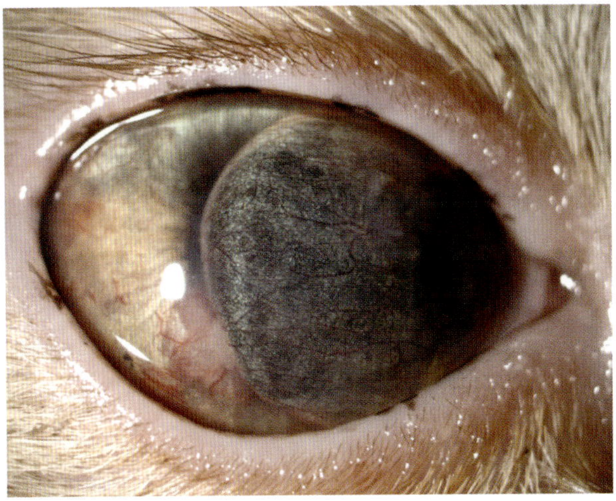

Iris bombé in a cat with traumatic uveitis. Note the bowing of the iris.

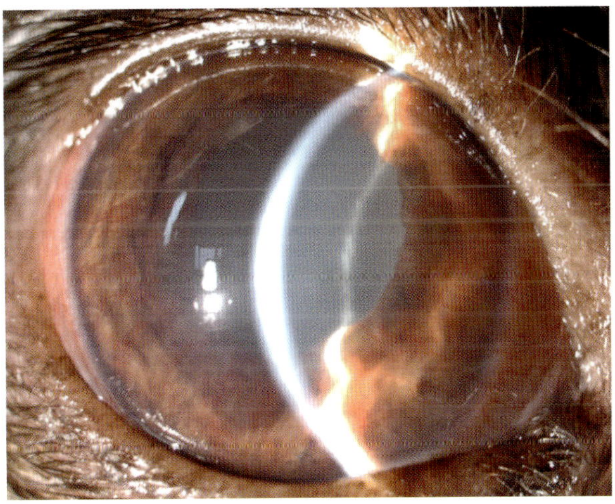

Canine patient with early iris bombé. Close-up of the iridal curvature and compromise of the anterior chamber. Slit-lamp picture.

i

Iris bombé is anterior bowing of the iris due to adhesion between the pupillary margin and the lens. When the whole pupillary margin is affected, the aqueous humour cannot flow from the posterior chamber (space between the lens and posterior surface of the iris) to the anterior chamber (space between the anterior surface of the iris and the cornea). This leads to glaucoma.

Uveitis

Sequelae

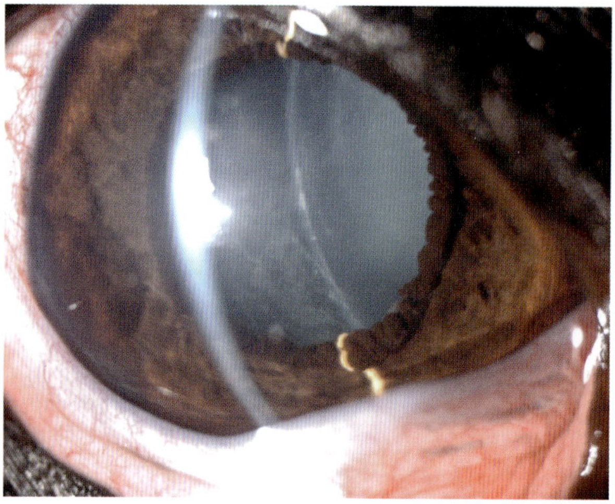

Ectropion uveae in a dog. Close-up of the eversion of the posterior iris epithelium following severe uveitis.

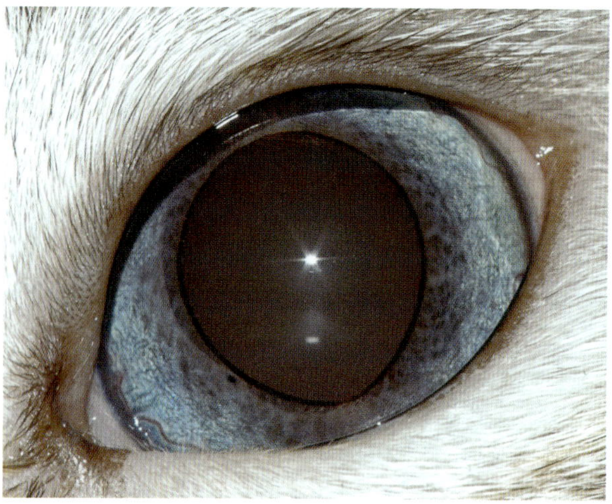

Ectropion uveae in a cat.

i | Eversions of uveal tissue (on the pupillary margin) and iridal atrophy secondary to uveitis are most common in dogs.

Uveitis

Sequelae

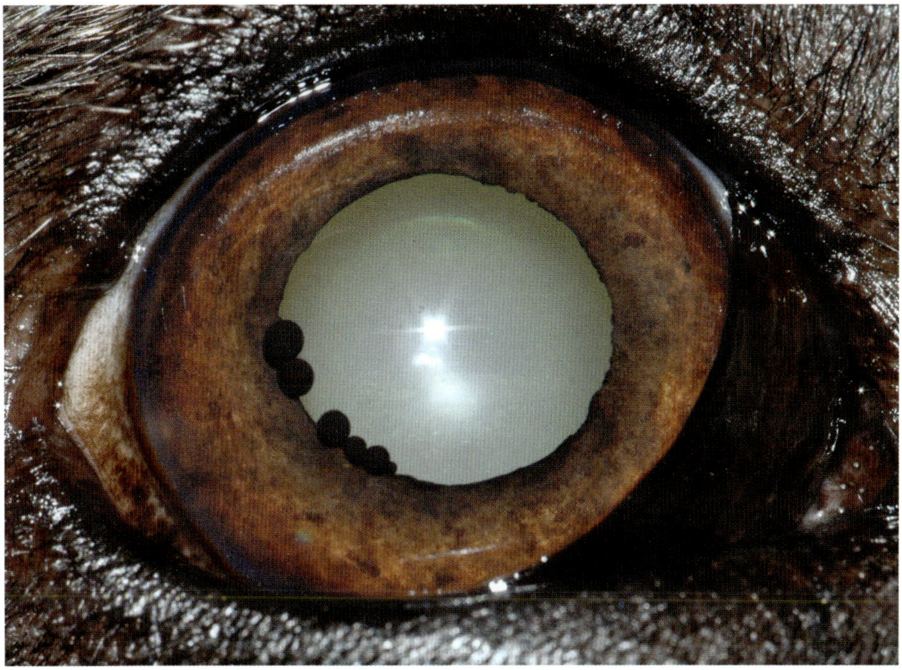

Iridal nodules in a six-year-old German Shepherd who had uveitis.
Nodules may appear on the pupillary margin following a uveal inflammatory reaction.

Important notes

- Iridal nodules are a sign of chronicity.

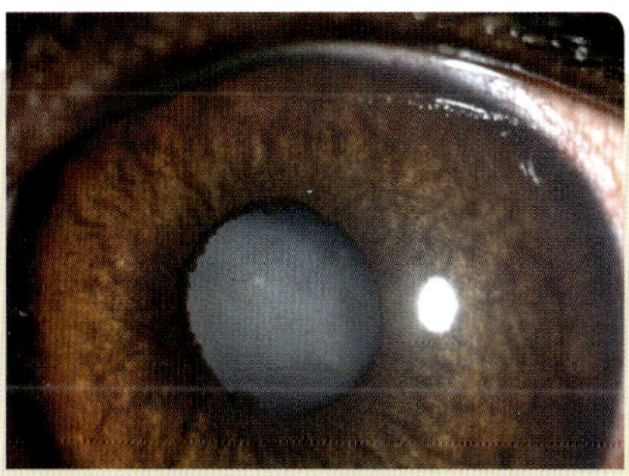

Iridal nodules and postuveitic ectropion uveae in a dog.

Uveitis

Sequelae

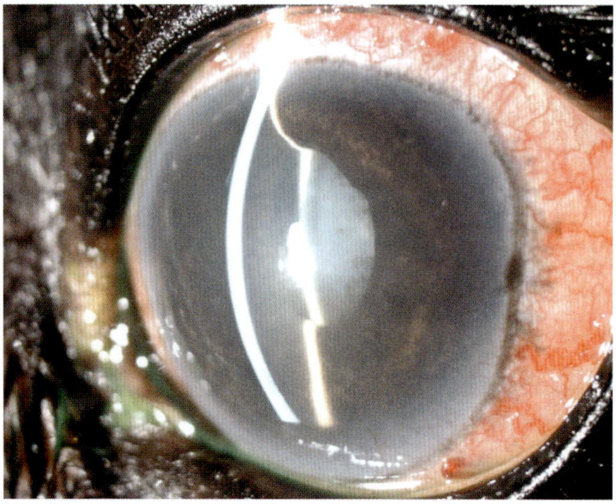

Glaucoma secondary to uveitis. Note the closure, the inflammatory component, and how the iris contacts the cornea (close-up with the slit lamp). The intraocular pressure when the picture was taken was 45 mmHg.

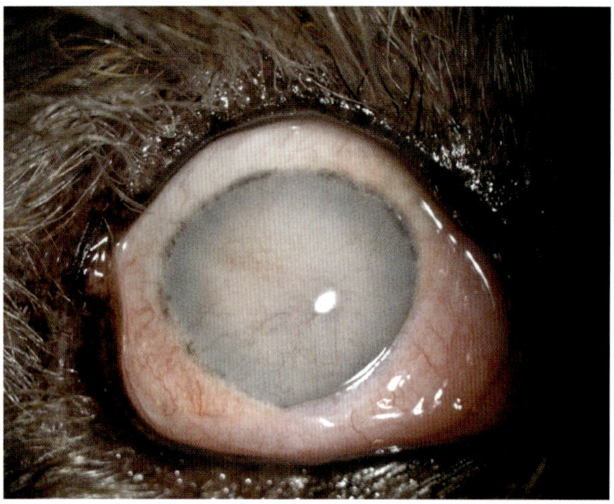

Phthisis bulbi (atrophy of the globe) in a patient who had repeated episodes of uveitis.

i | Glaucoma is the most severe complication of uveitis and carries a poorer prognosis for the patient's vision.

Uveitis

Sequelae

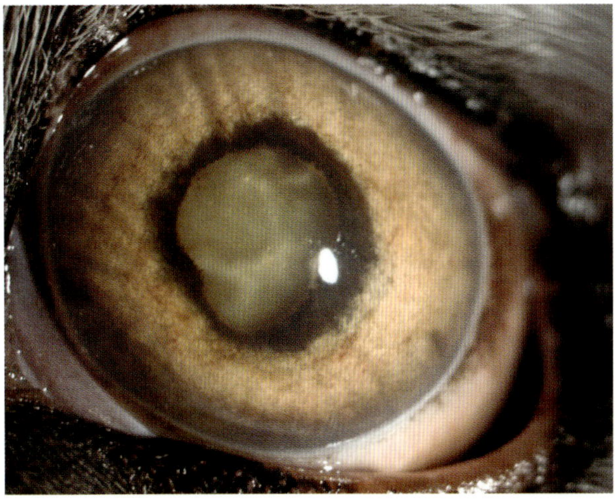

Postuveitic cataract in a Samoyed.
Patient with recurrent uveitis. Note the signs of the current inflammatory episode (rubeosis and oedema), as well as the posterior synechia and cataract resulting from prior uveitis episodes.

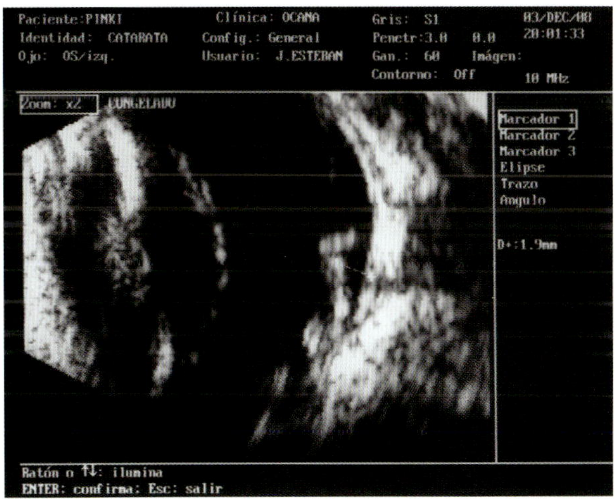

Retinal detachment has occurred behind the cataract.

Important notes

Ocular ultrasound may be used to examine ocular structures in cases where an opacity impedes ophthalmoscopic examination.

Iris cysts

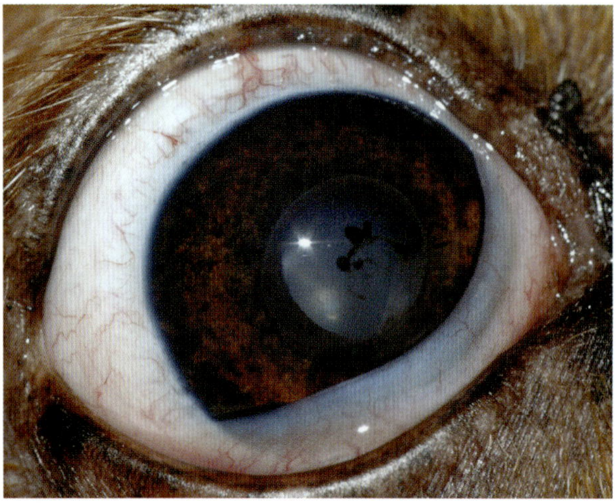

Iris cysts in an 11-year-old mixed-breed dog.
Note the large central one and the three small ventrally located ones.
Incidental finding in a routine consultation.

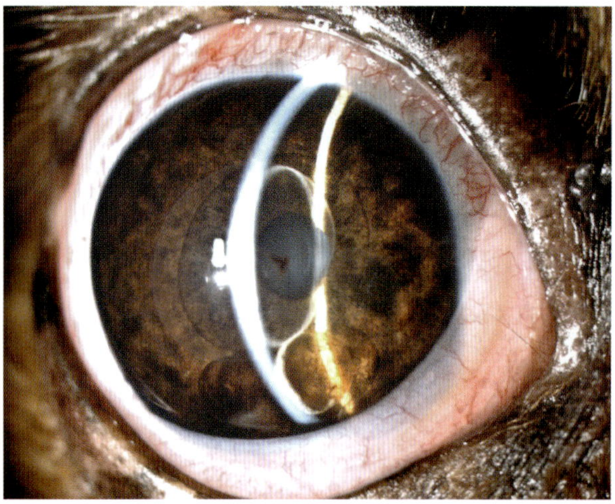

Slit-lamp picture of the patient shown above. Note the cysts in the anterior chamber. With the nictitating membrane at its lowest position, the fourth, smallest, cyst is visible.

i Benign fluid-filled formations floating in the anterior chamber or adhered to the pupillary margin.

Iris cysts

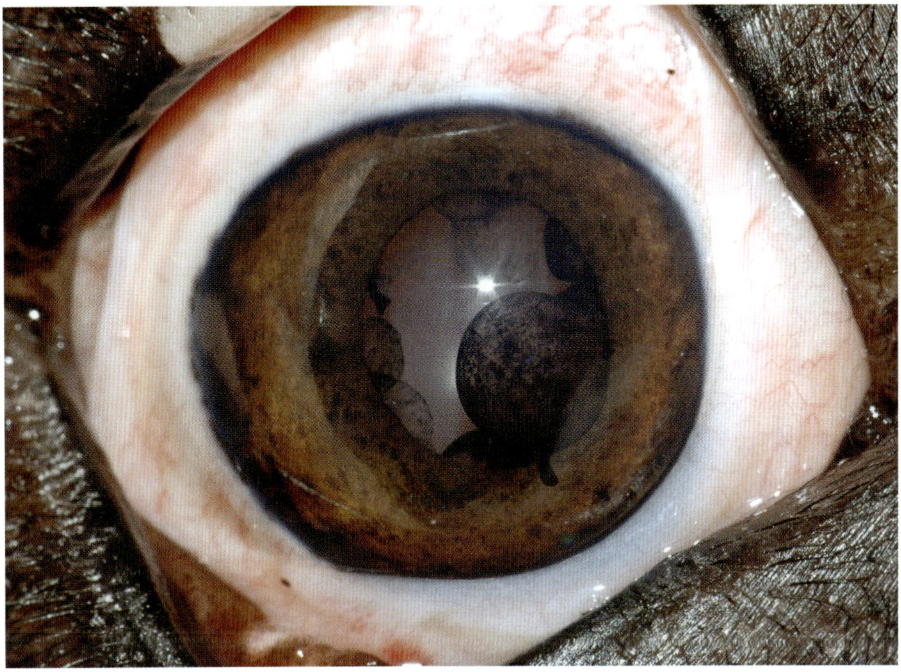

Multiple iris cysts in a Saint Bernard. Close-up of cysts moving from the posterior to the anterior chamber.

Interesting notes

- Iris cysts generally appear in older animals (mainly in dogs) and may be associated with uveitis.
- If they are numerous, we can remove them with paracentesis using a 25-gauge needle. They may also be ablated with lasers.

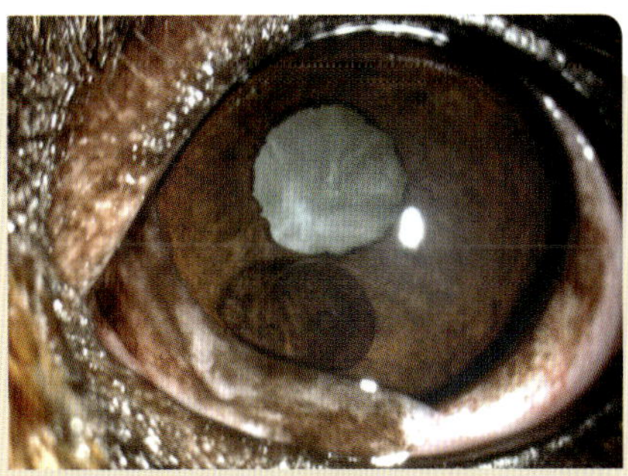

Uveal cyst in the anterior chamber of a dog. Smaller ones appear darker in colour, and as they grow, they lighten due to their walls thinning.

Iris cysts

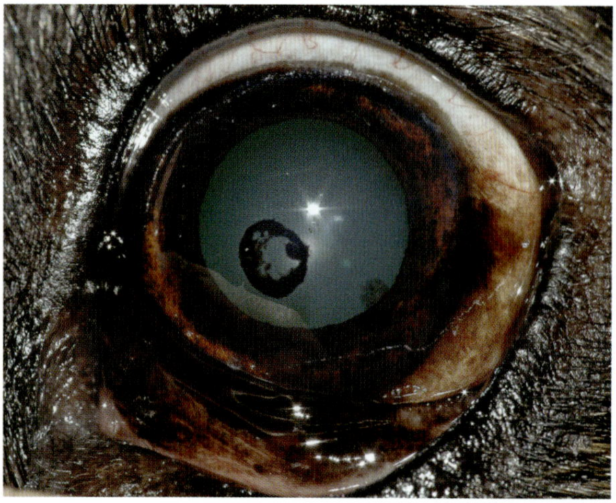

Remnants of a cyst wall lodged in the corneal endothelium. Thirteen-year-old canine patient, asymptomatic.

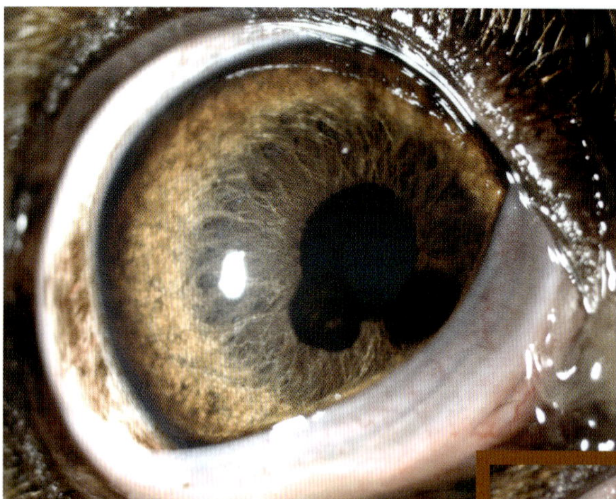

Cyst wall adhered to the corneal endothelium.

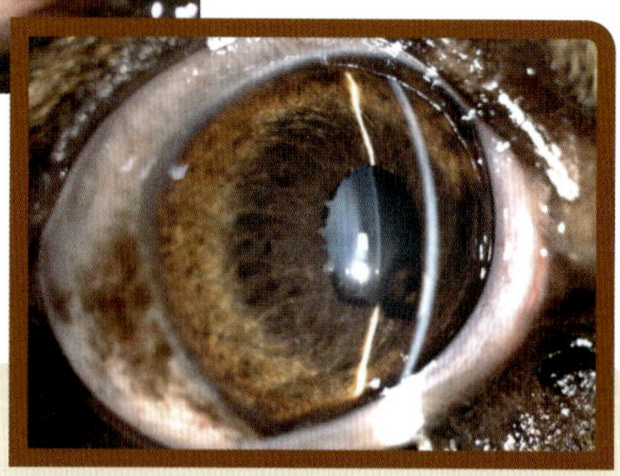

Slit-lamp picture of the patient shown above. Note the endothelial location of the cyst remnant.

- As cysts grow, they tend to burst.
- They do not often cause ocular injury or discomfort.

Neoplasms

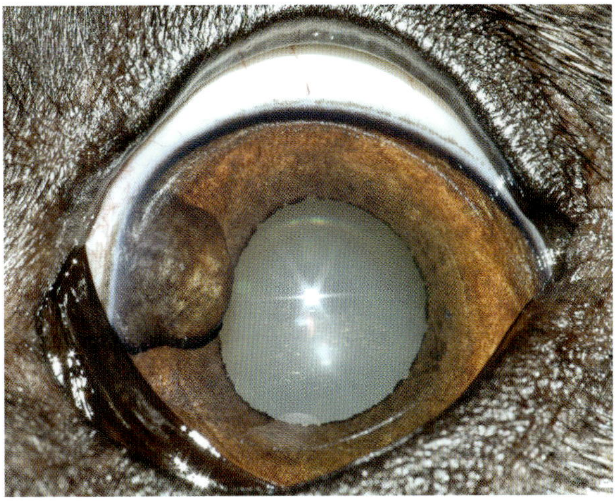

Uveal melanoma in an eight-year-old Labrador Retriever with a dark coat.

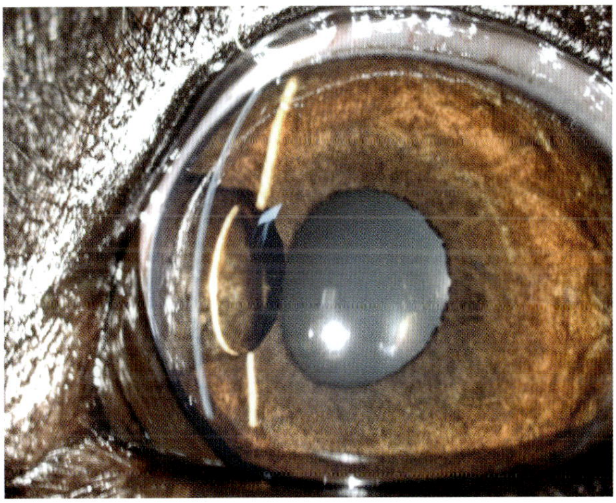

Slit-lamp picture of the patient shown above. Close-up of the mass causing a bulge in the iridal tissue.

- Uveal neoplasms may be PRIMARY (melanomas, adenomas, adenocarcinomas or sarcomas, among others), or METASTATIC.
- They are generally unilateral.

Neoplasms

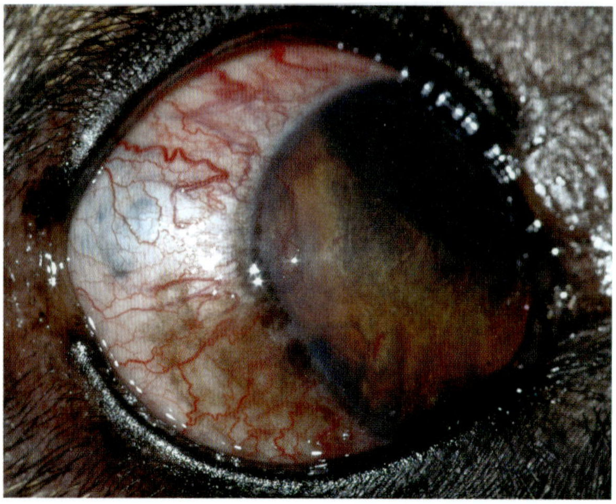

Intraocular neoplasm in an 11-year-old German Shepherd.

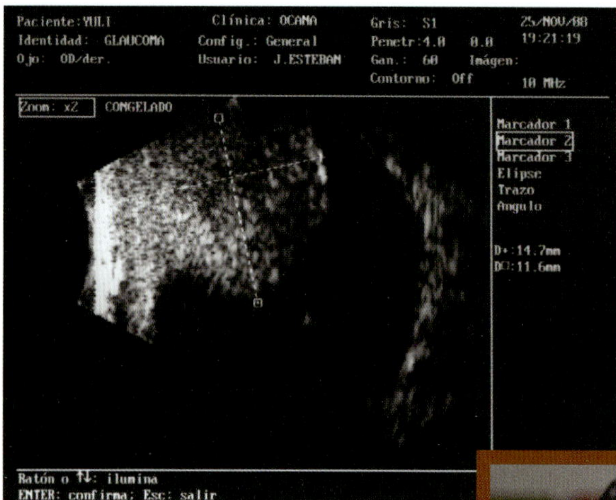

Ocular ultrasound reveals the full extent of the neoplasm. In this case, it is from the ciliary body.
Time since onset: three months.

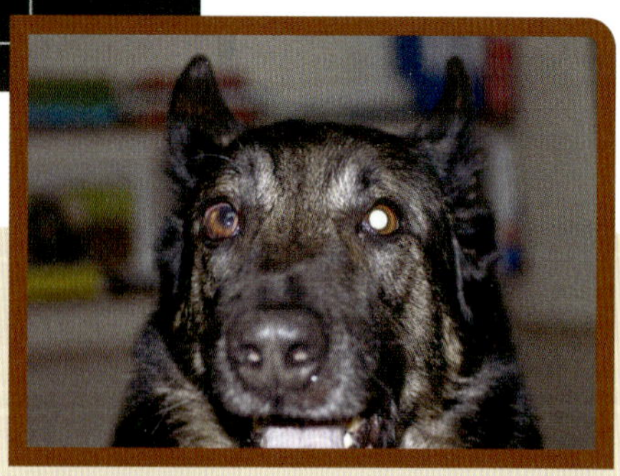

Note the difference between the affected and normal eyes.

Important notes

Glaucoma often occurs with intraocular tumours due to blockage of the iridocorneal angle, either by the mass or by inflammatory material.

Neoplasms

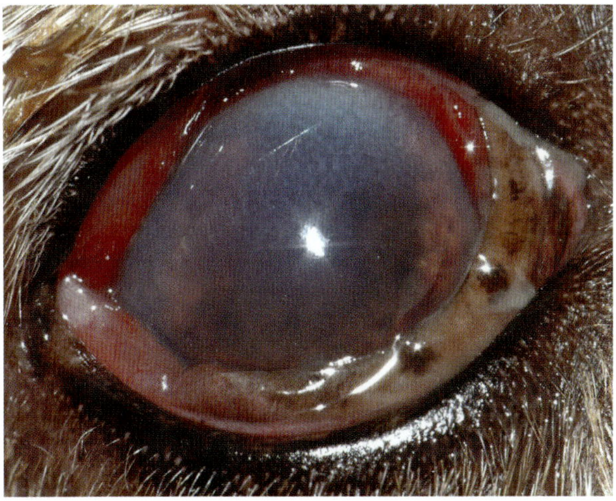

Ten-year-old Labrador Retriever.
Time since onset: thirty days of ocular discomfort with no response to treatment.
Glaucoma (48 mmHg) and subconjunctival haemorrhage.

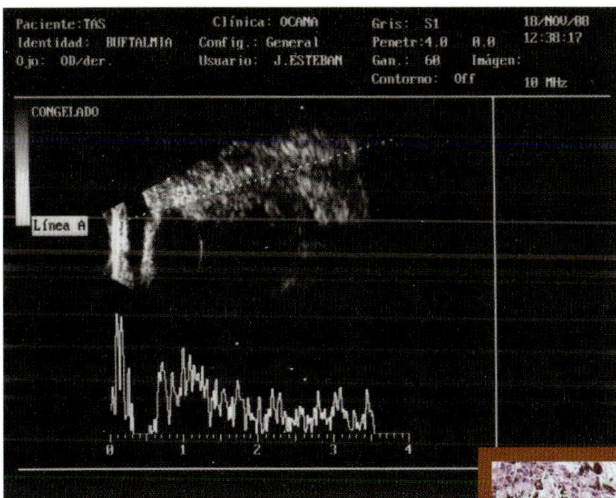

Ultrasound image compatible with uveal neoplasm. A/B-mode.

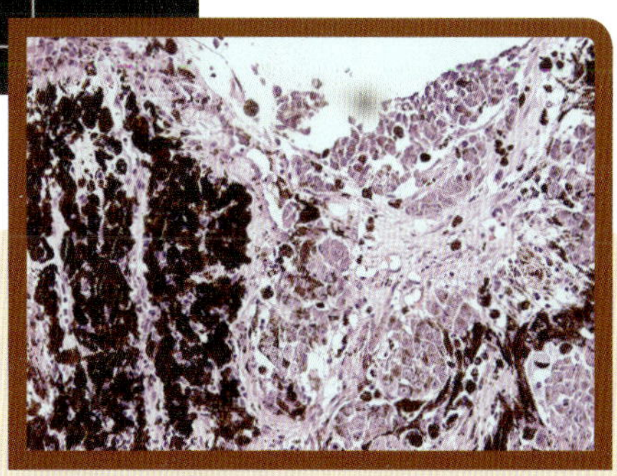

Pathological analysis of the patient's neoplasm. Ciliary body melanoma. Image courtesy of Andrés Calvo (Citopath).

Important notes

A/B-mode ultrasound assists in ultrasound-tissue correlation in the diagnosis of intraocular tumours. The simultaneous use of A- and B-modes shows peaks that are characteristic of uveal melanoma.

Neoplasms

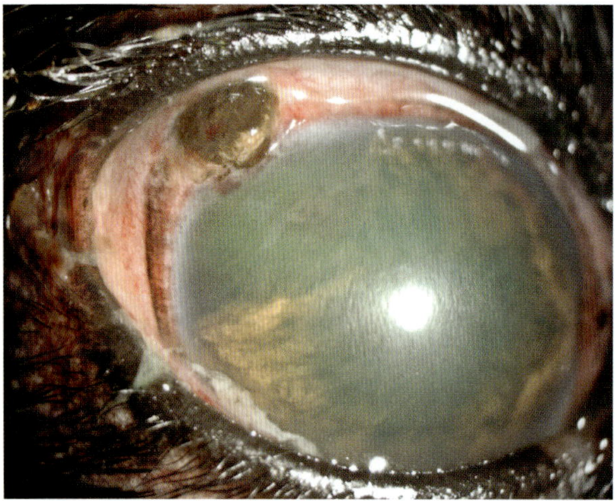

Scleral rupture with iris prolapse. Patient with ciliary body neoplasm.

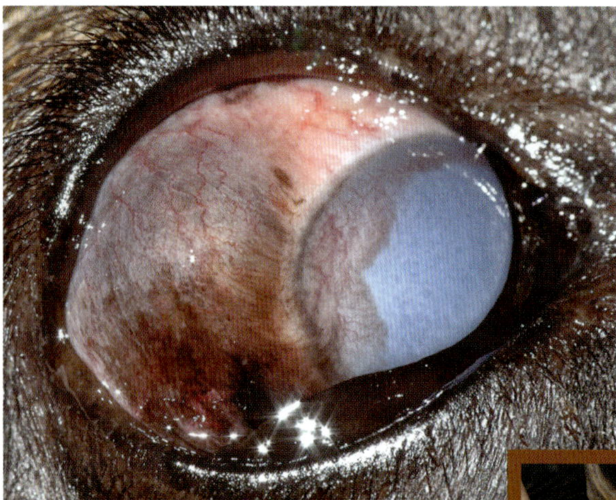

The tumour growth may distort the fibrous tunic of the eye.
Hypertensive uveitis secondary to an intraocular neoplasm.

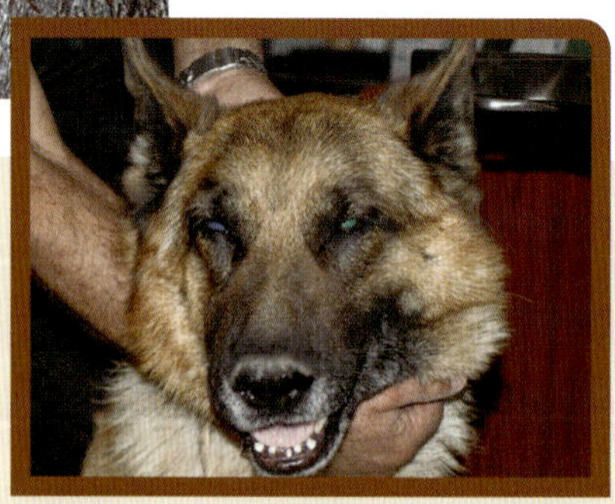

Patient pictured above, showing clear signs of pain (blepharospasm and photophobia).

Treatment

- If the tumour is small and the eye is visual, iridectomy and histopathological examination are advised.
- If the histopathology result (in the case above) is malignant, the tumour extends throughout the eye, or the eye is blind (glaucoma), EXENTERATION (with pathological examination) should be performed.

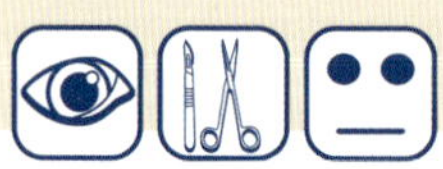

Neoplasms

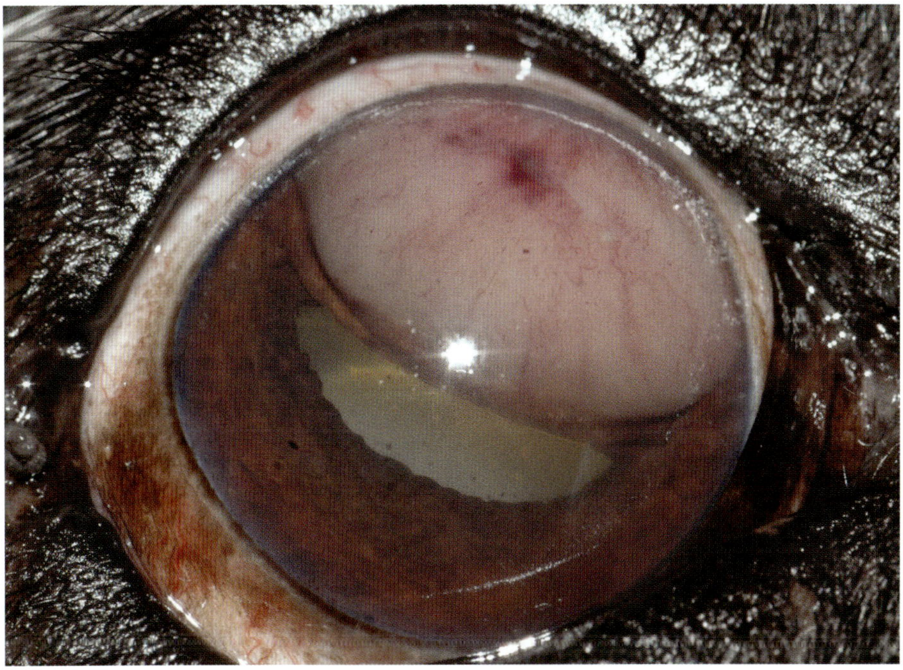

Uveal neoplasm in a nine-year-old Rottweiler. Right eye. First sign noted by the owner.

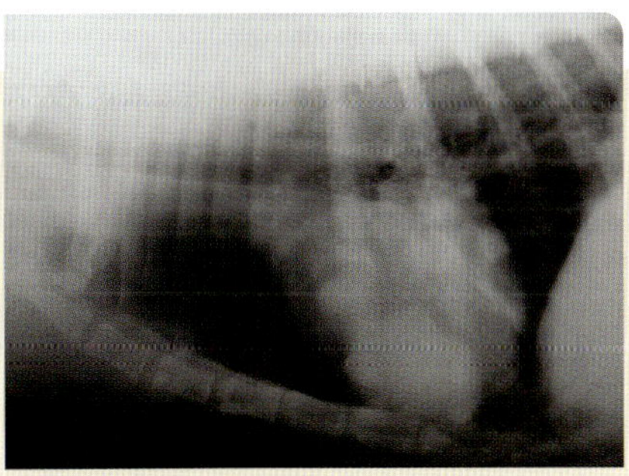

Thoracic radiograph of the patient (metastasis).

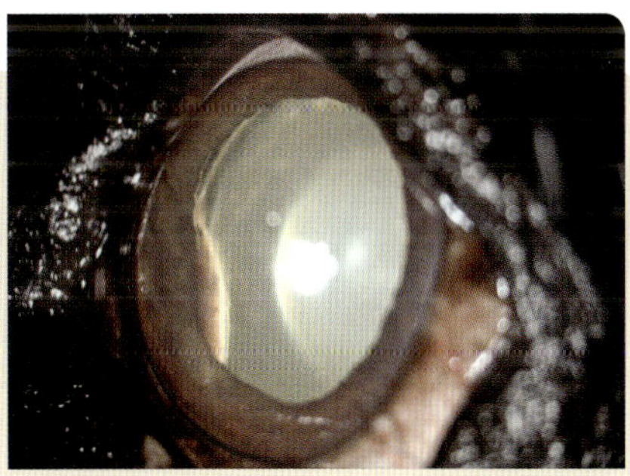

Patient's left eye.
Ciliary body neoplasm (using tropicamide to induce mydriasis).

Important notes

Prior to considering exenteration of an eye with an intraocular tumour, REMEMBER that the eye is connected to a patient. This dog had splenic haemangiosarcoma with metastasis to the liver, heart, lung, and eyes. She was euthanised a few days after the ophthalmological consultation.

Neoplasms

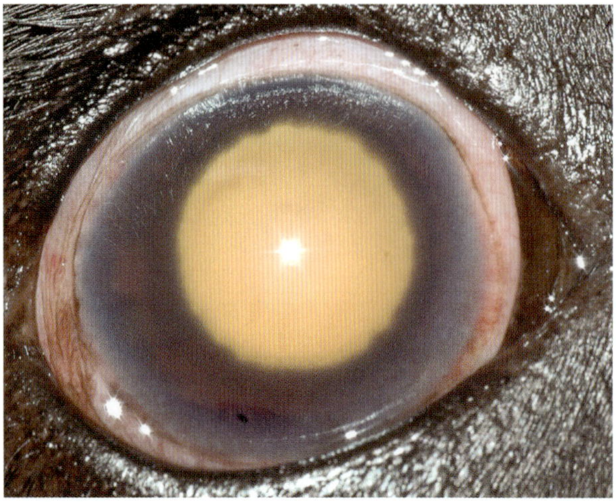

Corneal oedema (endothelial), iris rubeosis, and intraocular haemorrhage (hyphaema). Right eye.

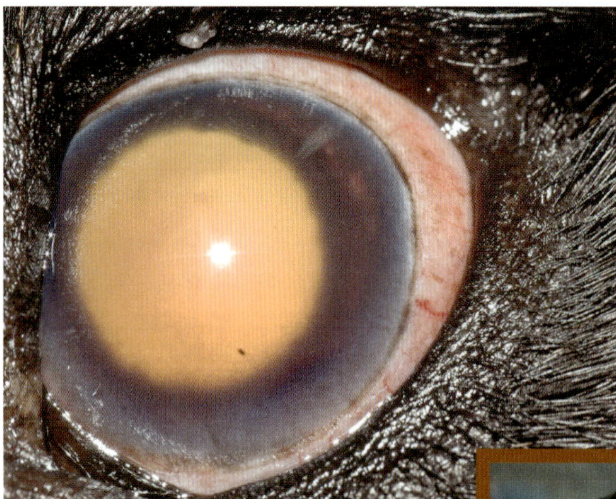

Left eye with similar signs.

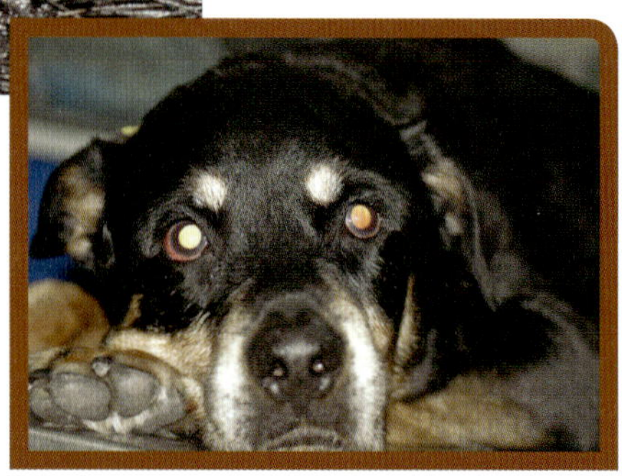

Our patient, an eight-year-old Rottweiler, was diagnosed with multicentric lymphoma by her regular veterinarian. Bilateral ocular signs 15 days later.

i Lymphoma is a neoplasm that commonly affects the eye (specifically the uvea) and carries a poorer prognosis (for both the patient's vision and survival).

Neoplasms

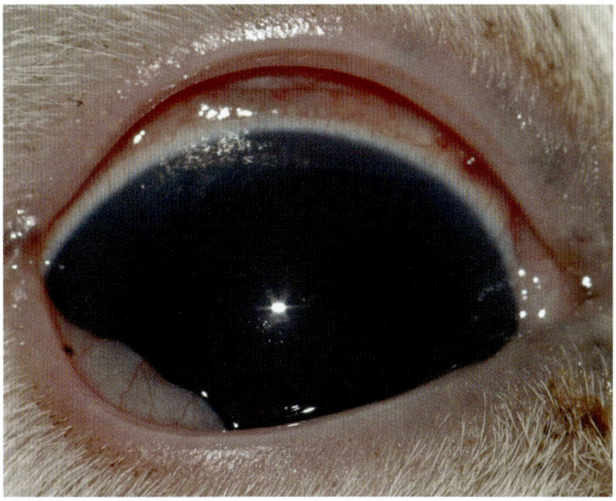

Diffuse melanoma of the iris in an 11-year-old Persian cat.
Glaucoma secondary to melanoma.
Conjunctival chemosis.

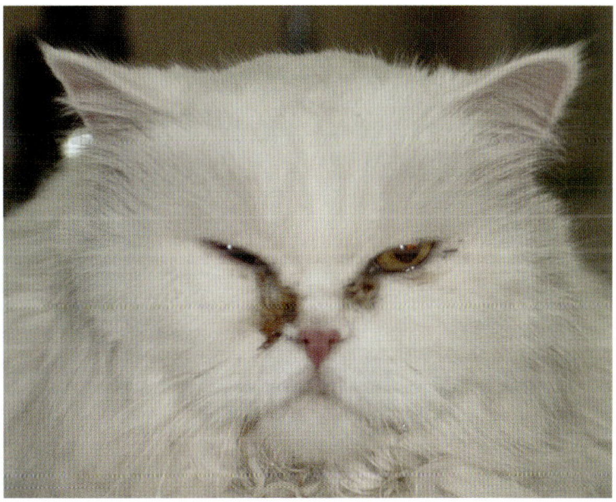

Ocular discomfort in our patient. Note the colour difference between the eyes.

Important notes

- Diffuse melanoma of the iris (a primary uveal tumour) may be malignant and tends to metastasise to the liver and lung.
- Early diagnosis and prompt surgical treatment are key to prolonging the patient's life.

Neoplasms

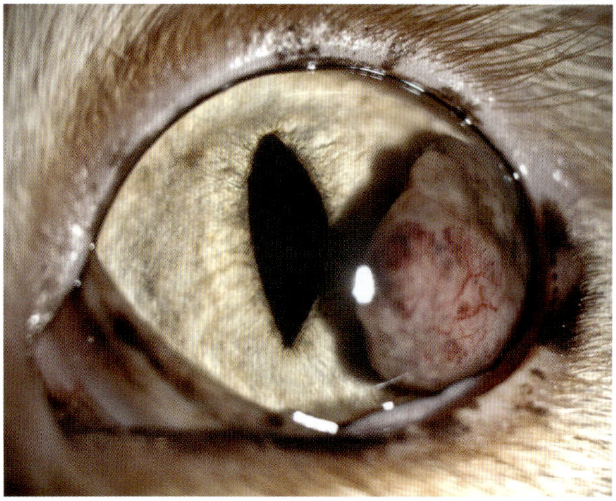

Uveal lymphosarcoma in a nine-year-old domestic shorthair cat.
These tumours are highly vascular and poorly pigmented.
Time since onset: two months.
Positive for FeLV.

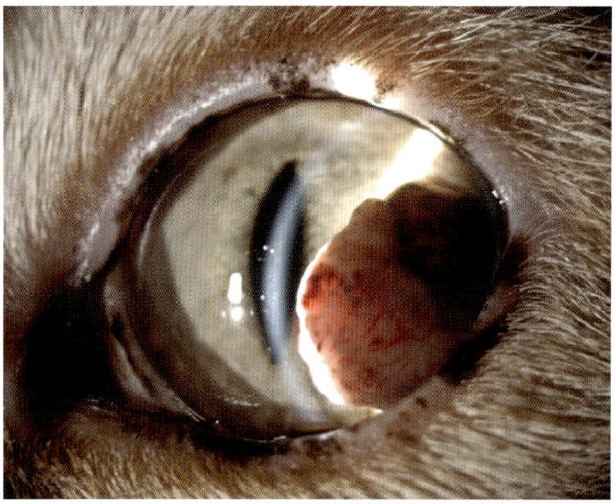

Slit-lamp picture. Close-up of the neoplasm. Note the space it occupies in the anterior chamber.

i Feline uveal lymphosarcoma is one of the most common metastatic intraocular tumours. It often affects the kidneys and/or intestine as well.

Iris atrophy

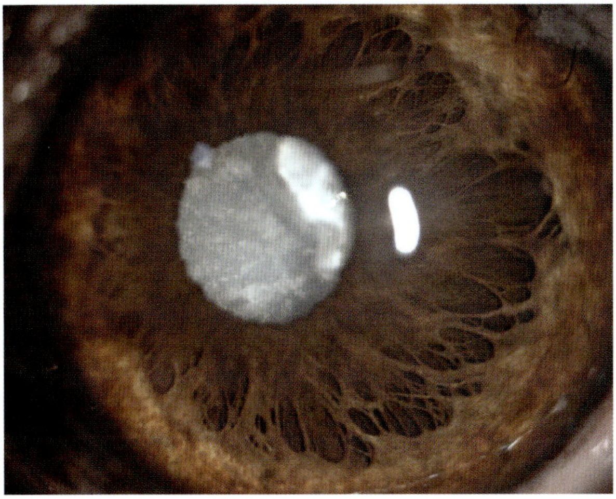

Age-related iris atrophy in a 15-year-old dog.
Note the loss of muscle in the external surface of the iris, revealing its posterior surface.

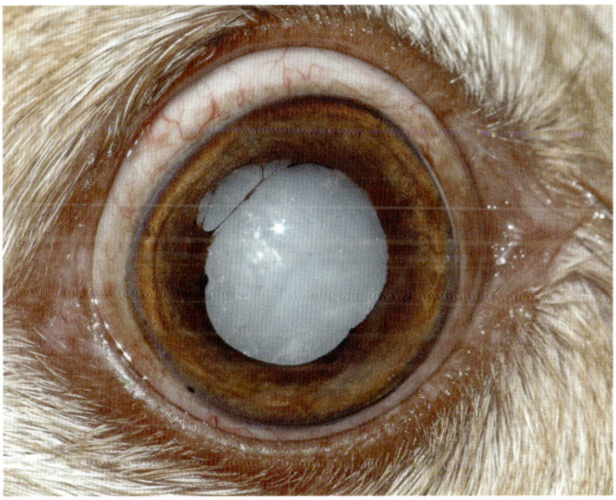

Atrophy of the uveal tissue.
In this patient, it produces an irregular pupillary margin.

This is a degeneration of the muscle tissue of the iris that occurs more frequently in older patients.

It may be age-related or associated with chronic uveitis.

Iris atrophy

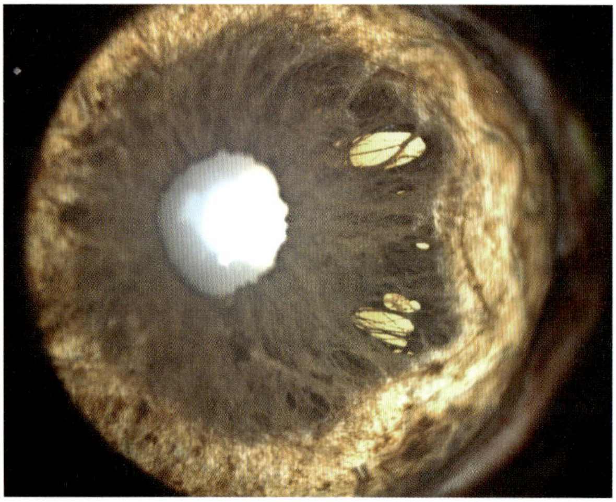

Partial age-related atrophy of the iris.
Sometimes actual holes are visible.
Picture taken with retroillumination.

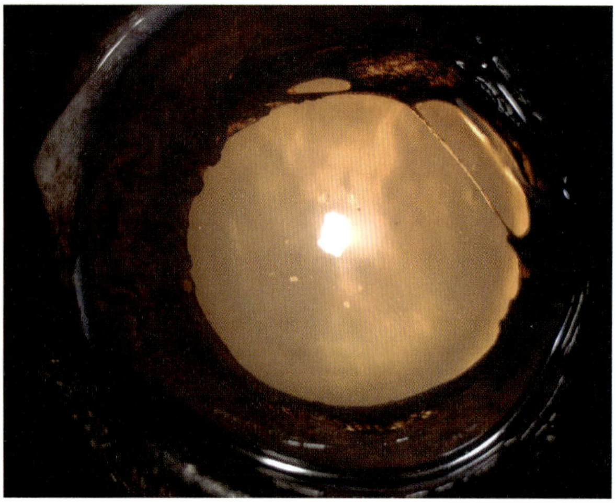

Under retroillumination, the light reflected in the tapetum shows the detail.
Iridal atrophy.

Breed predisposition

It is more common in dogs than in cats and mainly occurs in smaller breeds (Poodle, Yorkshire Terrier and Cocker Spaniel).

Iris atrophy

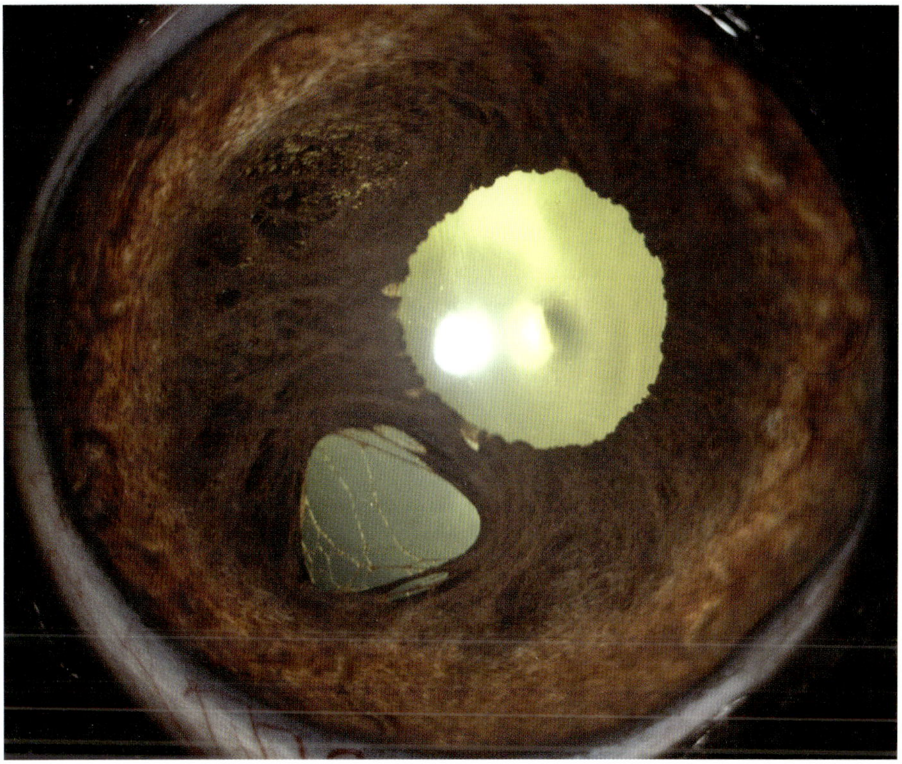

Age-related iris atrophy in a 10-year-old Cocker Spaniel.
Note the varying degrees of muscular degeneration:

- Partial (dorsotemporal to the pupil).
- Total (ventrotemporal to the pupil).
- Pupillary margin.

No treatment is available.

In advanced cases, the patient should not be taken outside on very sunny days as it may suffer photophobia.

Melanosis

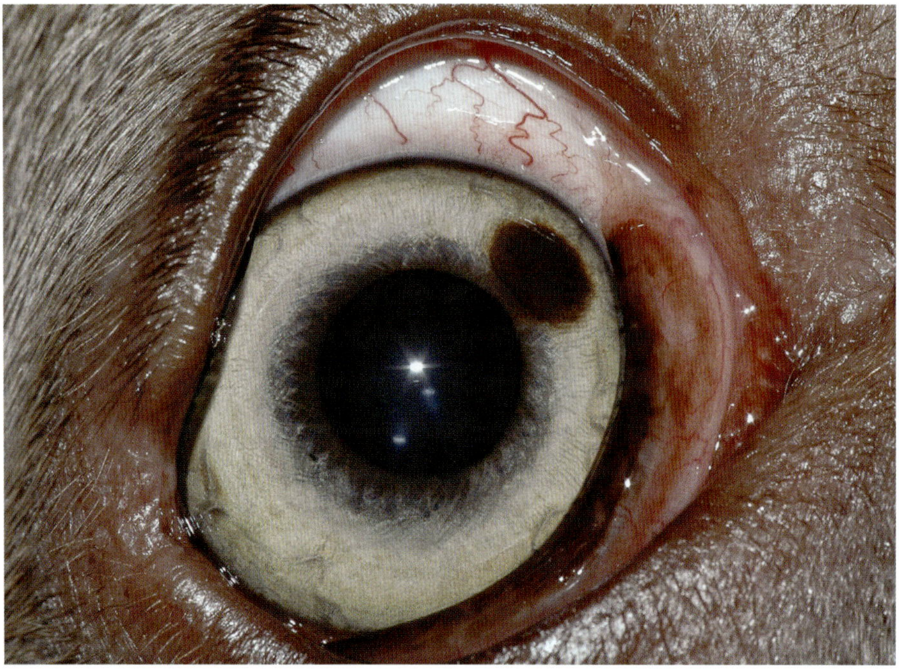

Iris melanosis in a six-year-old Weimaraner.
Close-up of the focus of melanotic pigment.
Time since onset: two years.
Asymptomatic.

i Benign melanosis, or nevus, is a benign lesion that develops from hyperpigmentation of uveal melanocytes.

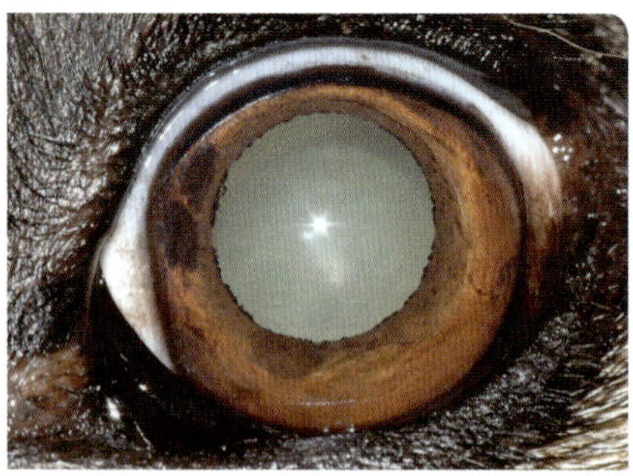

Benign melanosis in the nasal area of the iris.
Thirteen-year-old mixed-breed dog.

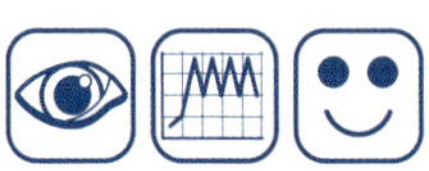

Melanosis

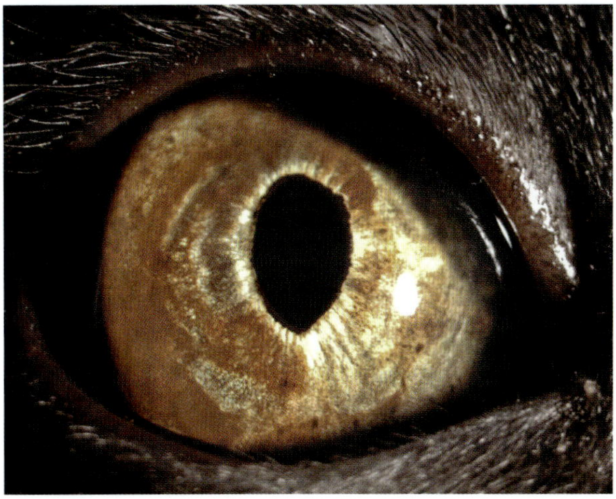

Benign melanosis in an 11-year-old black cat.

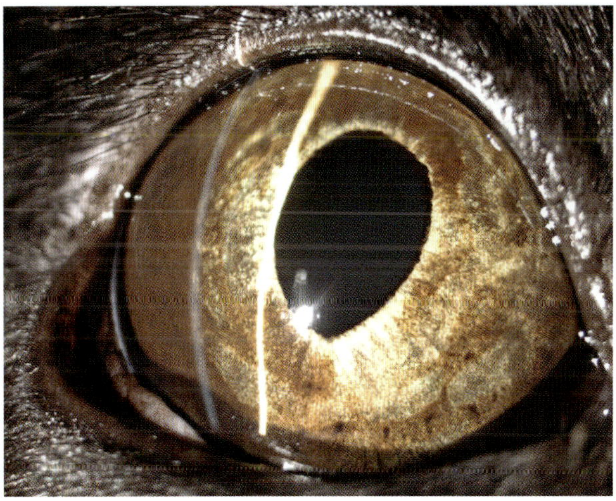

Slit-lamp picture of the patient shown above. The iris cross-section shows neither bulging into the anterior chamber nor uveitis (no Tyndall effect).

Important notes

- Closely monitor iridal melanin deposits in cats, as melanosis behaves quite distinctly from diffuse melanoma of the iris.
- Signs of uveitis (low IOP, Tyndall effect, blepharospasm) tend to develop over time in melanoma patients.

Melanosis

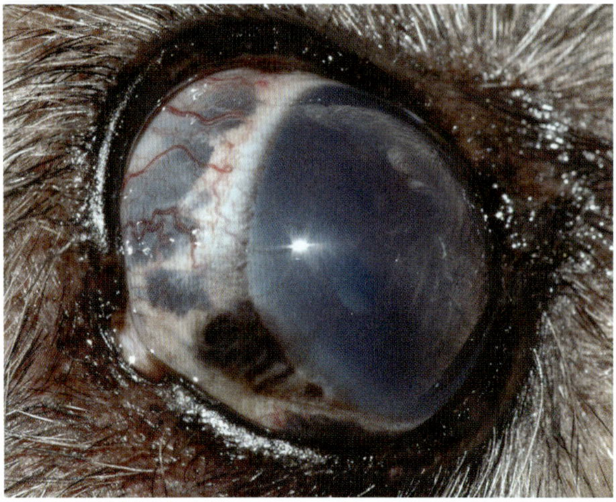

Uveal melanosis in a 10-year-old Labrador Retriever. Secondary glaucoma.

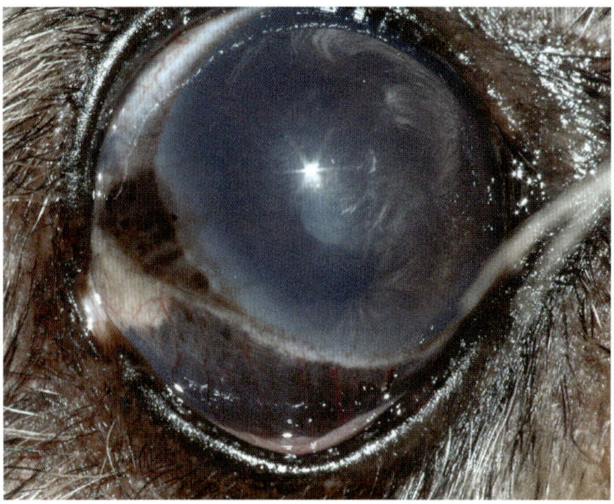

Patient pictured above. Close-up of pigment dispersion.

- Uveal melanosis in the Cairn Terrier is hereditary and likely autosomal dominant, with variable ages of onset and patterns of progression. It results in thickening and pigmentation of the iris. Pigment deposits may also appear in the sclera and the episclera.
- Pigment dispersion may cause closure of the iridocorneal angle, triggering glaucoma.

Hyphaema

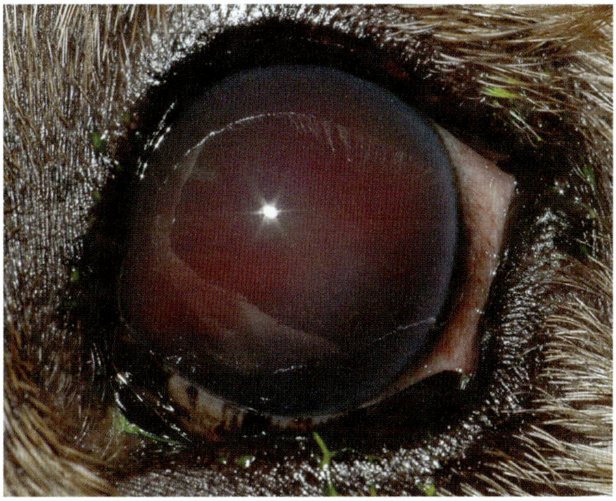

Hyphaema in a Golden Retriever.
Time since onset: 24 hours.
Ocular trauma.

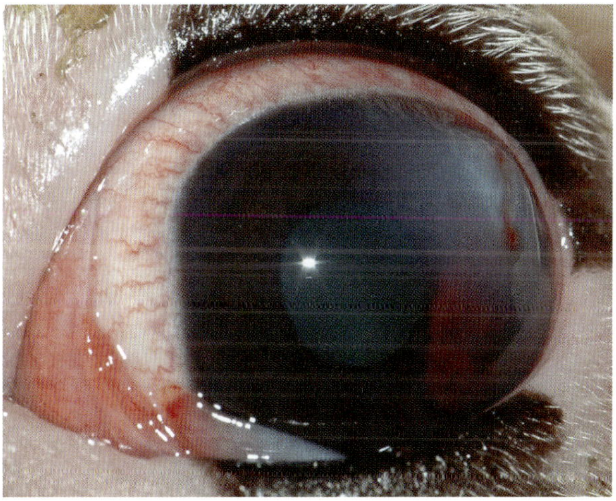

Hyphaema in a French Bulldog who was scratched by a cat. The claw perforated the cornea and damaged the iris.

i

Haemorrhage in the anterior chamber.

The main causes are trauma, neoplasms, retinal detachment, and uveitis. Certain systemic diseases (ehrlichiosis, hypertension, coagulopathies, or lymphomas) may also give rise to a secondary hyphaema.

Hyphaema

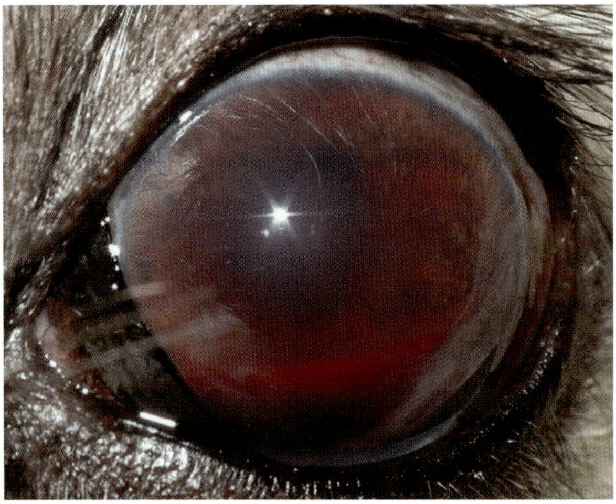

Post-traumatic hyphaema after 72 hours.
A horizontal band delimiting the hyphaema is visible in the ventral part of the anterior chamber based on where the red blood cells precipitate.

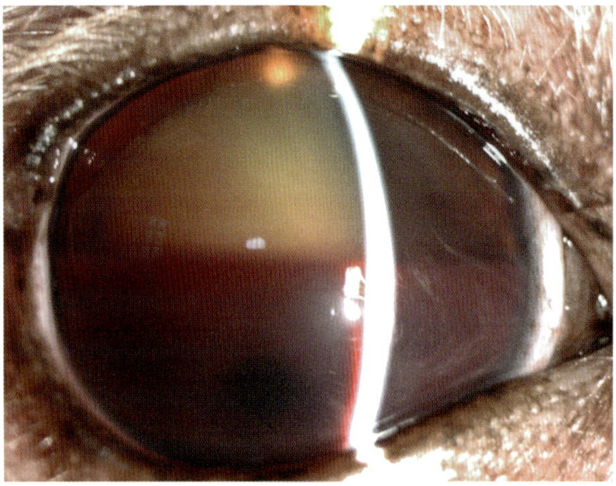

Close-up of the settled blood (48 hours later). Slit-lamp and retroillumination pictures.

Contraindicated

- DO NOT PERFORM PARACENTESIS to remove the blood.

Treatment

- Apply topical corticosteroids (if no corneal ulcer is present): 1 % prednisolone acetate.
- Add subconjunctival and systemic corticosteroids.
- Tropicamide (topical) is preferable to atropine in order to minimise the risk of glaucoma.

Hyphaema

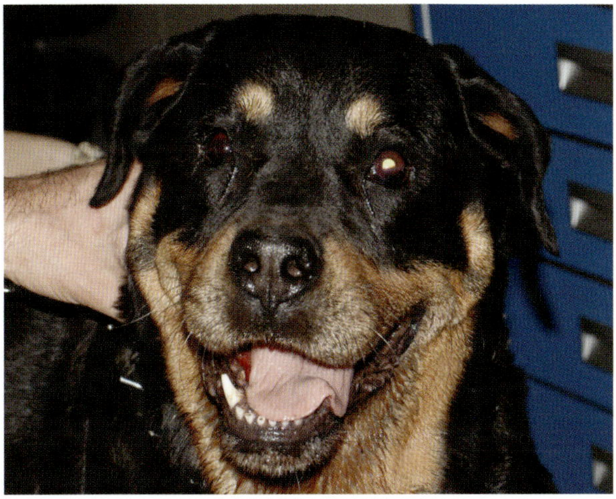

Eight-year-old Rottweiler with bilateral hyphaema. Lymphoma.

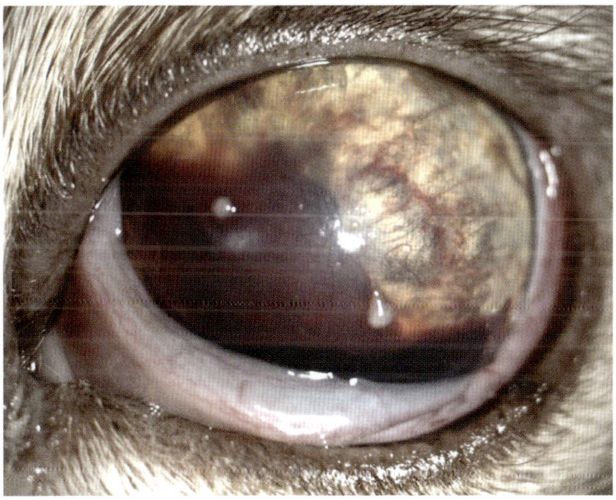

Cat with FIP presenting with bilateral hyphaema. The left eye was more severely affected.

Important notes

Always suspect systemic diseases in cases of bilateral hyphaema.

Hyphaema

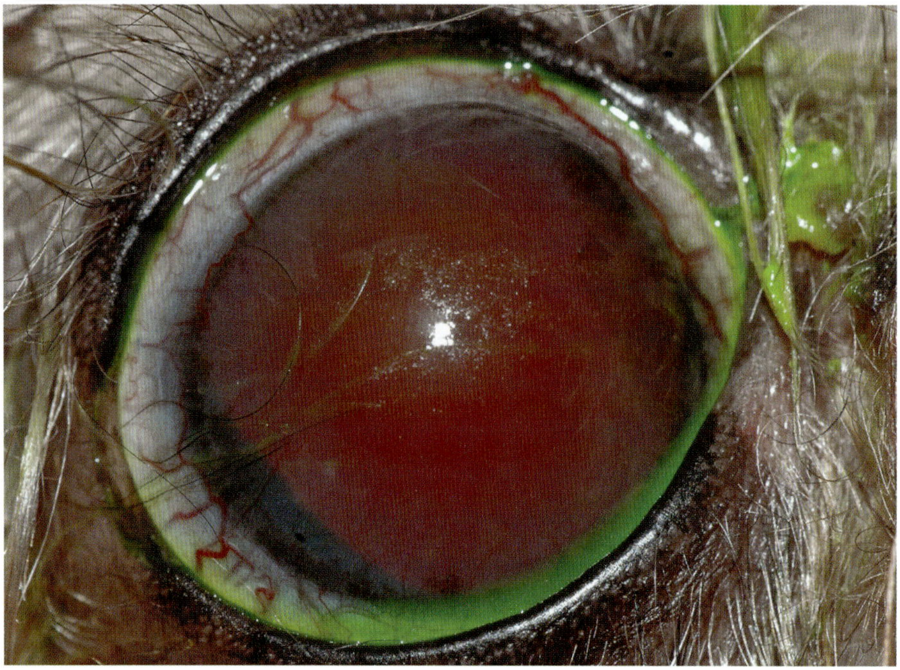

Glaucoma secondary to hyphaema.
Note the congested episcleral vessels.
IOP: 56 mmHg.

Important notes

- The main complication of unresolved hyphaema is closure of the iridocorneal angle and secondary GLAUCOMA.

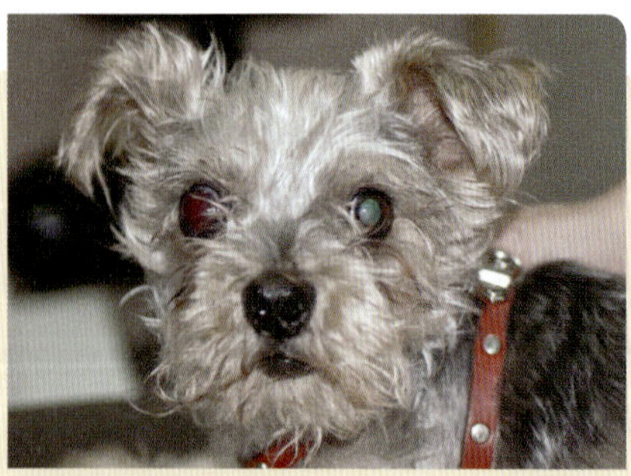

Patient pictured above.
Note the buphthalmic eye due to glaucoma.
Blind eye.

Lens

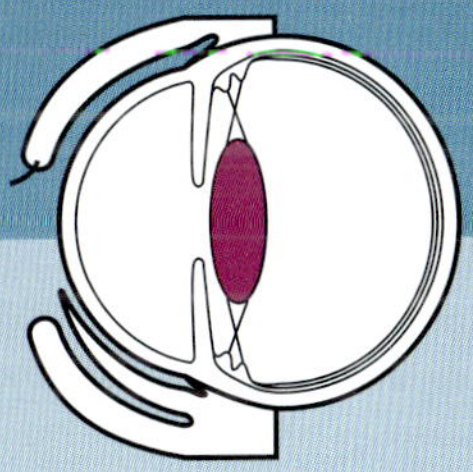

Microphakia

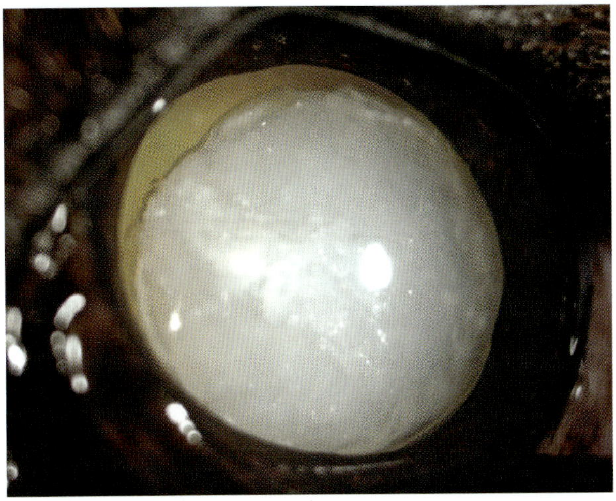

Microphakia in a five-year-old Catalan Sheepdog. A cataract is also present.
The margin of the lens is visible because the lens is smaller than normal.

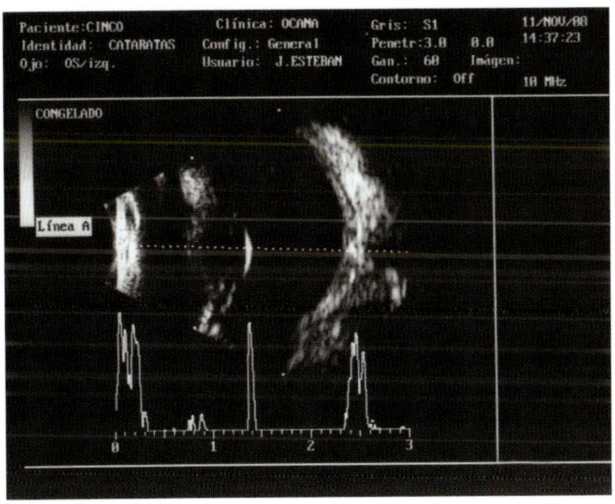

A/B mode ultrasound of the patient.
Close-up of the microphakia and the cataract.

i

An abnormally small lens. This is a congenital developmental anomaly. It is often accompanied by other intraocular alterations.

It has been described in the Rottweiler, the Catalan Sheepdog, and the Old English Sheepdog, among other breeds.

Coloboma

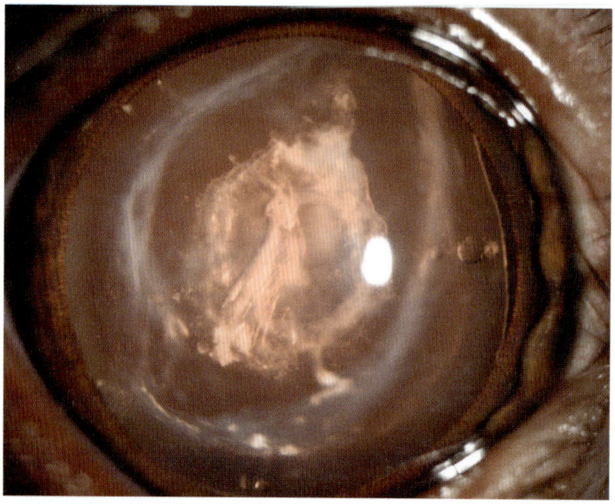

Medially-located lens coloboma in a dog. This is associated with a congenital cataract.
The ciliary processes are clearly visible. The patient's eye is mydriatic (using tropicamide).

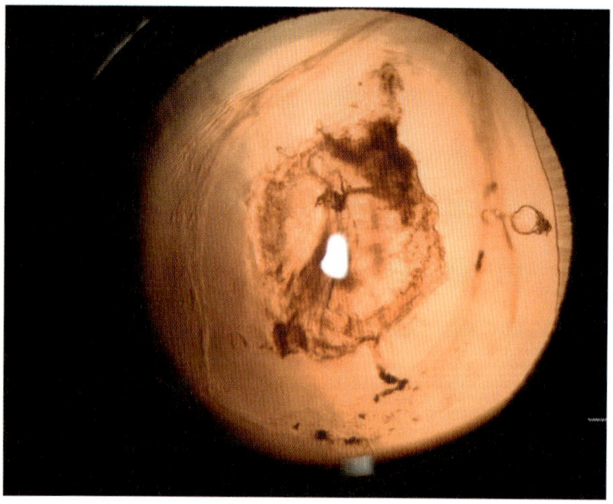

This picture of the patient was taken with retroilllumination. Close-up of the coloboma and of the zonular fibre attachments.

A coloboma is a congenital developmental defect of the lens. This is a partial lack of lens tissue (hypoplasia), usually located at its equator.

It is generally associated with cataracts.

Nuclear sclerosis

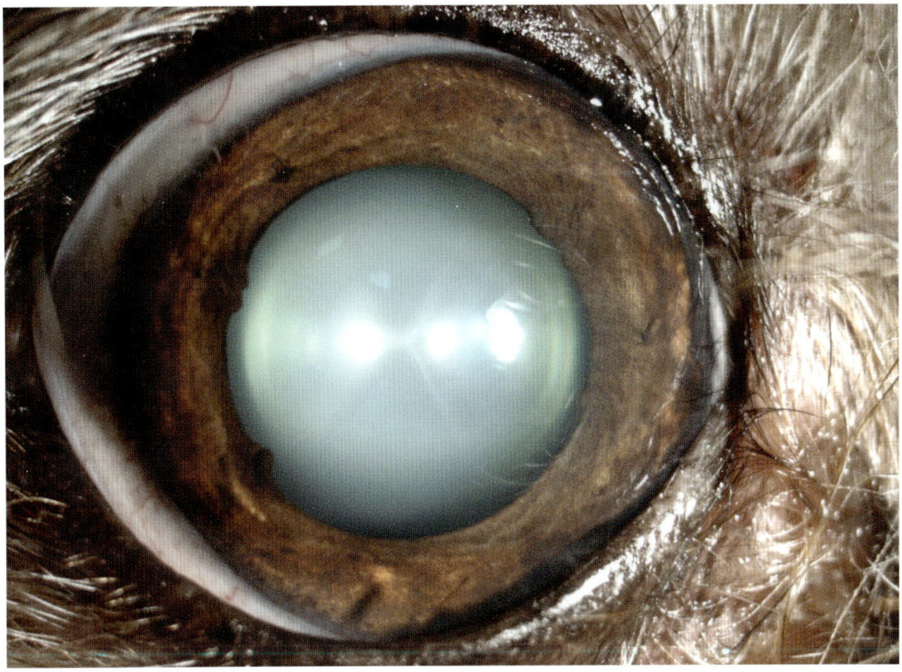

Nuclear sclerosis of the lens in a 14-year-old dog.
Note the yellowish-green reflection of the ocular fundus.

Important notes

- Do not confuse nuclear sclerosis (age-related degeneration) of the lens with a cataract.
- Sclerosis is OPALESCENCE and a cataract is an OPACITY.
- It starts from six years of age in dogs and 10 years of age in cats.

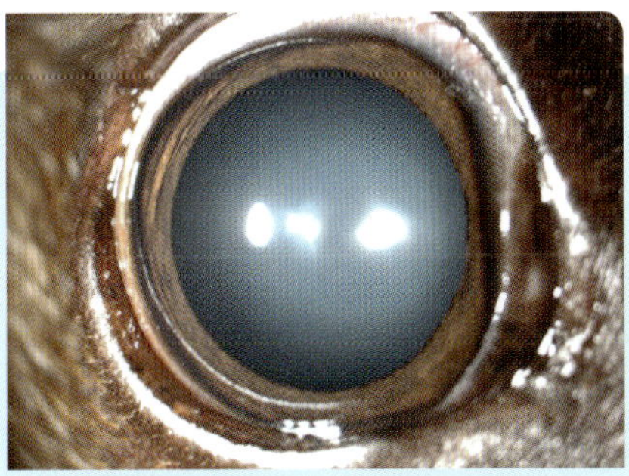

Age-related degeneration of the lens.
Close-up of the three Purkinje-Sanson images.

Nuclear sclerosis

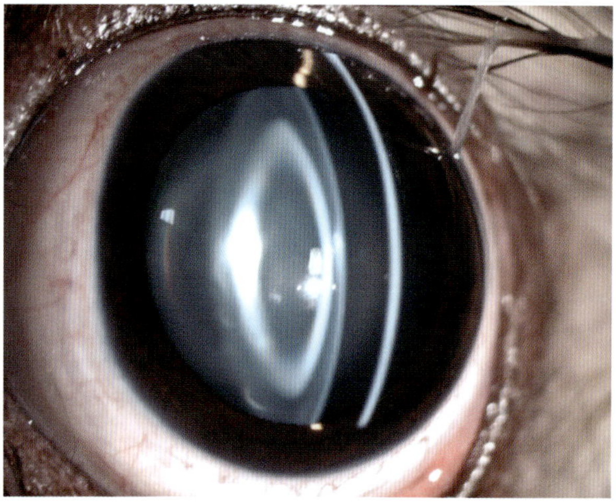

Nuclear sclerosis in a nine-year-old Shih-Tzu.
The slit lamp can reveal early nuclear sclerosis.

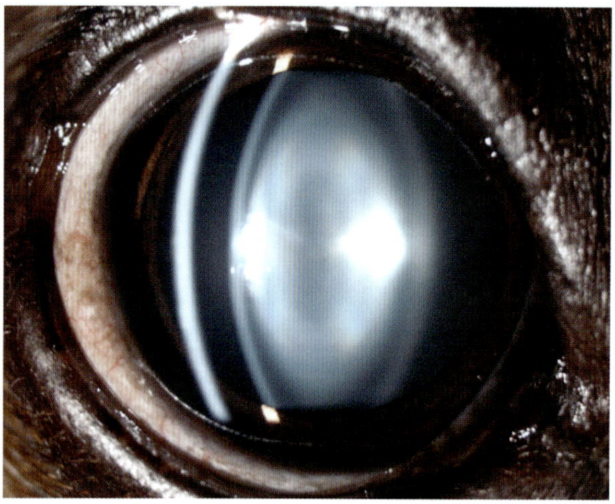

Advanced nuclear sclerosis. Generalised nuclear opalescence.

- The patient's pupils MUST BE DILATED in order to properly examine the lens.
- Nuclear sclerosis does not require surgical treatment unless age-related cataract develops concurrently.

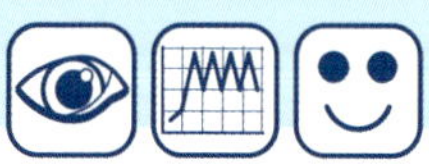

Cataracts

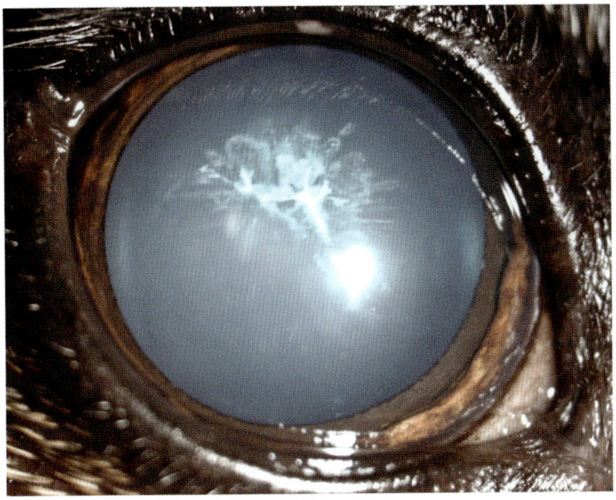

Incipient cataract in a three-year-old dog. Polar location.

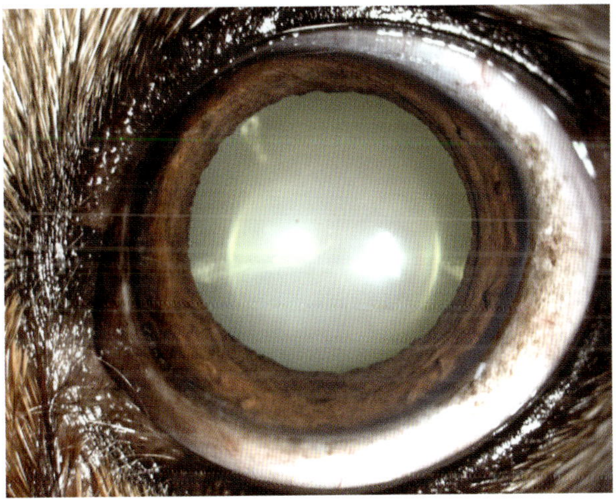

Incipient, or early, cataract in a 14-year-old dog, associated with nuclear sclerosis. Equatorial location.

Important notes

Patients with incipient cataracts have:

- NO visual deficit.
- A tapetal reflection.
- A smooth anterior lens capsule.

PUPILS MUST BE DILATED DURING THE EXAMINATION.

Cataracts

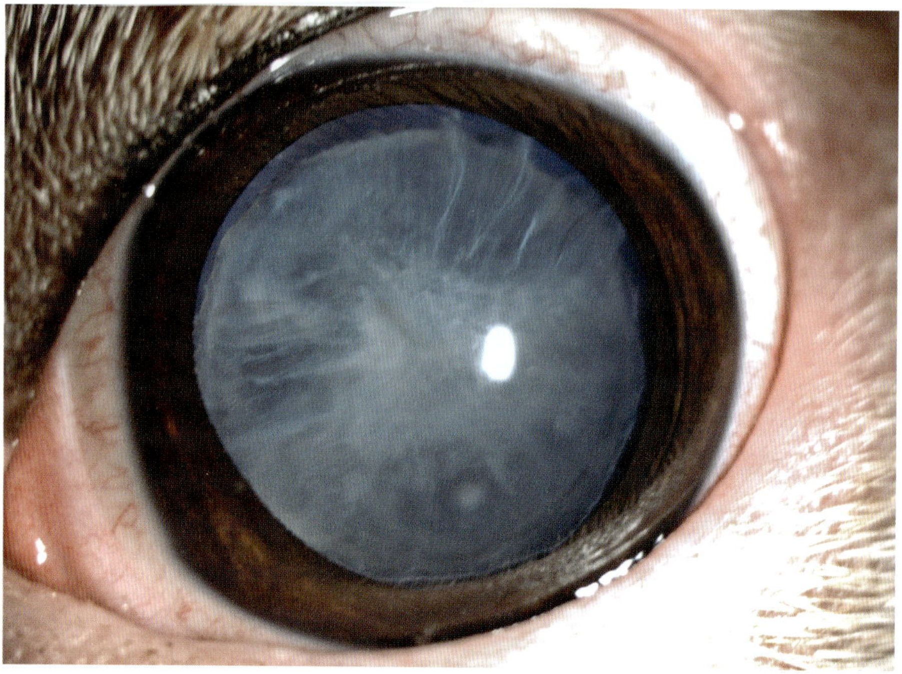

Immature cataract in a French Bulldog.

- In the second phase of cataract progression:
  - The patient has some degree of visual deficit.
  - There is still, however, some tapetal reflection.
  - The anterior capsule remains smooth.
  - The lens may be intumescent from rapid fluid absorption. This sometimes reveals the suture lines of the lens (see picture).

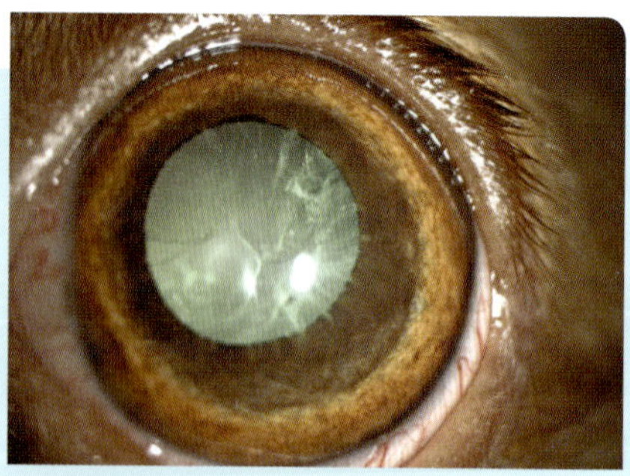

Immature cataract
in a six-year-old mixed-breed dog.
Rapid progression: six days.
Close-up of the Y-shaped anterior suture line of the lens.

Cataracts

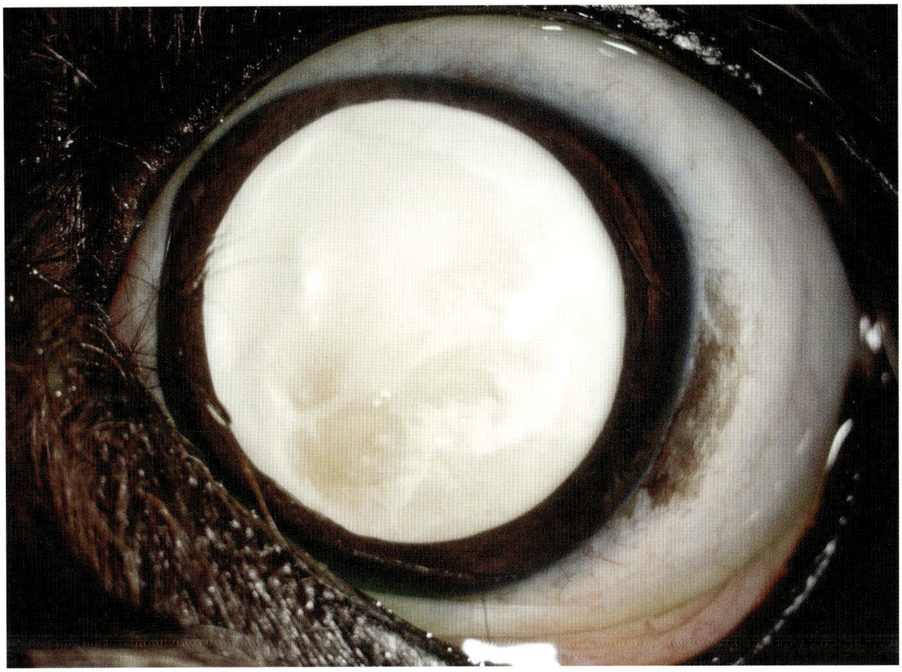

Mature cataract. Blind eye.

Important notes

Patients with mature cataracts have:

- No tapetal reflection.
- There is a visual deficit.
- A smooth anterior lens capsule.

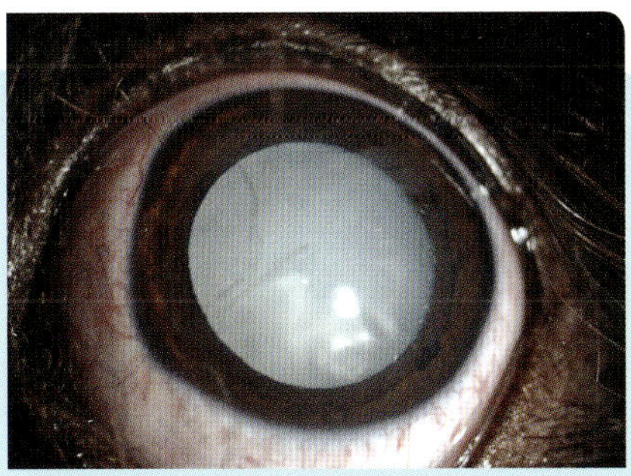

Mature cataract in an 11-year-old dog. Close-up of leukocoria (white pupil). Generalised lens opacity.

Cataracts

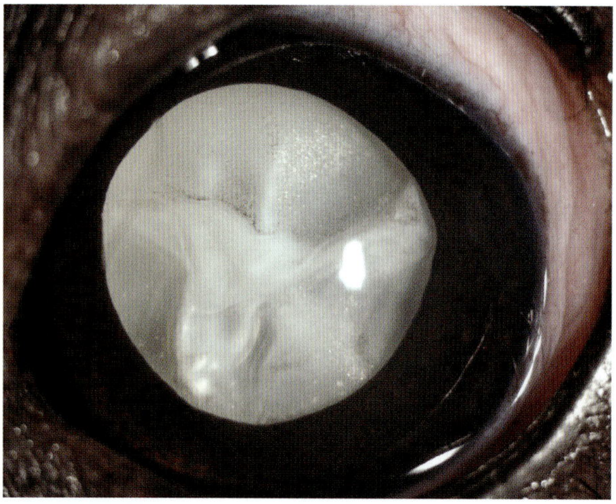

Hypermature cataract in a 13-year-old dog.
Time since onset: one year.
Note the areas of greater opacity (cellular density).

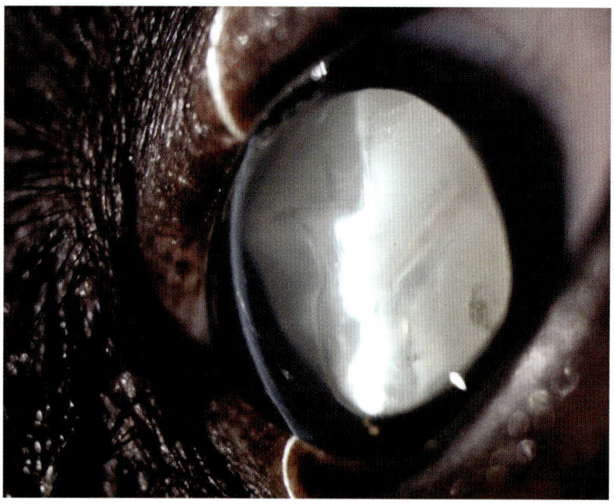

Wrinkling of the anterior capsule in a **hypermature** cataract. Slit-lamp picture of patient shown above.

Important notes

Patients with hypermature cataracts have:

- NO appreciable tapetal reflection (except in advanced stages of resorption).
- A wrinkled anterior lens capsule.

Cataracts

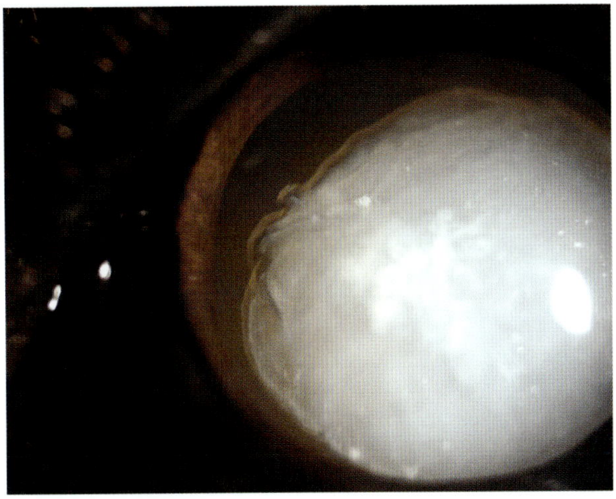

Hypermature cataract. Wrinkling of the anterior lens capsule.

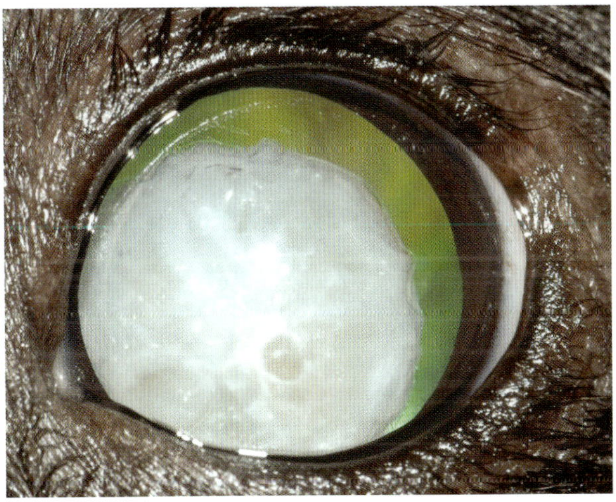

Hypermature cataract during resorption. The tapetal reflection is visible.

Interesting notes

In some hypermature cataracts that are very advanced, the tapetal reflection is visible because of the cortical degeneration of the lens.

Cataracts

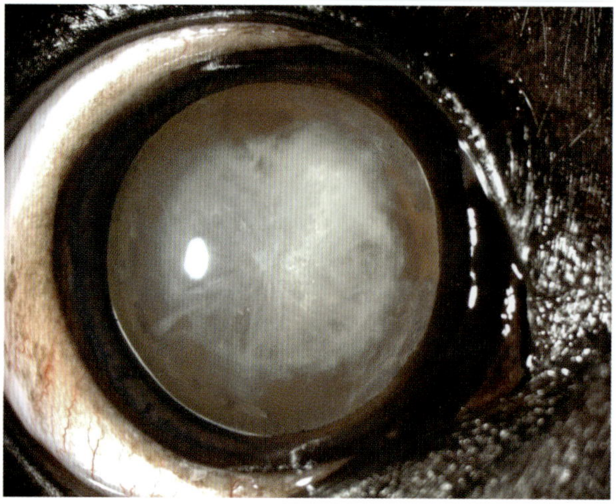

Congenital cataract in an eight-month-old Shih-Tzu. This cataract is associated with microphakia.

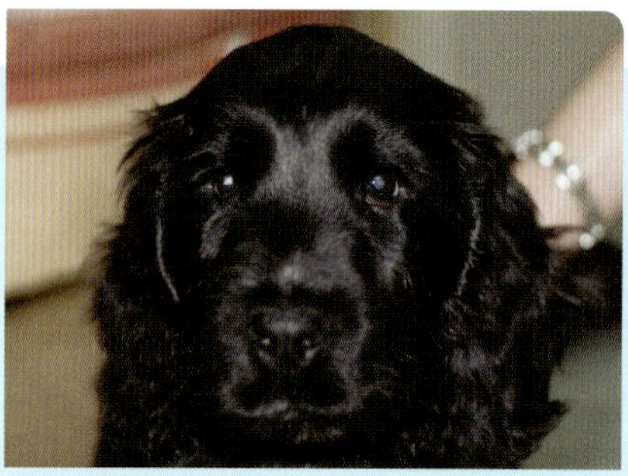

Three-month-old English Cocker Spaniel. Congenital bilateral cataract.

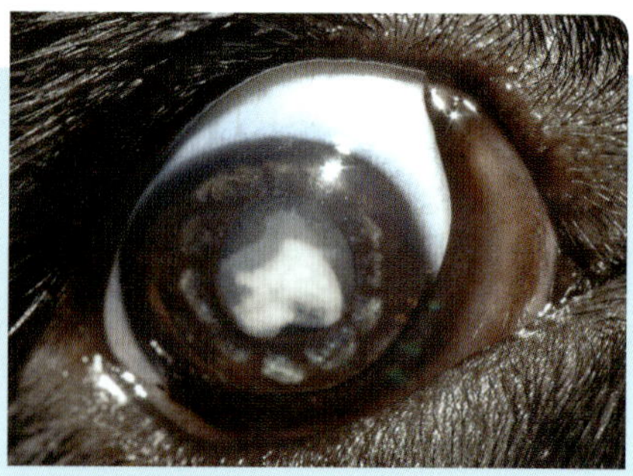

Close-up of the right eye of the patient pictured above.

Breed predisposition

- Congenital cataracts are described in Retrievers (Labrador and Golden), some Spaniels (Cocker, Springer), Old English Sheepdogs and West Highland White Terriers.
- These are present from birth and may have a hereditary component.
- This type of cataract is often accompanied by other alterations such as PPM (persistent pupillary membrane, microphakia, microphthalmia, etc.).

Cataracts

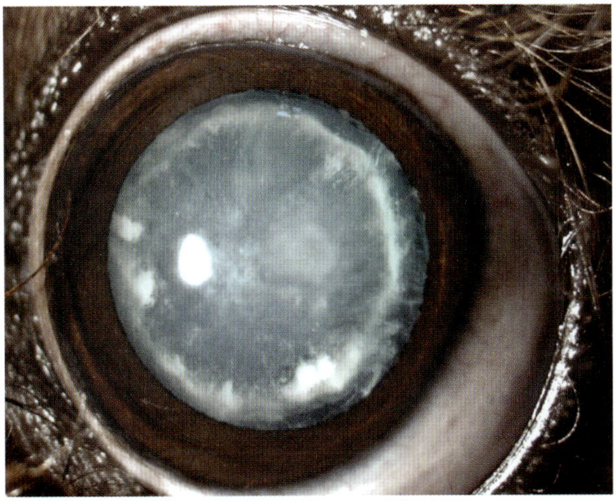

Juvenile cataract in a five-year-old dog. Progressive cataract that started at three years of age and in the immature phase.

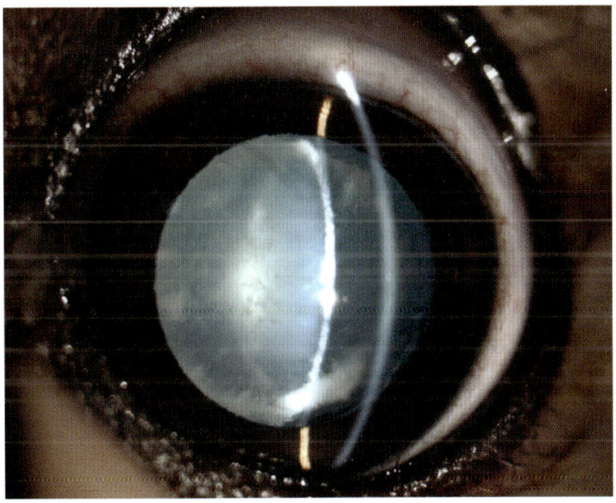

Cortical location of the cataract.

Interesting notes

Juvenile cataracts are generally progressive, bilateral in presentation, and most frequently originate in the cortex.

Breed predisposition

German Shepherds and Miniature Schnauzers are the most frequently affected.

Cataracts

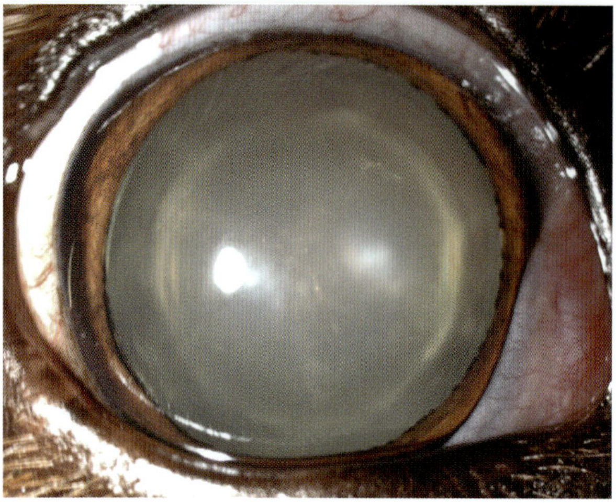

Age-related cataract, incipient, in a 15-year-old mixed-breed dog.
This patient has a cataract in the anterior part of the lens (note the Y-shape) along with nuclear sclerosis.

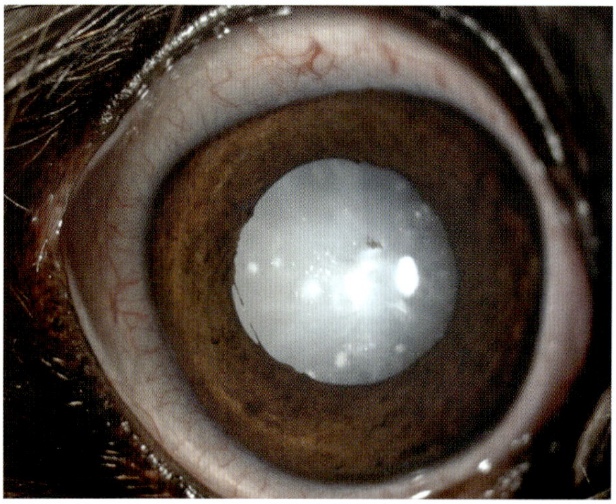

Age-related, hypermature cataract in a 14-year-old dog, accompanied by iridal atrophy.

Surgery is often indicated for age-related cataracts except in cases of simultaneous retinal degeneration or keratoconjunctivitis sicca.

Age-related cataracts sometimes occur with iris atrophy or vitreal degeneration.

Cataracts

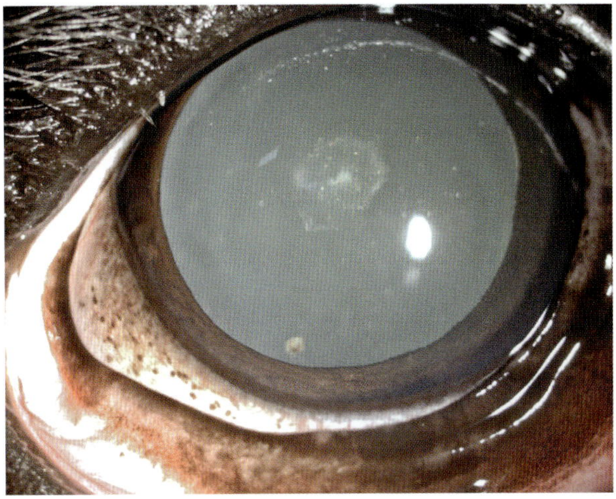

Anterior polar **capsular** cataract in a one-year-old Boxer.

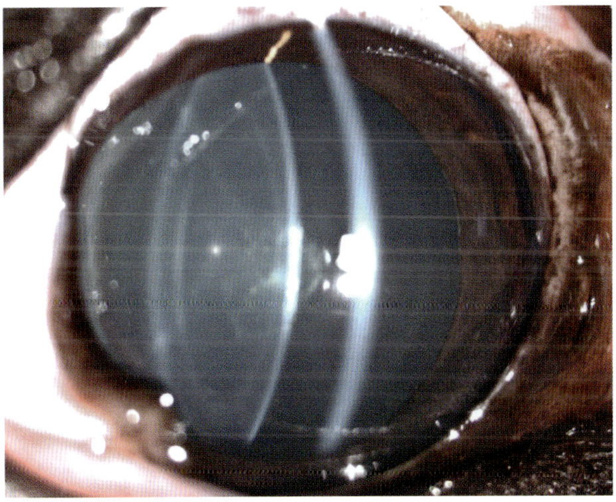

The slit lamp reveals the opacity in the axial area of the anterior capsule.

Cataracts are categorised by their location:

- Capsular (anterior or posterior).
- Subcapsular (anterior or posterior).
- Cortical (anterior or posterior).
- Nuclear.

Cataracts

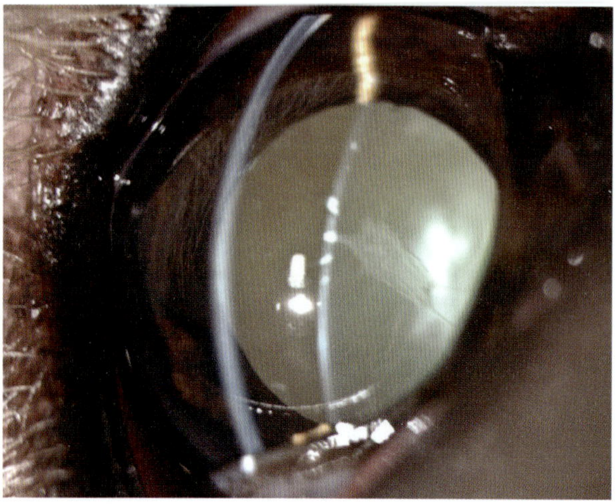

Focal **anterior capsular** cataract in a two-year-old Cocker Spaniel.
Congenital cataract.

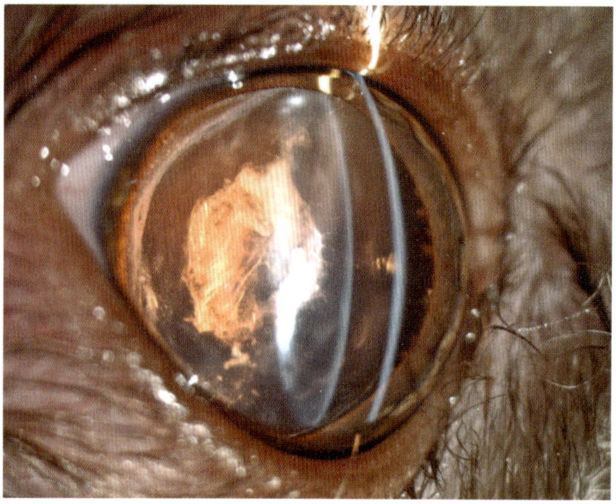

Congenital **posterior capsular** cataract associated with persistent hyperplastic primary vitreous.

Important notes

In order to precisely locate the cataract:

- FULLY DILATE THE PUPIL (with mydriatic drugs).
- USE THE SLIT LAMP.

Cataracts

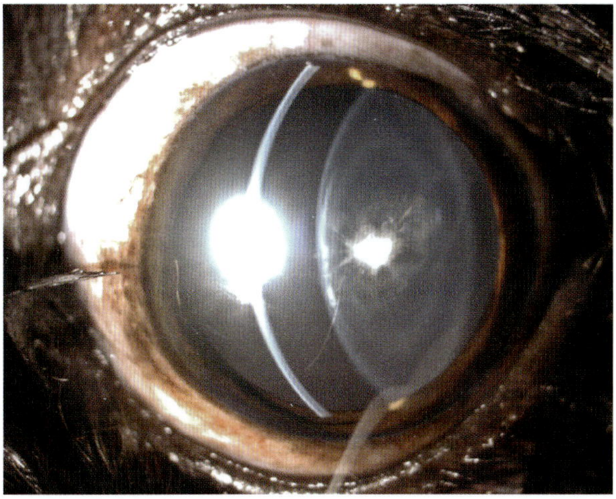

Anterior **subcapsular** cataract in a dog.
Close-up of the lesion with a slit lamp. Focal cataract.

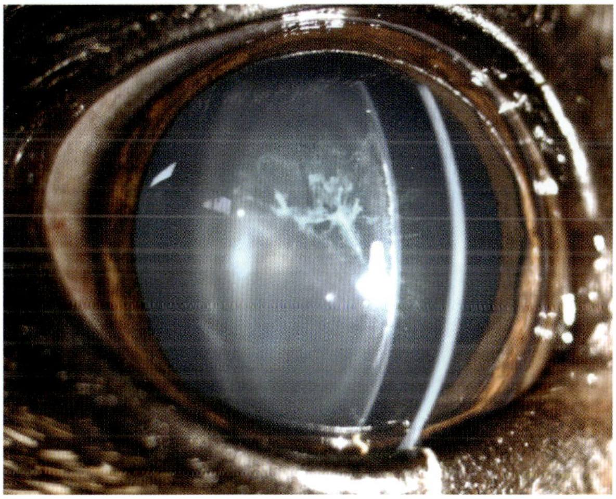

Anterior **subcapsular** cataract.
Use the frontal view of the Y-suture for orientation in localising cataracts.

i | Subcapsular cataracts tend to be progressive.

Recommendation

In interpreting slit-lamp pictures, consider the frontal view along with the optical cross-section.

Cataracts

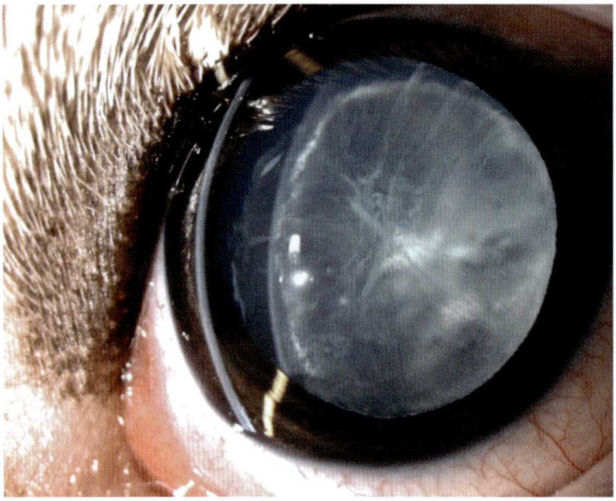

Anteroposterior view of a **cortical** cataract in a hypothyroid patient. The slit lamp enables us to confirm the cortical location of this immature cataract.

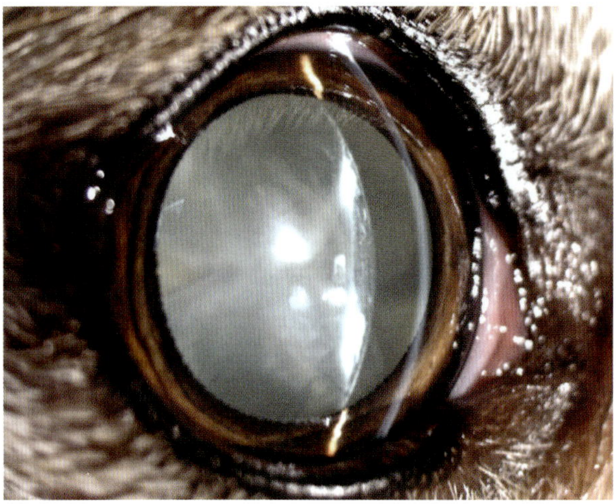

Cortical subcapsular diabetic cataract in a seven-year-old dog. Acute presentation: eight days since onset.

i

Cortical cataracts are often associated with metabolic and endocrine diseases (hypocalcaemia, diabetes, Cushing's syndrome, or hypothyroidism).

Cortical cataracts with a hereditary component have also been described (Golden Retriever, American Cocker Spaniel).

Cataracts

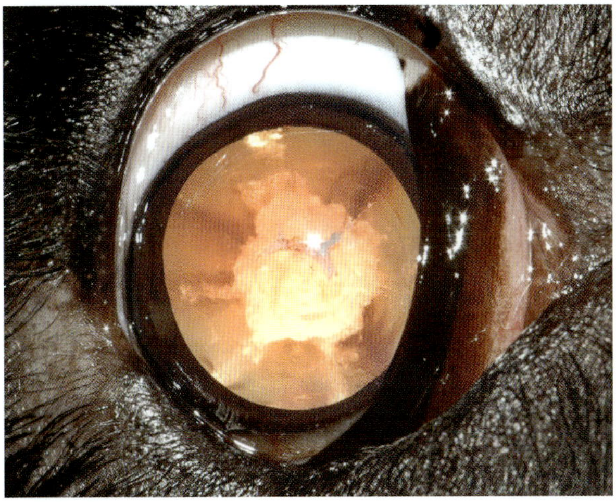

Cortical cataract in a Cocker Spaniel.
Arranged in spokes.

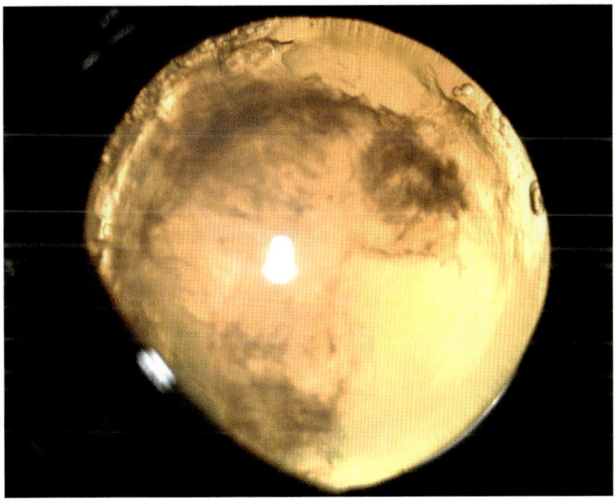

Cortical cataract with a vacuolar shape in the equatorial zone. Picture taken using retroillumination.

i

Vacuoles, spokes, and fissures are commonly seen in cortical cataracts.

Cortical cataracts may affect the anterior, posterior, or equatorial area of the lens.

Cataracts

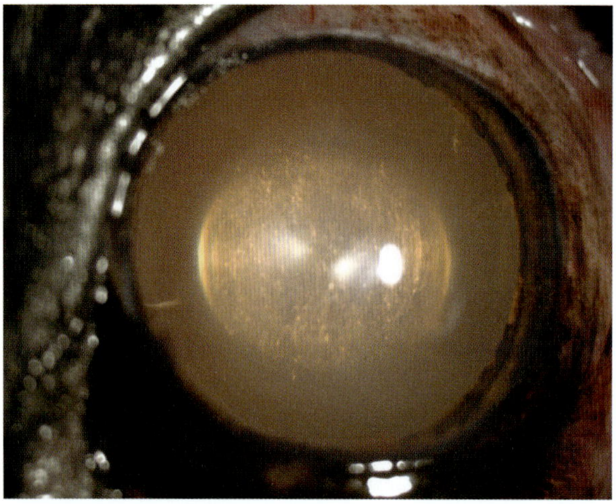

Age-related **nuclear** cataract in a Cocker Spaniel. Incipient phase.

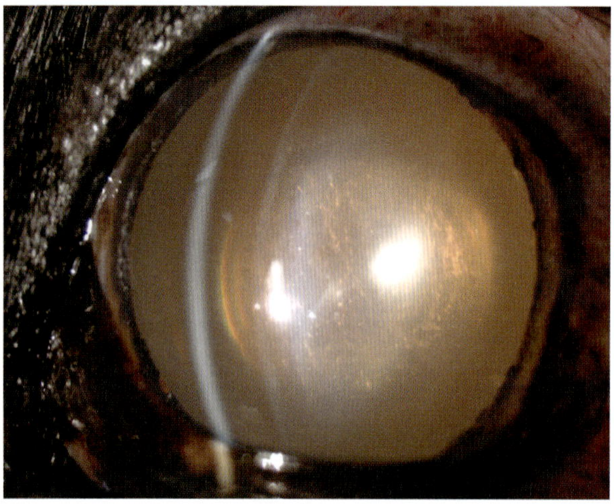

Slit-lamp picture of the cataract in the patient pictured above. **Nuclear** location.

Interesting notes

Nuclear cataracts do not tend to be progressive in older patients, and in incipient phases they do not cause severe visual deficits.

Cataracts

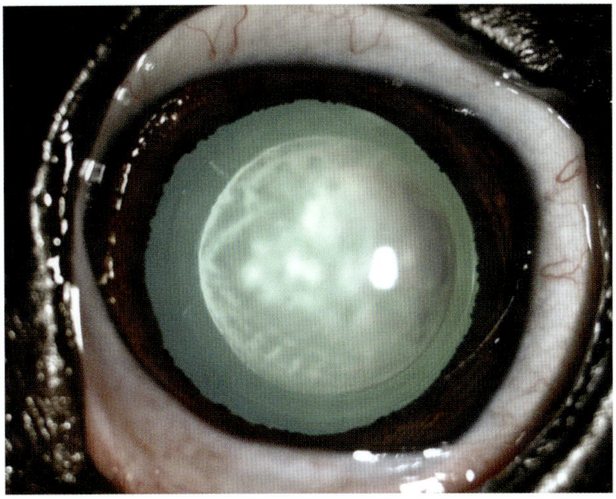

Nuclear congenital cataract in a three-year-old Boxer.

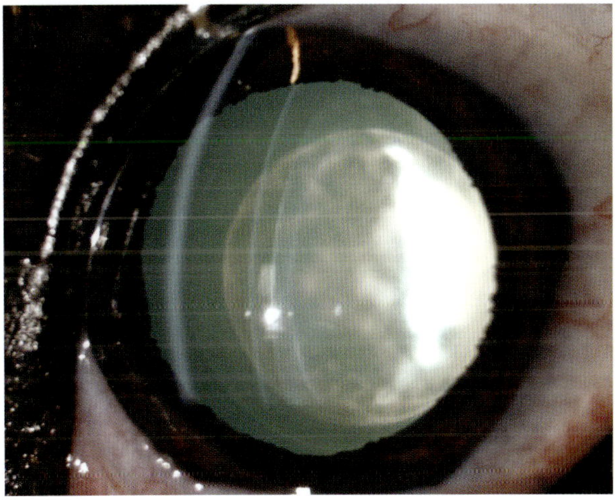

Close-up of the **nuclear** location of the opacity (immature cataract), under mydriasis. Patient pictured above.

i

Nuclear cataracts are typically congenital.

They tend to present bilaterally, though they may be in different phases of progression.

Cataracts

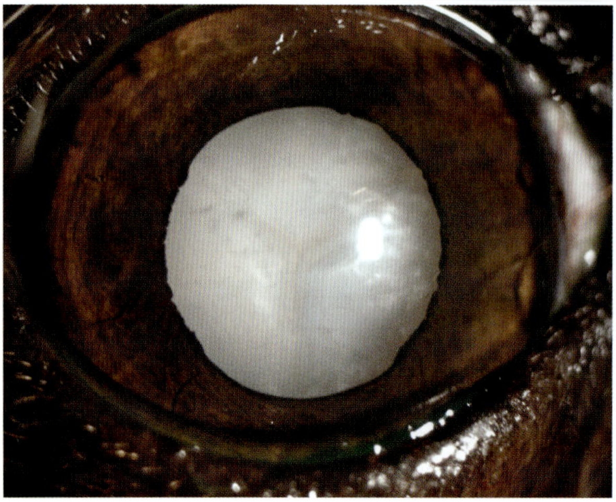

Diabetic cataract in an eight-year-old dog.
Intumescent lens.

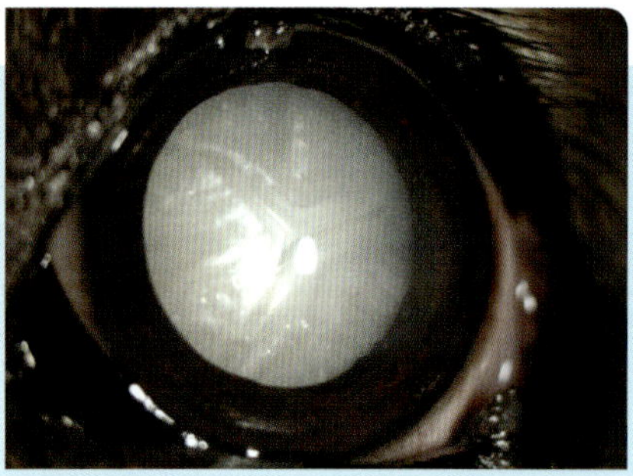

Mature **diabetic** cataract with loss of lens material. Close-up of the leak into the anterior chamber.

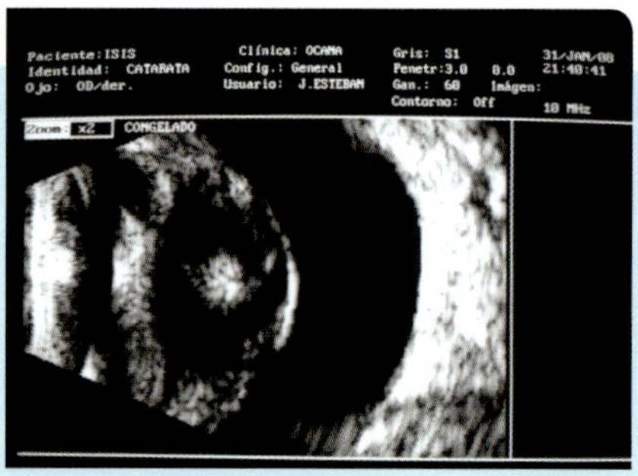

Ocular ultrasound.
Close-up of the lens size in an intumescent diabetic cataract.

Important notes

- Diabetic cataracts are always bilateral. They progress quickly and are often intumescent.
- They originate from the lens equator and are caused by sorbitol precipitation.
- Diabetic cataract surgery should be performed as promptly as possible because the risk of phacolytic uveitis is high.

Cataracts

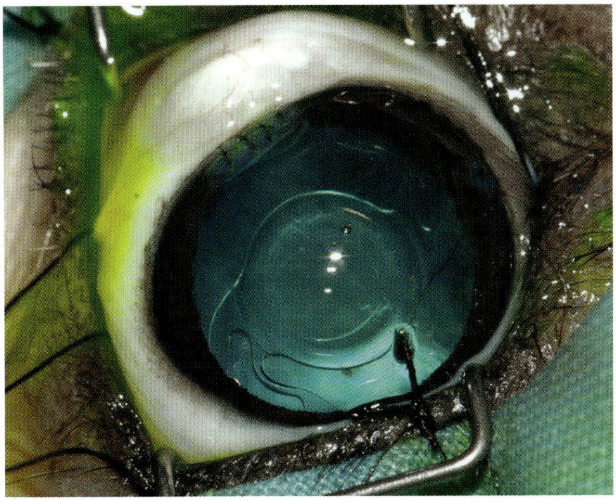

Cataract surgery by phacoemulsification and implantation of an intraocular lens (IOL). In surgery.

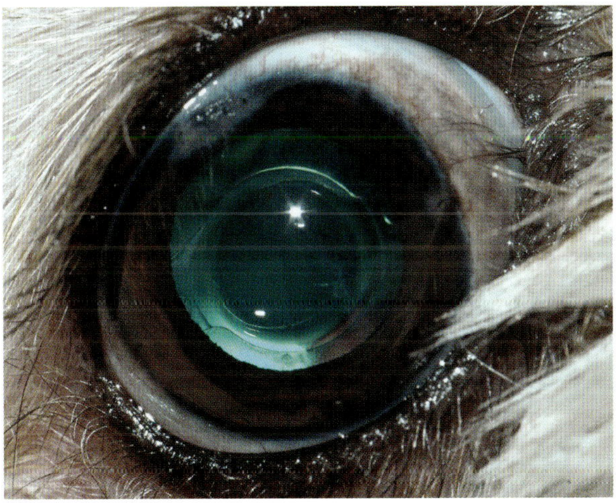

Patient pictured above, 30 days postoperatively. Close-up of the IOL position in the capsular sac. Note the tapetal reflection.

Important notes

- Surgery is currently the treatment of choice for cataracts.
- The most common technique is phacoemulsification, but extracapsular surgery may be needed in some cases.
- Good patient selection is critical to a successful outcome.

Cataracts

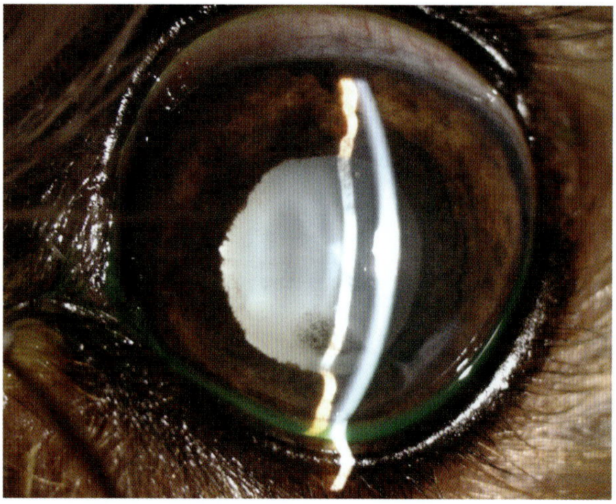

Traumatic capsular and anterior cortical cataract in a dog that was scratched by a cat. Note the corneal scar.

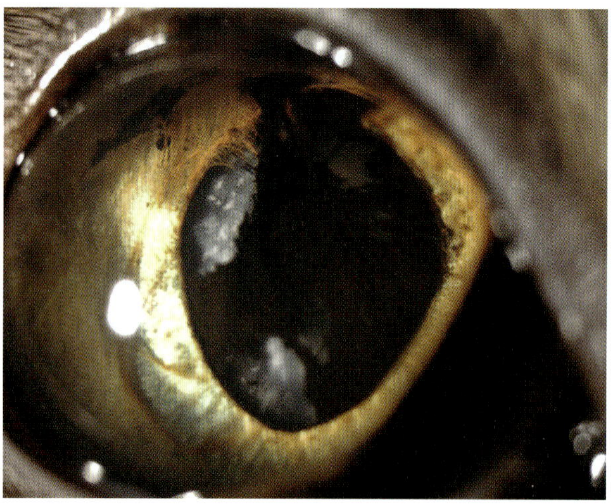

Post-traumatic cataract in a Maine Coon cat resulting from a pellet wound. Hypermature cataract. Uveal tissue remnants appear on the anterior lens capsule.

i | Any direct trauma to the lens that damages the capsule or induces cellular disorganisation will lead to a cataract.

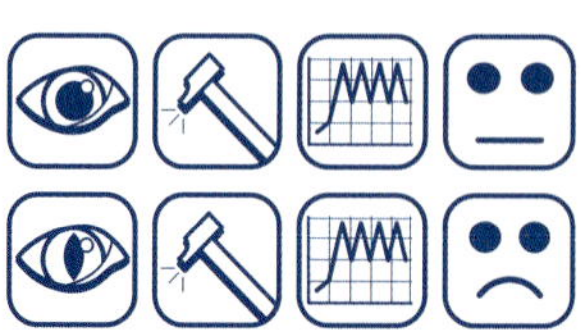

Cataracts

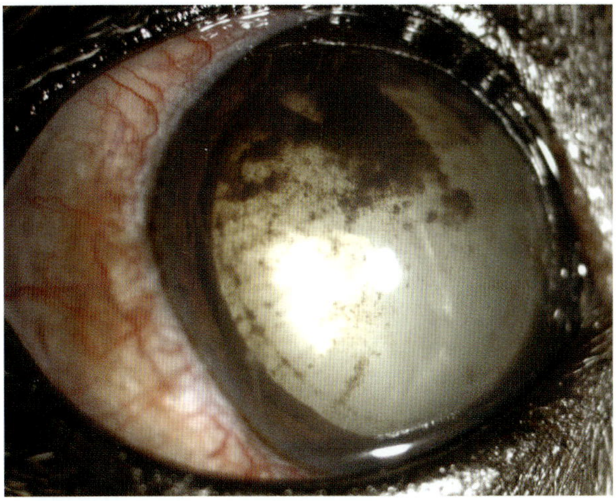

Postuveitic mature cataract in a dog. Close-up of inflammatory material deposits on the lens.

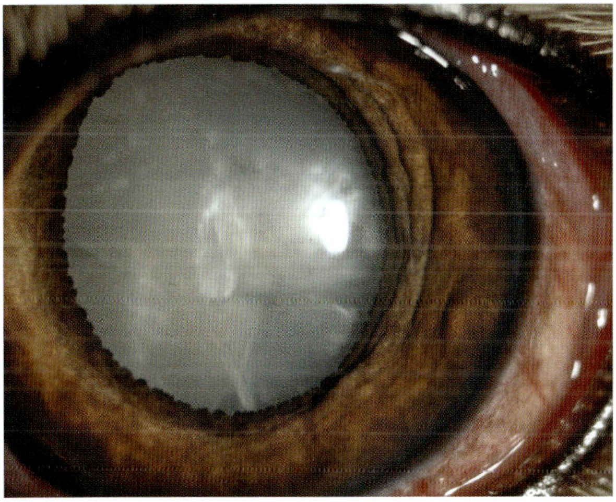

Postuveitic mature cataract.

Interesting notes

Any change in the composition of the media in contact with the lens (aqueous or vitreous humour), may give rise to a cataract.

Contraindicated

Surgery is not indicated for cataracts associated with uveitis. Intraocular inflammation must first be treated, followed by a detailed examination of all intraocular structures to determine if an intervention is possible. These patients are at very high risk of glaucoma or retinal detachment.

Cataracts

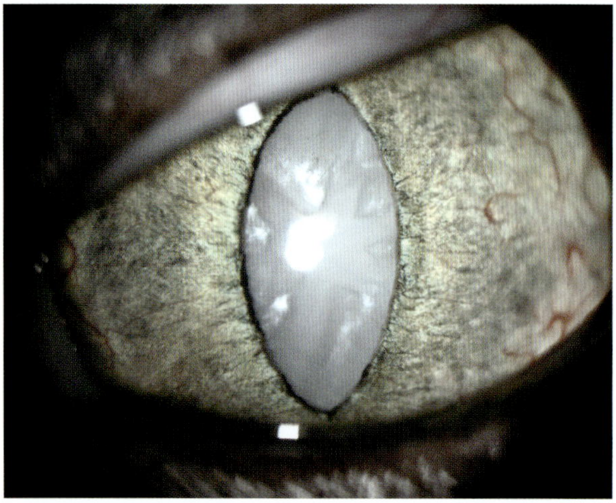

Mature cataract secondary to FIV-induced uveitis in a cat.

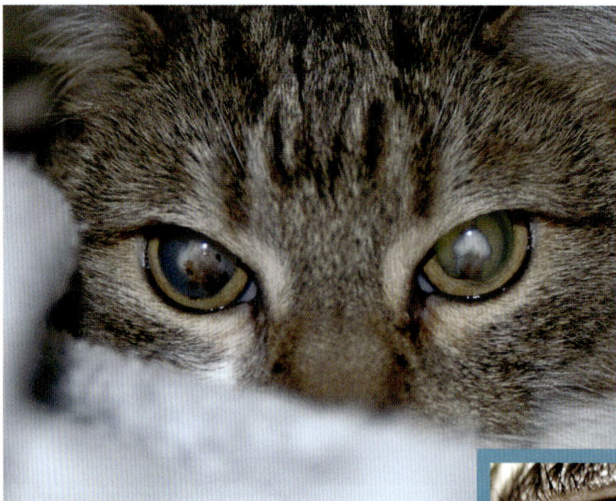

Cat with bilateral cataracts secondary to uveitis.

i

Cataracts are less common in cats than in dogs.

Most feline cataracts are secondary to intraocular inflammation, as congenital cataracts are rare (see picture).

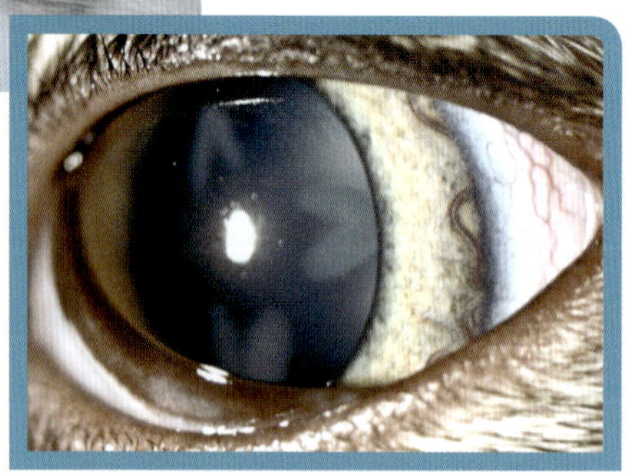

Congenital bilateral cataract in a kitten.

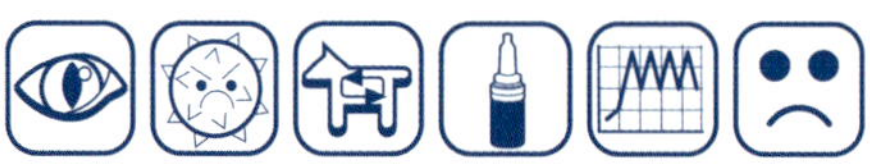

Lens subluxation

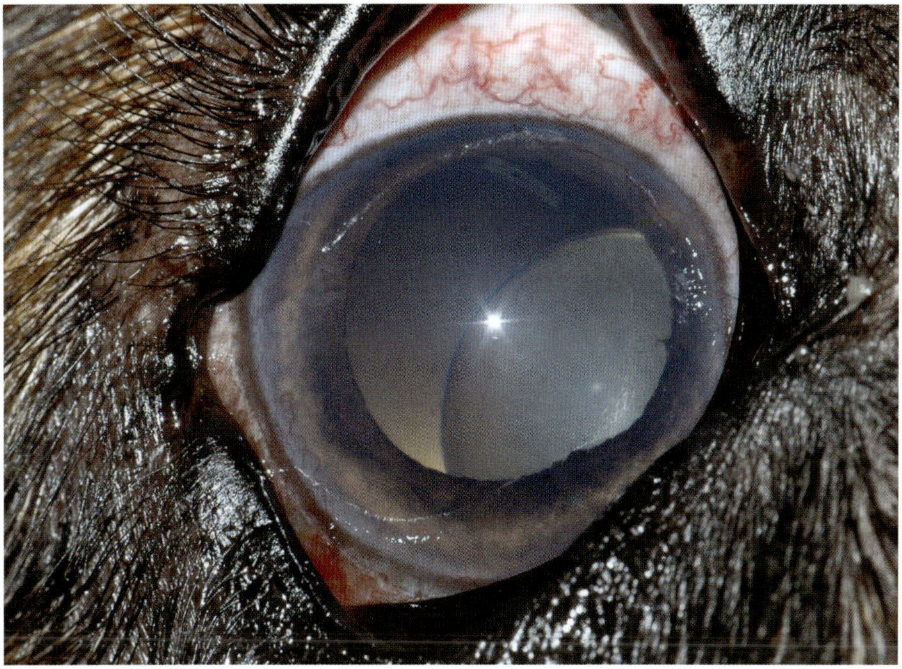

Lens subluxation in a dog following an ocular trauma.
Close-up of the aphakic crescent.

i

This is a partial lens displacement (anterior or posterior) from its normal position.

Ocular trauma, cataracts, chronic uveitis, and glaucoma predispose patients to this lens disease.

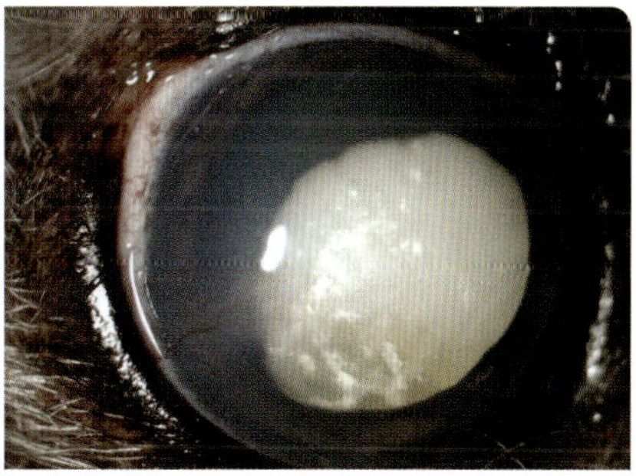

Lens subluxation. Hypermature cataract.

Lens subluxation

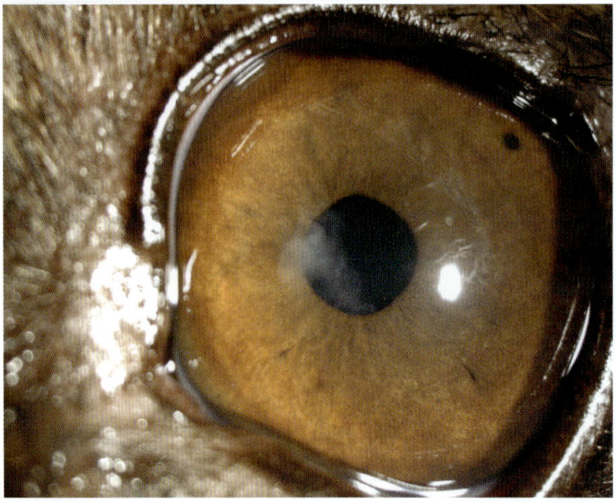

The presence of vitreous in the anterior chamber is an early sign of lens subluxation. Close-up of vitreous flowing through the pupil.

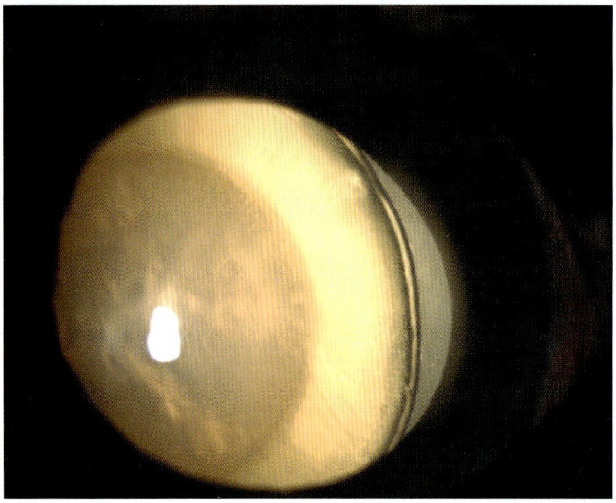

The aphakic crescent is readily visible using retroillumination in this patient with lens subluxation.

Important notes

The early signs of lens subluxation are as follows:

- Vitreous humour in the anterior chamber.
- Aphakic crescent: space between the pupillary margin and lens equator through which the ocular fundus is visible.
- Iridodonesis: abnormal trembling motion of the iris due to the loss of support.

Lens subluxation

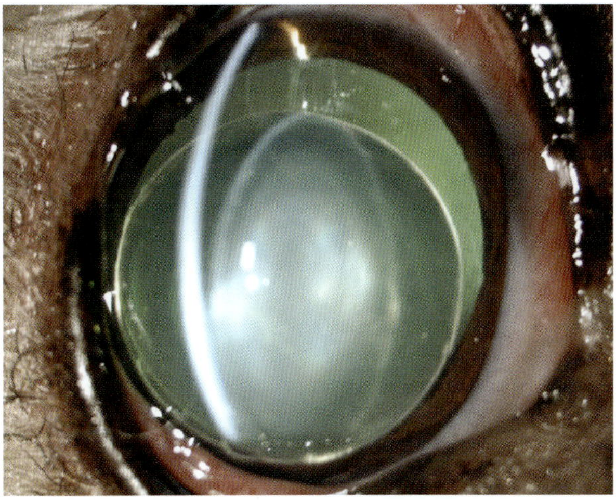

Anterior lens subluxation.

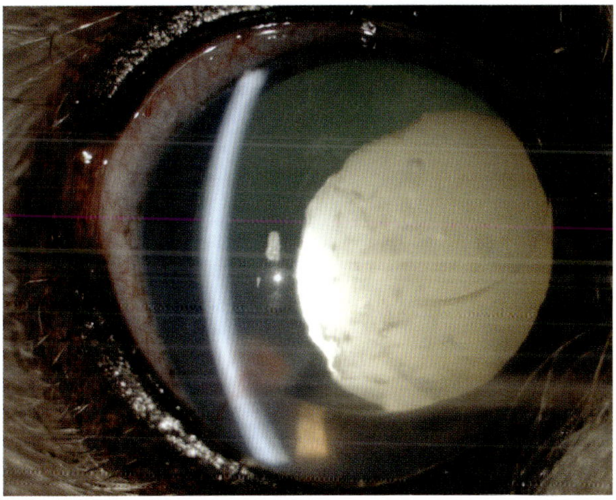

Posterior lens subluxation.

- The slit lamp reveals the lens displacement.
- In an anterior subluxation, the anterior chamber is narrower than normal.
- In a posterior subluxation, the anterior chamber is deeper than normal.

Lens luxation

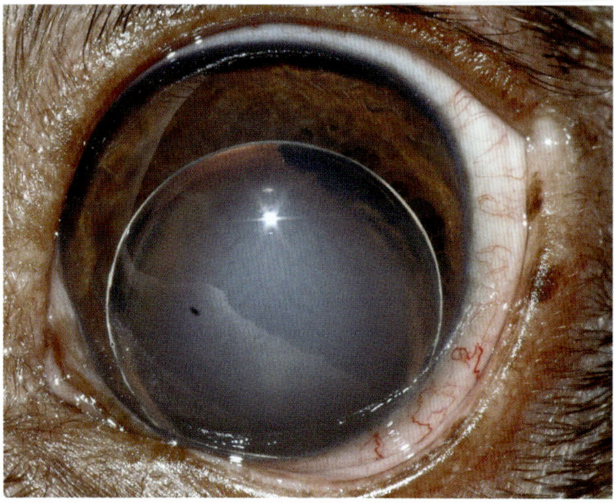

Anterior luxation of the lens, traumatic, in a 14-year-old dog. The lens is in the anterior chamber, in front of the iris. Time since onset: 12 hours.

Lens luxation (complete displacement) occurs upon rupture of all the zonular fibres that anchor the lens. The causes are similar to those of subluxation.

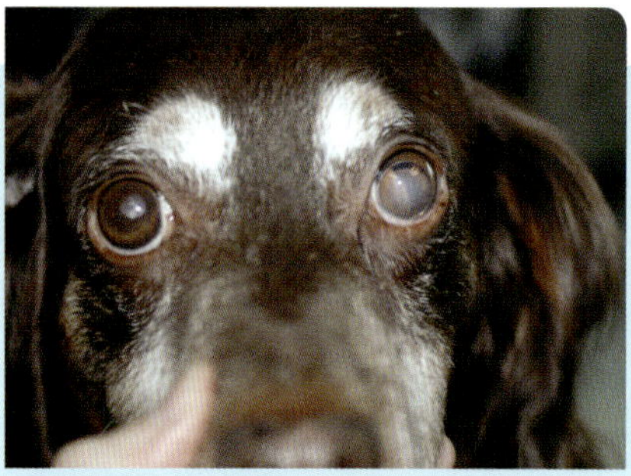

The left eye of this patient is pictured above. Note the contrast with the right eye (normal).

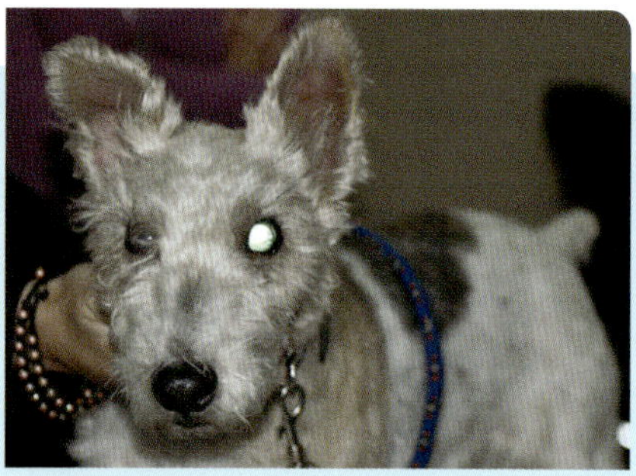

Fox Terrier with **anterior luxation** of the lens in the left eye.

Important notes

- Terrier breeds (Fox, Jack Russell, Welsh, and Tibetan) and mixes are predisposed.

Lens luxation

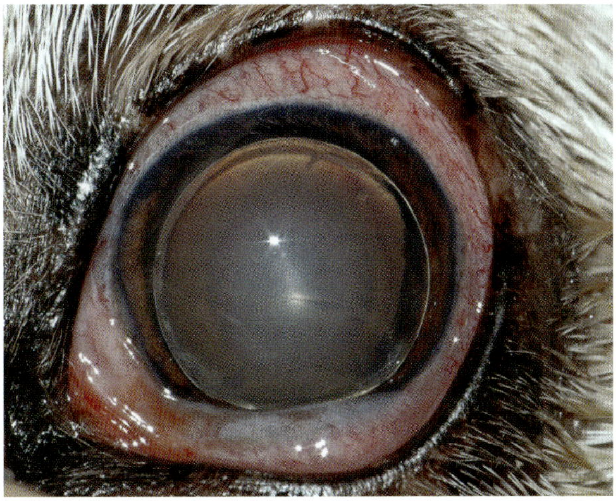

Anterior lens luxation.
Time since onset: four days.

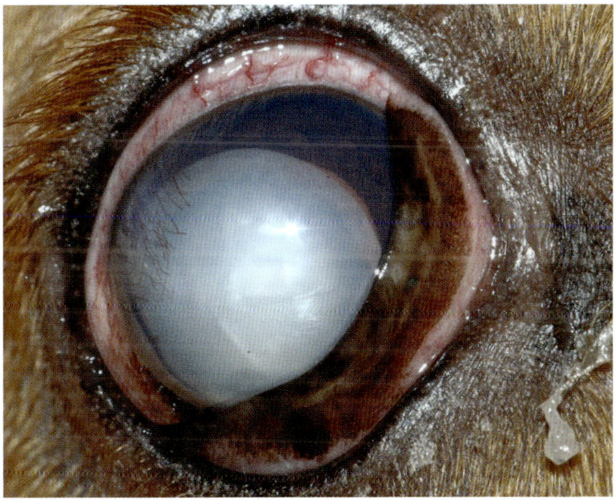

Anterior lens luxation.
Time since onset: 20 days.
Secondary glaucoma: IOP of 36 mmHg.

Important notes

- Anterior lens luxation is considered a SURGICAL EMERGENCY, mainly in dogs, due to the risk of rapid onset (few hours) of glaucoma and endothelial damage.
- Intracapsular lens extraction is the technique of choice.
- A luxated lens tends to develop cataracts over time.

Lens luxation

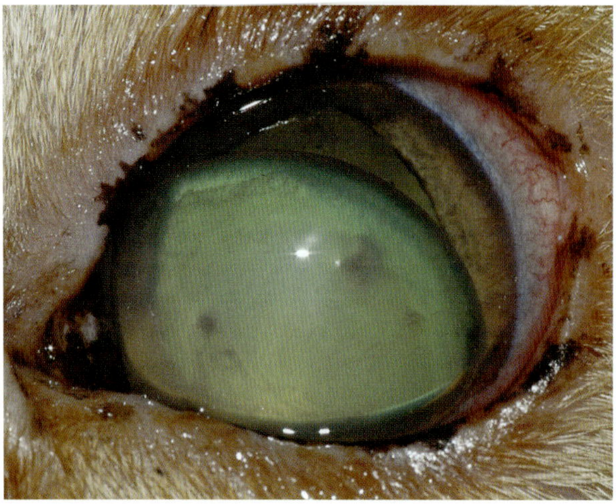

Anterior lens luxation in a cat (left eye).
Time since onset: two months.

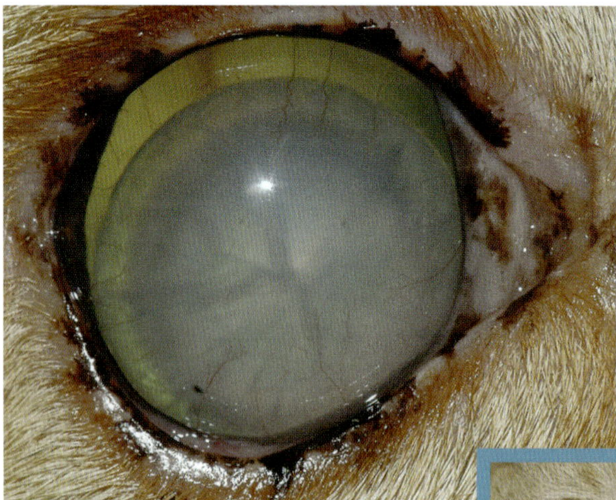

Anterior lens luxation in the right eye of the same patient.

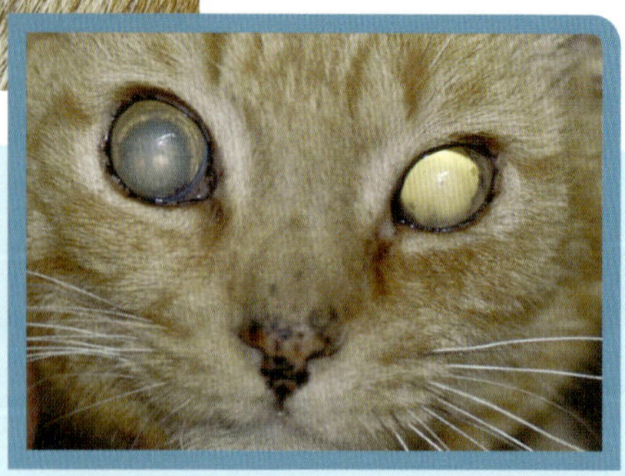

Our patient.

- Always consider UVEITIS in cats with anterior lens luxation, even more so if the luxation is bilateral.
- The risk of glaucoma is lower than in dogs because the anterior chamber is wider and the iridocorneal angle more open.
- Surgical treatment is advised.

Lens luxation

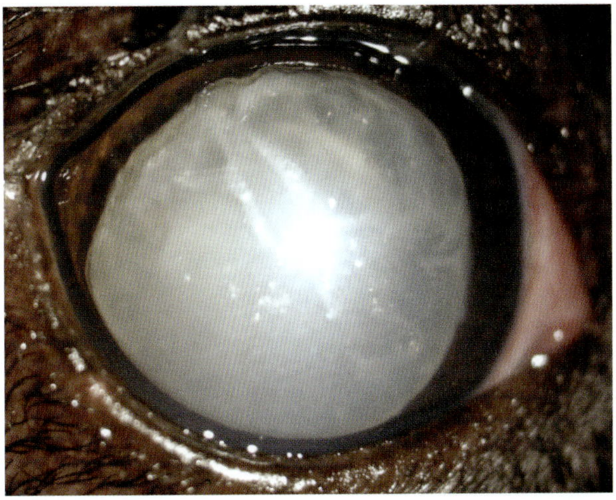

Anterior lens luxation associated with a hypermature cataract.
Eleven-year-old Cocker Spaniel.

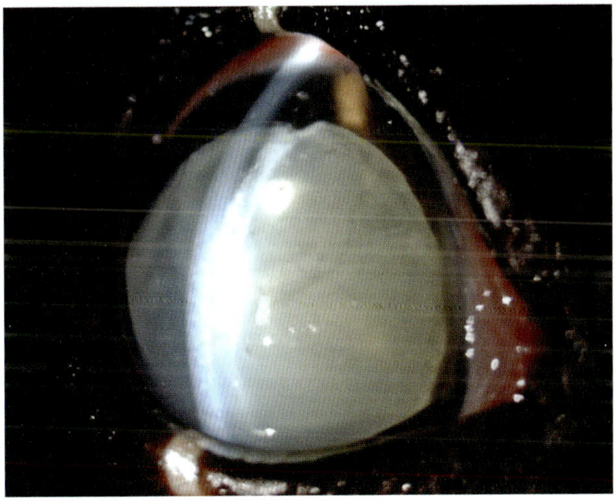

Slit-lamp picture of the patient pictured above. Close-up of athalamia (absence of anterior chamber) and corneal oedema (of endothelial origin) secondary to an anterior luxation.

Contraindicated

DO NOT USE ATROPINE in a patient with an anterior lens luxation. It will increase the risk of glaucoma.

Lens luxation

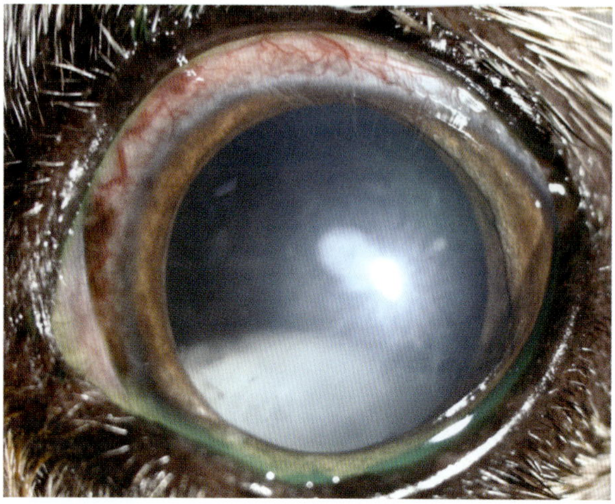

Posterior lens luxation in a dog.
Through the pupillary aperture, the lens can be seen within the vitreous.

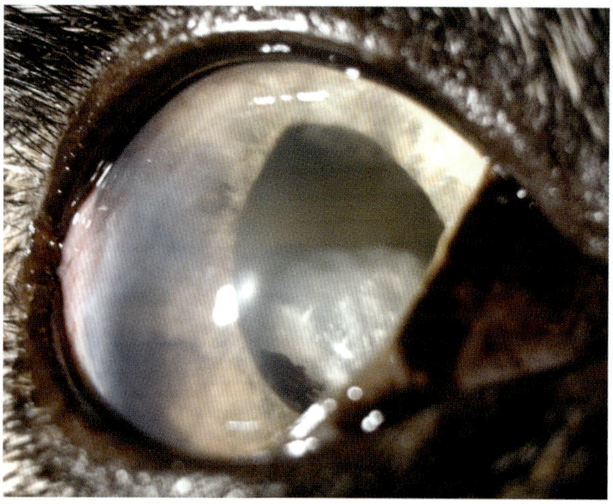

Posterior lens luxation in a cat that suffered a facial trauma.

When the lens falls towards the vitreous, miotic agents can be used to prevent anterior luxation.

The prognosis for vision is better than in an anterior luxation.

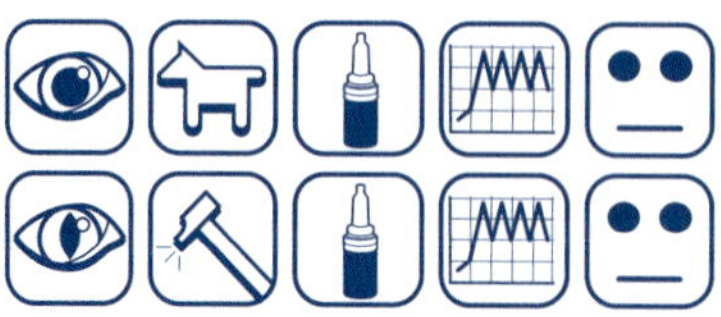

Lens luxation

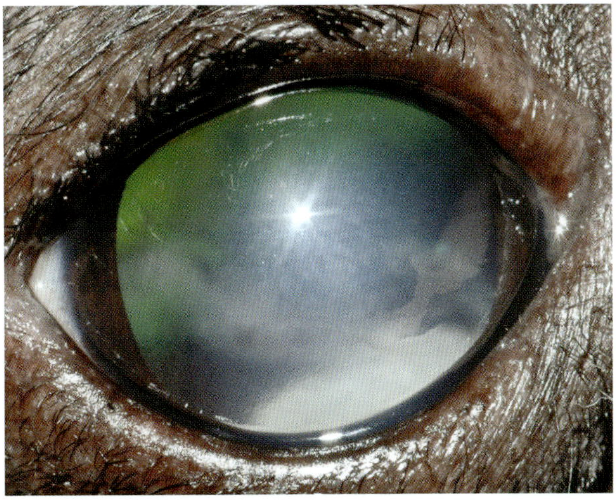

Posterior lens luxation.

Close-up of the anterior vitreous next to the posterior lens capsule.

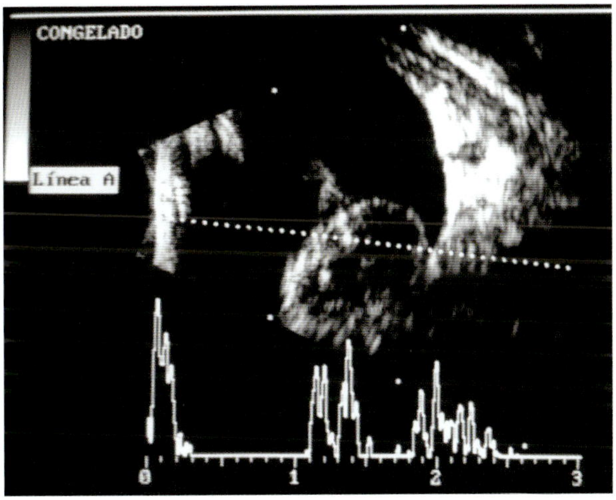

A/B mode ocular ultrasound of the patient pictured above. Note the opaque lens in the vitreous and the hyaloideocapsular ligament remnants.

Patients with unilateral lens luxation who belong to predisposed breeds should have their other eye regularly monitored because of the risk of bilateral luxation.

Thus, be sure to explain this condition to the owner.

Ocular fundus

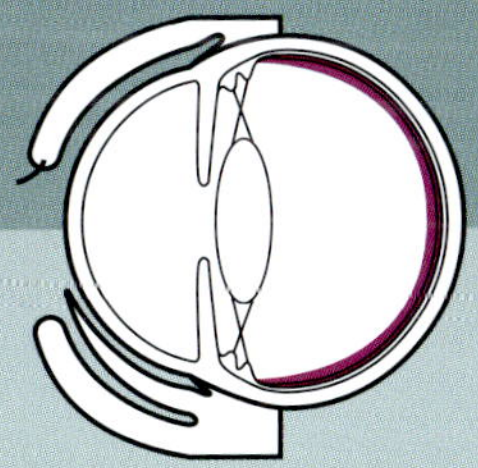

Normal ocular fundus

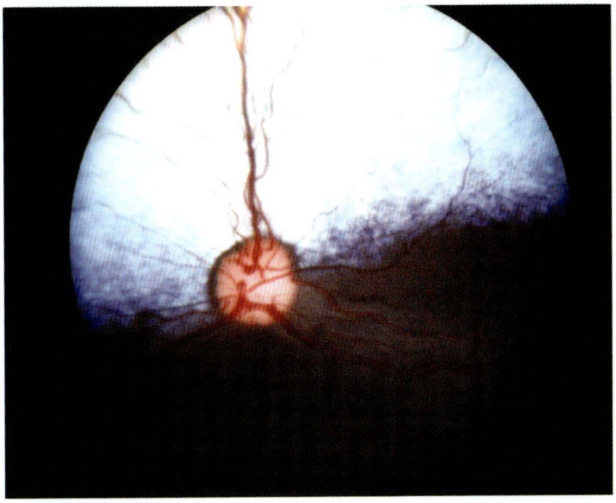

Normal left eye in a medium-sized dog (13-kg mixed-breed).

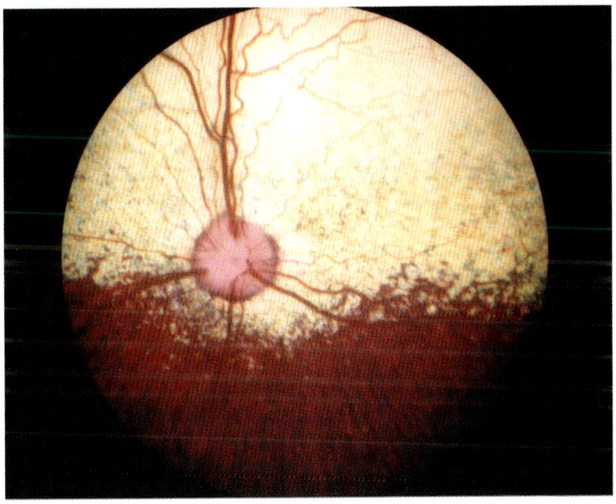

Tigroid fundus in a dog. Left eye. The choroid vessels are visible through the poorly pigmented tissue.

Important notes

In dogs:

- The optic papilla is round or triangular (depending on the myelin concentration) and contains a venous circle.
- The position of the optic papilla does not change, but the size of the tapetum changes.
- There are 15–20 retinal arterioles and 3–5 retinal veins.

Normal ocular fundus

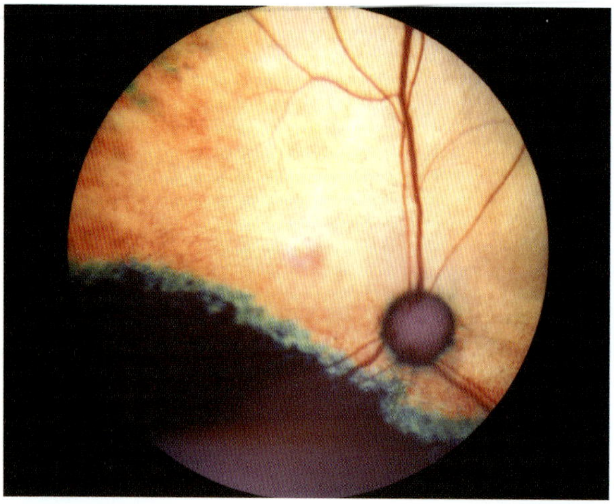

Domestic shorthair cat, right eye.

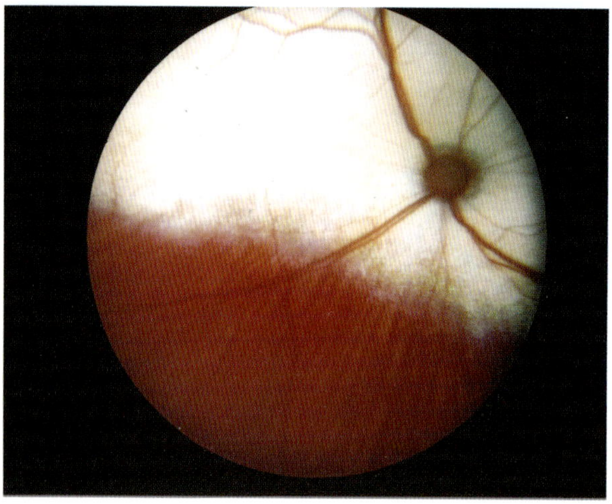

Siamese cat. Tigroid fundus. Left eye.

Important notes

In cats:

- The optic papilla is always round, avascular, and poorly myelinated.
- There are 6–13 retinal arterioles and 3 primary retinal veins.
- As in dogs, there is no central retinal artery.

Retinal detachment

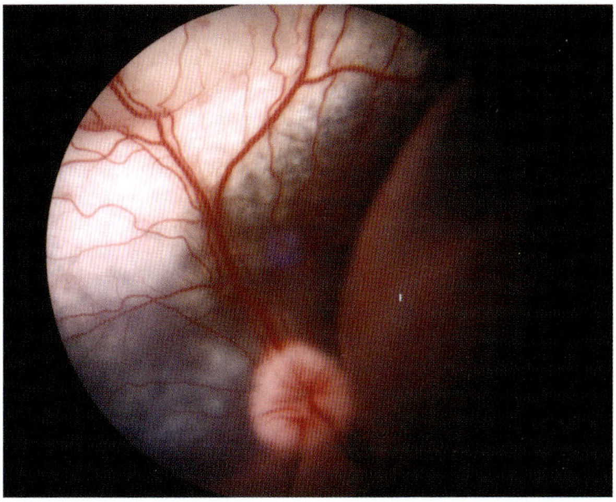

Bullous retinal detachment in a dog.
The dorsotemporal area of the left eye is affected.

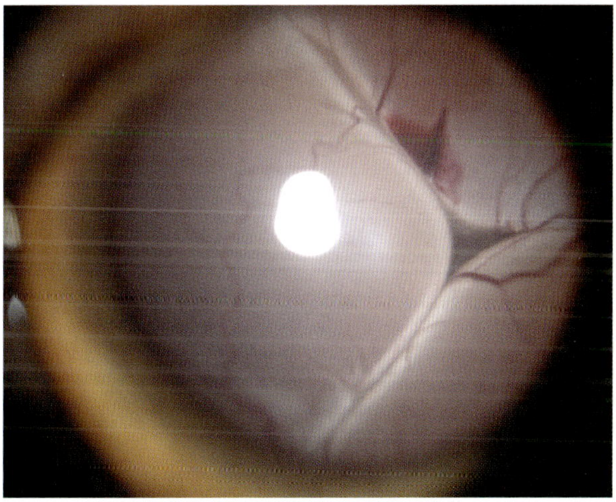

Complete bullous retinal detachment in a dog with arterial hypertension. There is an obvious intraretinal haemorrhage.

i This is a separation of the neuroretina from the retinal pigmented epithelium.

The most common causes of retinal detachment are as follows:

- Posterior uveitis.
- Arterial hypertension.
- Trauma.
- Retinal degeneration.

Retinal detachment

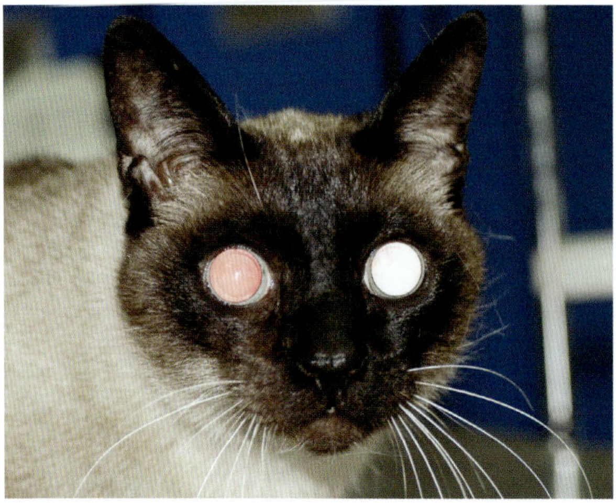

Areflexive mydriasis is one of the most common clinical signs of retinal detachment.

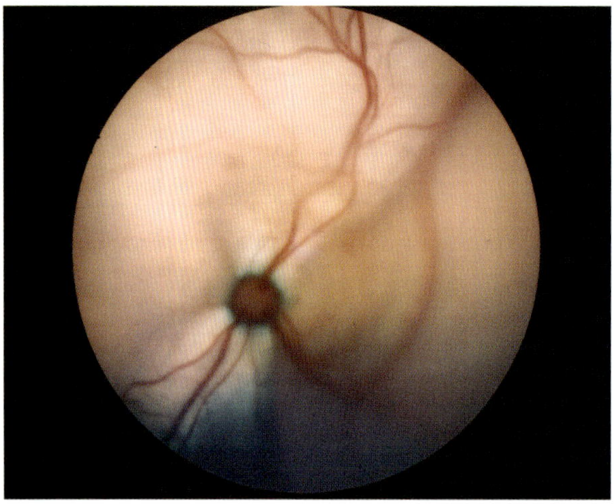

Exudative retinal detachment in a cat with arterial hypertension.

Important notes

- The inability to get the complete ocular fundus in focus using a direct ophthalmoscope may indicate a retinal detachment. If the direction of the blood vessels also changes, this is diagnostic.

Retinal detachment

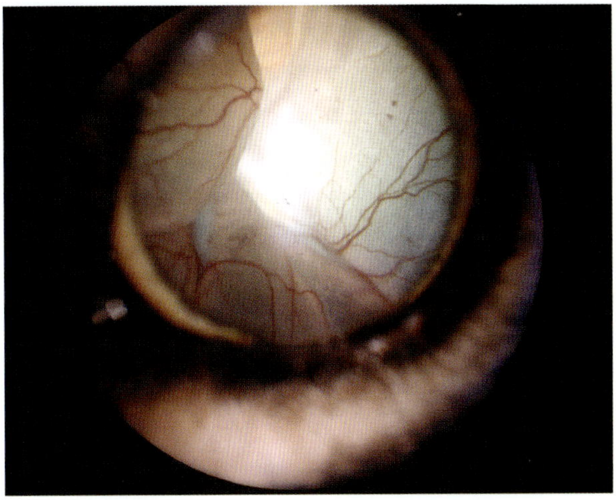

Retinal detachment is visible with a penlight; ophthalmoscopy is unnecessary.
Close-up of the retinal folds.

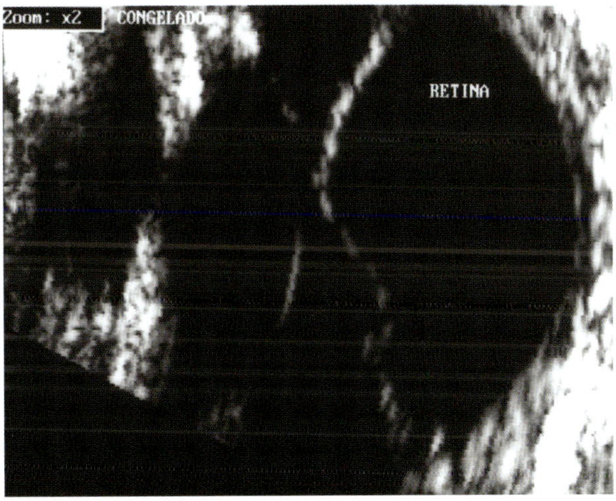

Exudative retinal detachment. B-mode ultrasound (bidimensional).

Important notes

- Ocular ultrasound is very useful in diagnosing retinal detachment, especially in case of a corneal or lens opacity.
- The ultrasound above shows a hyperechoic band with an anechoic space behind it.

Retinal detachment

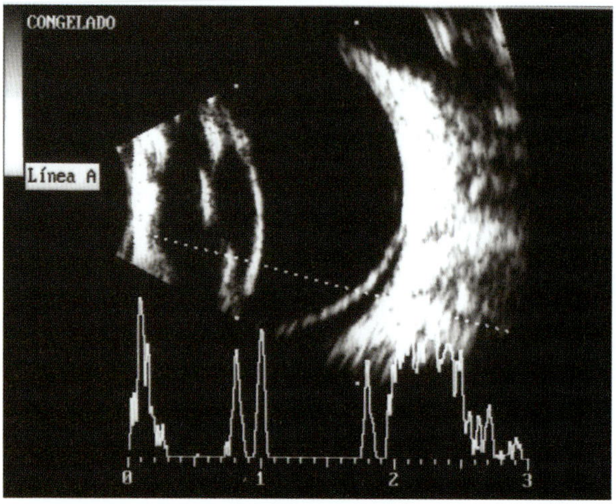

Partial retinal detachment along with a cataract in a dog.
A/B mode ultrasound.

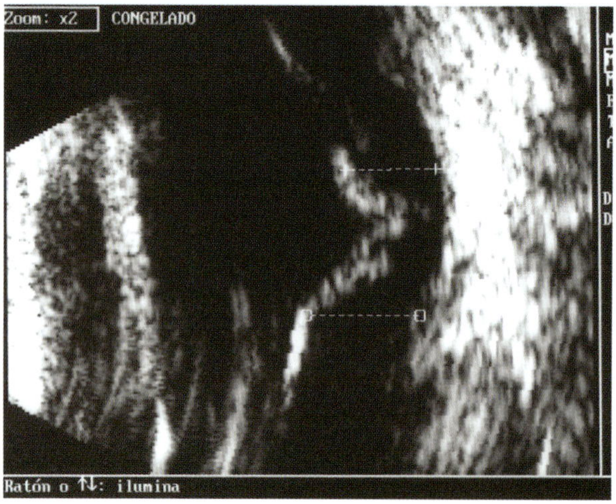

Bullous retinal detachment in a dog.
Close-up of the detachment.
B-mode ultrasound.

Important notes

- A-mode ultrasound of retinal detachment shows high-amplitude peaks. Simultaneous use of A and B modes permits examination of the area of interest.
- In exudative and bullous detachments, the retina remains attached to the ora serrata and the optic disc (see picture above).

Retinal detachment

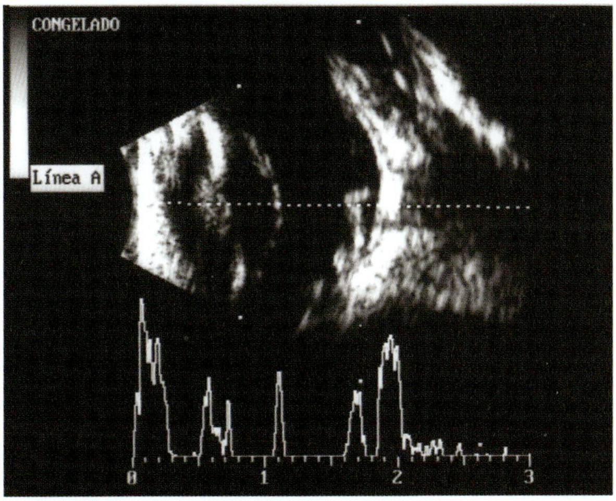

Retinal detachment with separation from the ora serrata.
A/B mode ultrasound shows a high-amplitude double peak corresponding to the dorsal retina collapsed ventrally.

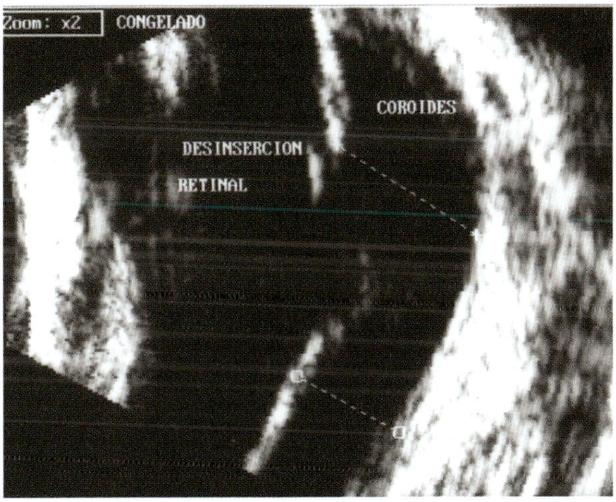

In severe posterior uveitis, retinal detachment may be accompanied by choroid detachment.

i In complete detachments, the retina often forms a V shape in the vitreous due to its points of attachment. It may assume different shapes when it detaches from the ora serrata.

Retinal haemorrhage

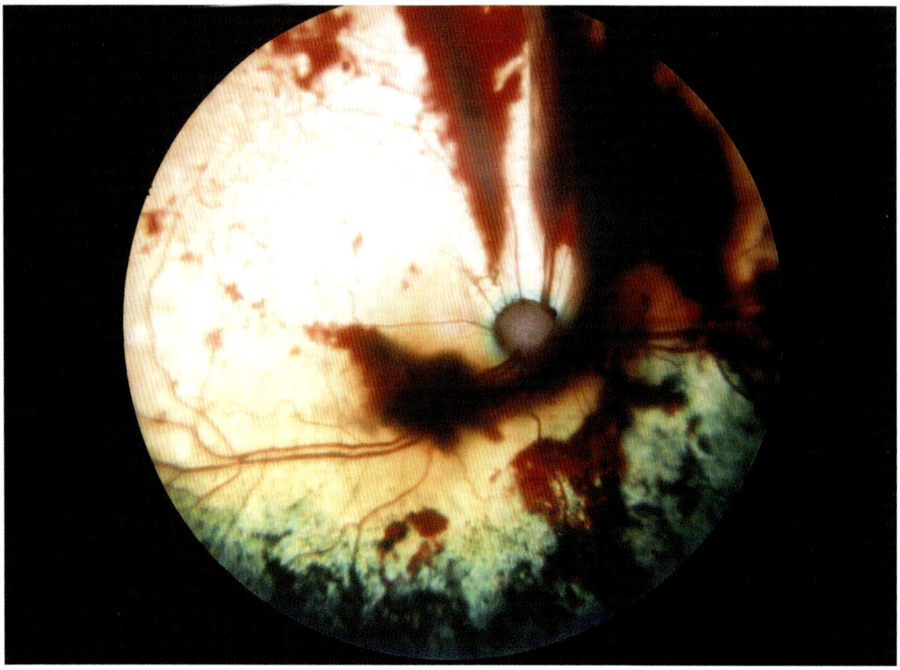

Very severe retinal haemorrhage in a cat with arterial hypertension.

i

Systemic arterial hypertension is the main cause of retinal haemorrhage in cats. Chronic renal failure, in most cases, and hyperthyroidism are the diseases that trigger hypertension.

All senior profiles should check renal and thyroid function.

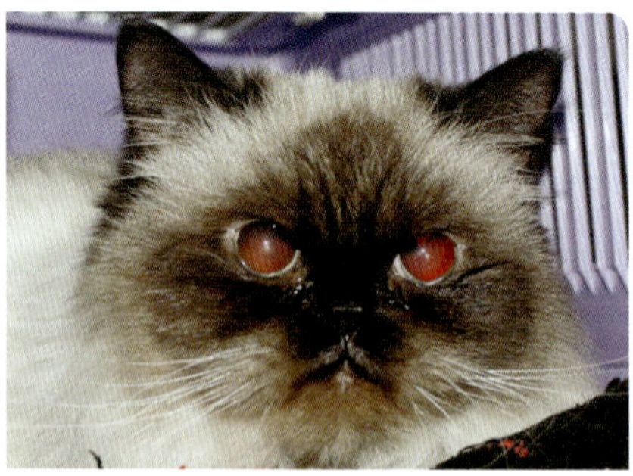

Cats with ocular effects of arterial hypertension often present with areflexive mydriasis and retinal haemorrhages.

Retinal haemorrhage

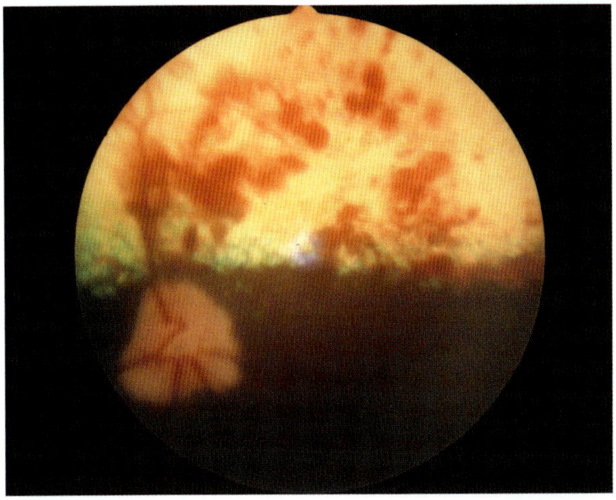

Retinal haemorrhage in a Cocker Spaniel with lymphoma.

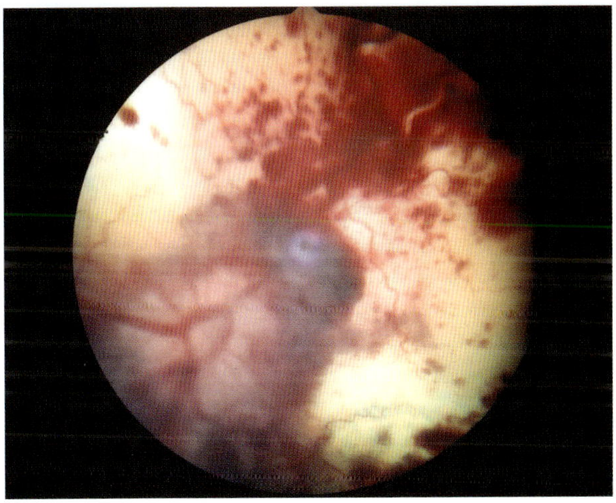

Very severe retinal haemorrhage in a dog with *Ehrlichia*.

The most common causes of retinal haemorrhage in dogs are as follows:

- Coagulopathies.
- Infectious diseases: *Ehrlichia*.
- Neoplasms.
- Hyperviscosity syndrome.
- Immune-mediated diseases: haemolytic anaemia, immune-mediated thrombocytopaenia.
- Systemic arterial hypertension.

Retinal haemorrhage

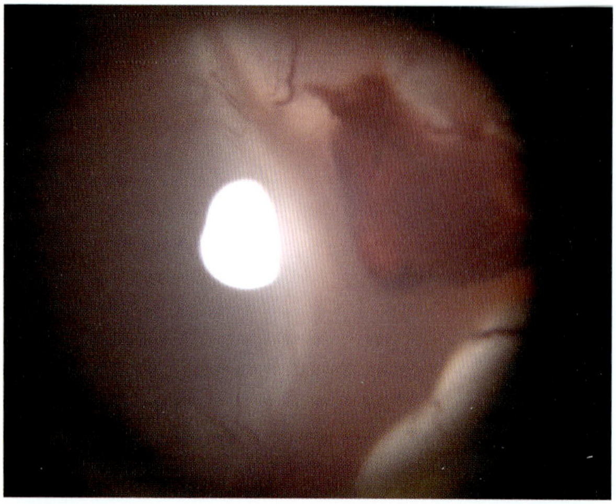

Preretinal haemorrhage in a dog, associated with bullous retinal detachment.
This type of haemorrhage assumes a boat-keel shape.

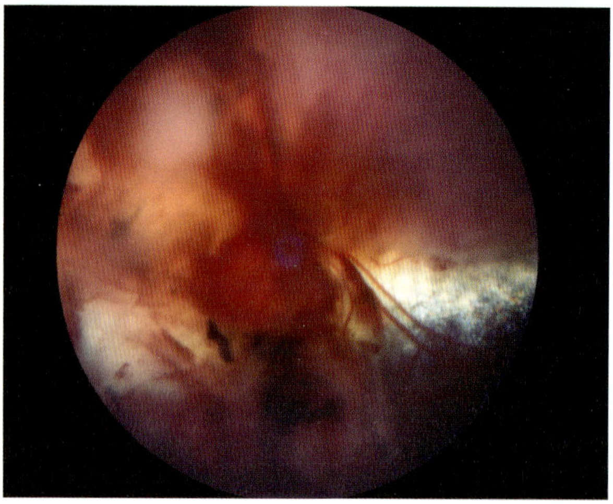

Retinal haemorrhage (pre-, intra-, and subretinal) along with retinal detachment in a cat with systemic arterial hypertension.

- Retinal haemorrhages are categorised by location:
  - Superficial intraretinal (flame-shaped).
  - Deep intraretinal.
  - Preretinal (boat keel–shaped).
  - Subretinal (shadow-shaped).

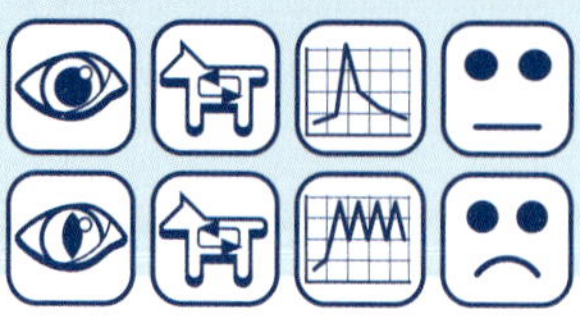

Retinal dysplasia

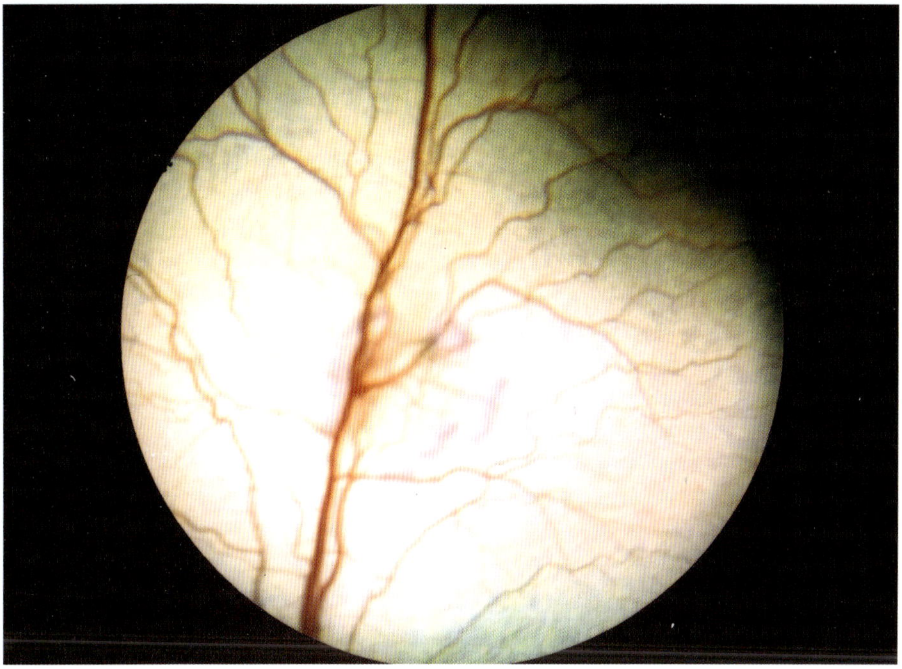

Retinal dysplasia in a Golden Retriever puppy.
Close-up of the neuroretinal folds.

Congenital, hereditary retinal disease characterised by the presence of neuroretinal folds that are separated from the pigmented epithelium.

- It generally occurs in the tapetal region.
- Retinal dysplasia may be regional or multifocal, and the vision effects depend on the retinal areas involved.

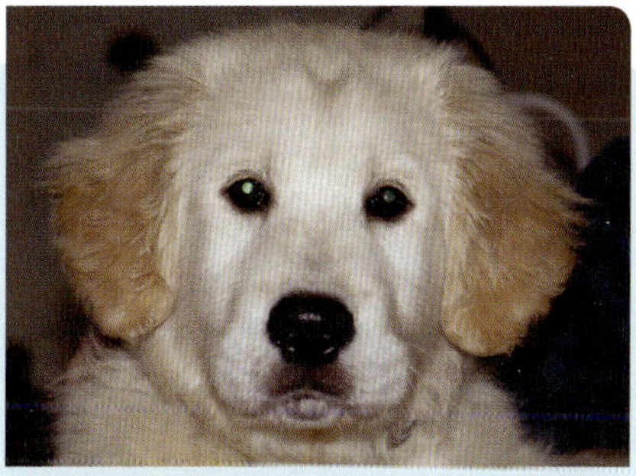

Our patient.

Optic nerve hypoplasia

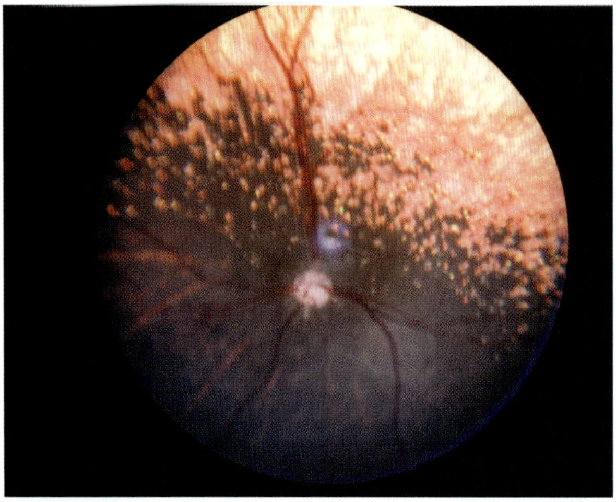

Optic nerve hypoplasia in the left eye of a Shih-Tzu.
Note the small size of the optic nerve head.
It is accompanied by areflexive mydriasis.

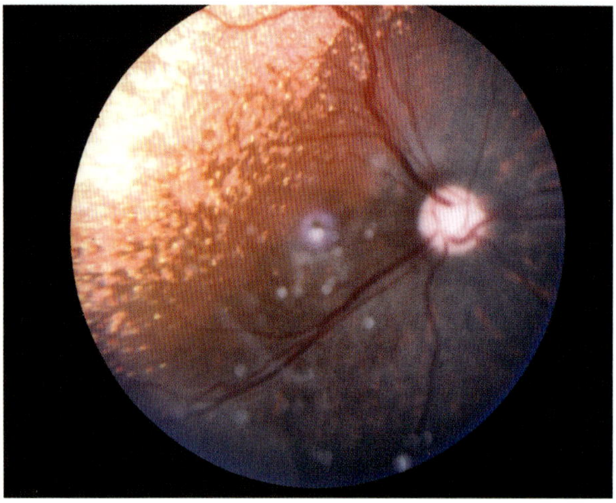

Normal right eye of the patient pictured above.
Normal-sized optic disc.

Important notes

- Optic nerve hypoplasia is a congenital disease that causes blindness, in contrast to micropapilla, which does not affect the patient's vision.
- It may occur with microphthalmos and presents unilaterally or bilaterally.

Optic neuritis

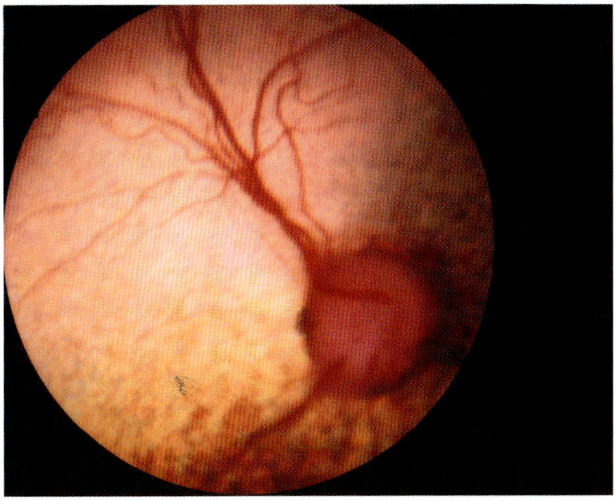

Optic neuritis in a dog with distemper.
Vascular congestion of the optic papilla and oedema are the most prominent signs on retinography.

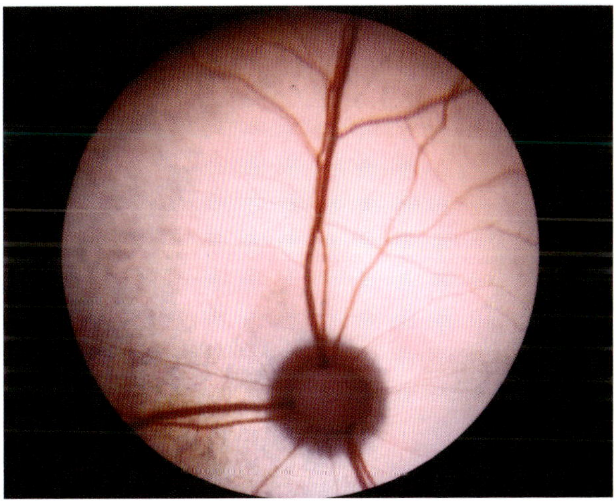

Optic neuritis in a cat with FIP.

The most common causes of optic neuritis are as follows:

- Infectious (canine distemper, feline infectious peritonitis).
- Traumatic.
- Neoplastic.
- Immune-mediated.
- Reticulosis of the CNS.

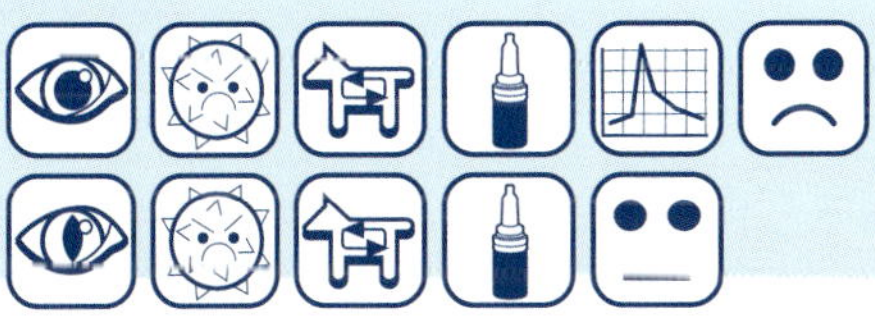

Optic neuritis

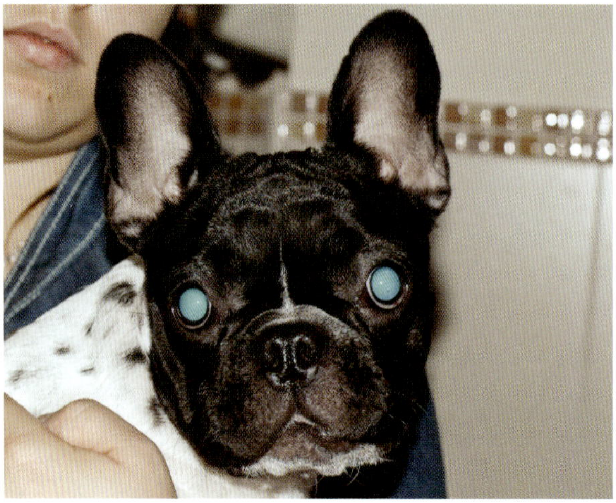

French Bulldog with bilateral areflexive mydriasis.
Acute blindness.
Time since onset: 24 hours.

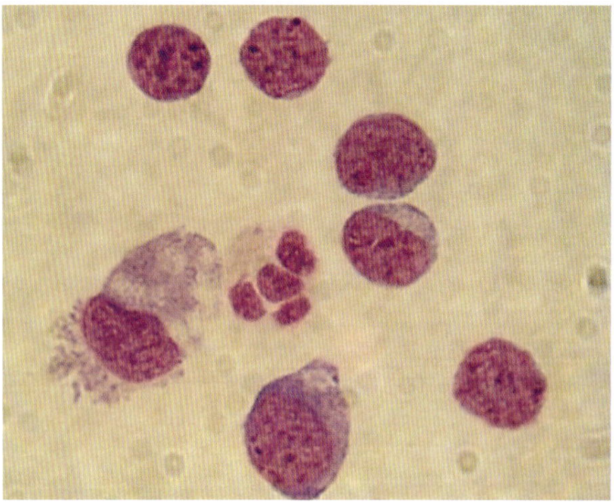

Cerebrospinal fluid cytology of the patient pictured above.
Granulomatous meningitis.
Mononuclear pleocytosis.
Picture courtesy of Dr Valentina Lorenzo.

Important notes

- Forms of optic neuritis that affect the optic nerve along its trajectory (retrobulbar or intracraneal) are not observable using direct ophthalmoscopy because the ocular fundus appears normal.
- Some types of optic neuritis are associated with meningitis or meningoencephalitis.

Retinal degeneration

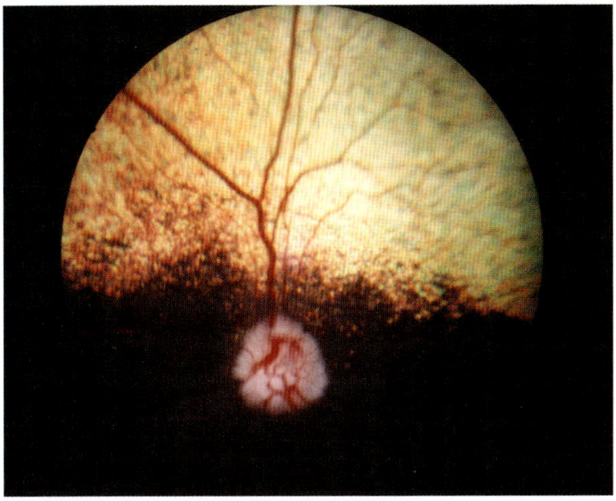

Ocular fundus of a dog in the initial phase of retinal degeneration.
Note the narrowing of the retinal arteries.
Patient with a visual deficit in the dark.

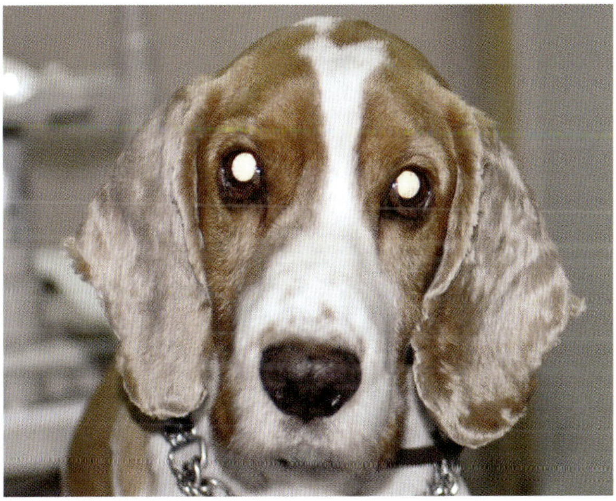

Tapetal hyperreflectivity is another clinical sign characteristic of retinal degeneration.

Progressive degeneration of retinal photoreceptors has a hereditary component in certain breeds (Cocker Spaniel, Miniature Poodle, and Labrador Retriever) and the most common clinical signs are:

- Narrowing of retinal vessels.
- Tapetal hyperreflectivity.
- Pale optic papilla.
- Changes in pigment distribution.

Retinal degeneration

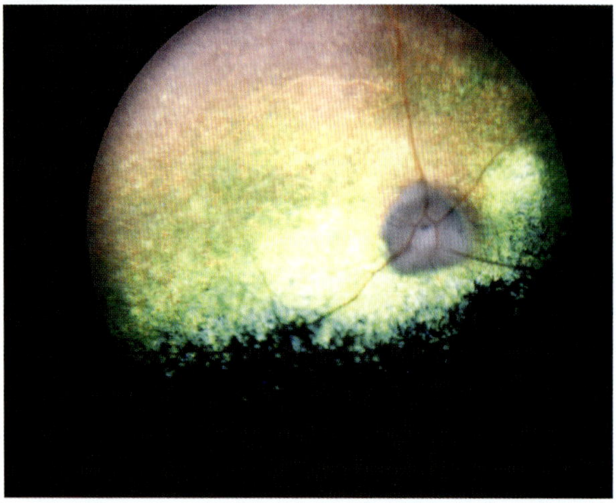

Severe retinal degeneration. Close-up of the narrowed retinal vessels and the greyish aspect of the optic papilla.

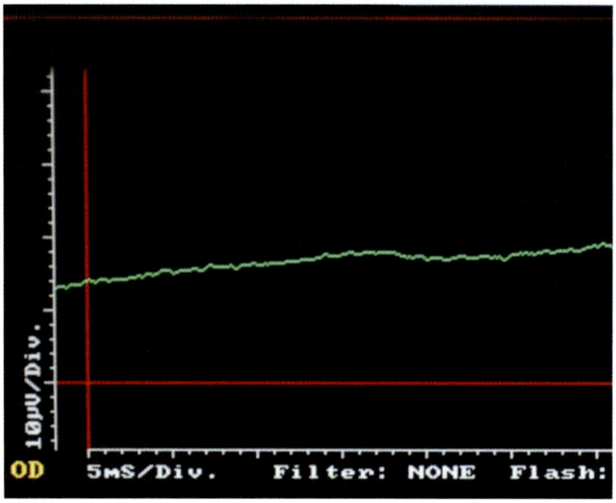

Flat electroretinogram from a dog with retinal photoreceptor degeneration. End stage of the disease.

Important notes

- No cure exists for this bilateral degenerative disease of the retina.
- Early diagnosis and the use of nutritional supplements (selenium, vitamin E) for the retina may help the patient.

Globe and orbit

Enophthalmos

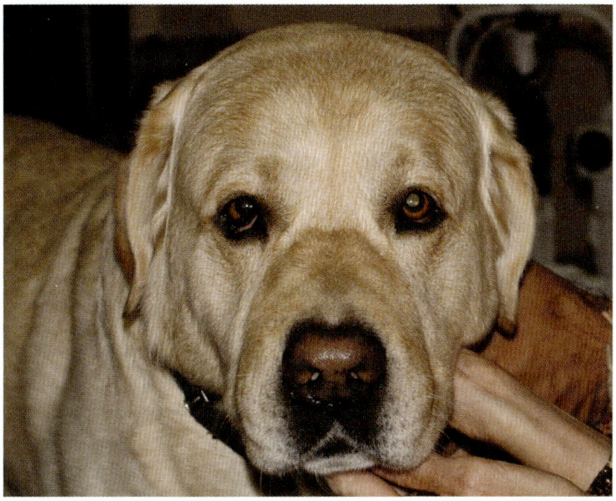

Labrador Retriever with enophthalmos of the right eye.
Protrusion of the nictitating membrane.
Horner's syndrome.

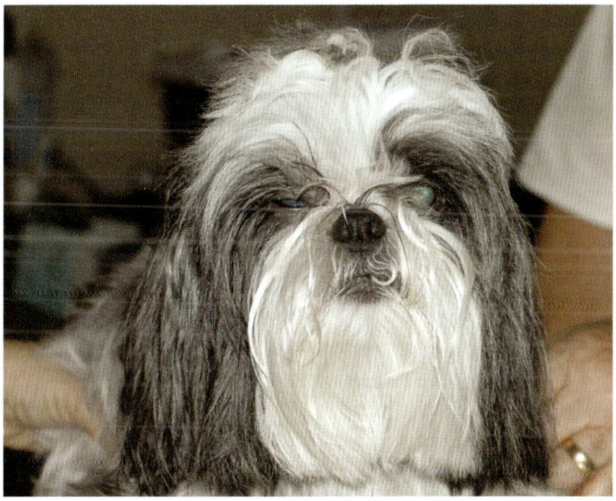

Enophthalmos of the right eye in a Shih-Tzu with a corneal ulcer.

This is a normal-sized globe that is sunken within the orbital cavity.

Interesting notes

Enophthalmos may result from pain in patients with uveitis or corneal ulcers, in conjunction with neurological conditions (Horner's syndrome), from states of dehydration, or be observed incidentally in dolicocephalic dog breeds.

Exophthalmos

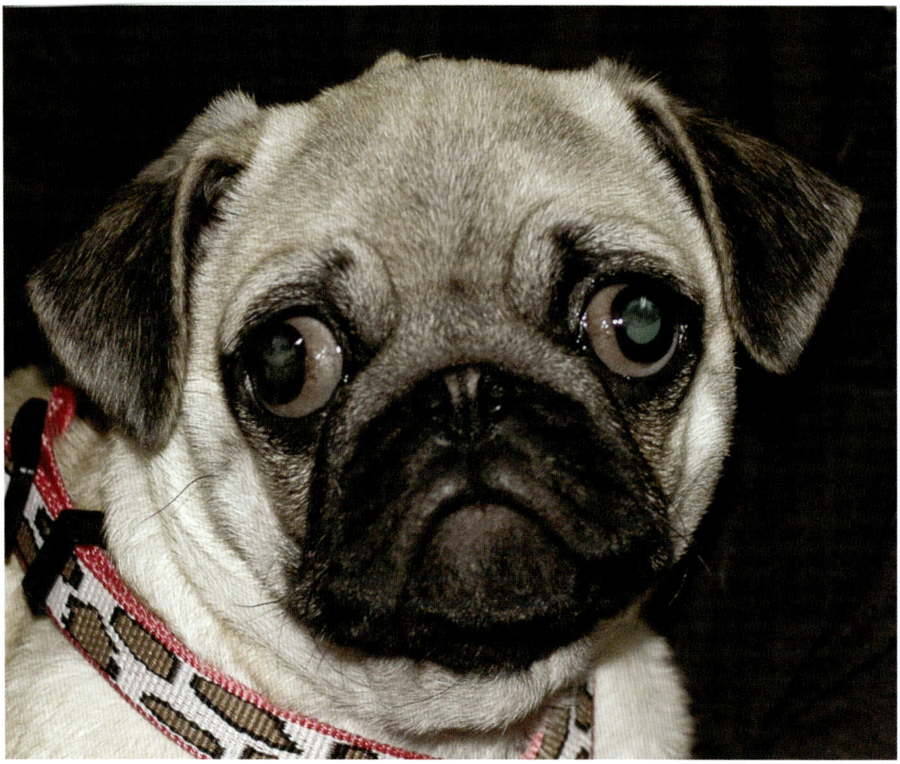

Bilateral exophthalmos in a Pug. Excessive exposure of the globes.

i | Normal-sized globe placed more externally in the orbital cavity.

Interesting notes

Exophthalmos is part of the anatomical conformation of brachycephalic breeds (Pug, Shih-Tzu, Lhasa Apso, Pekingese, French Bulldog, etc.).

Exophthalmos

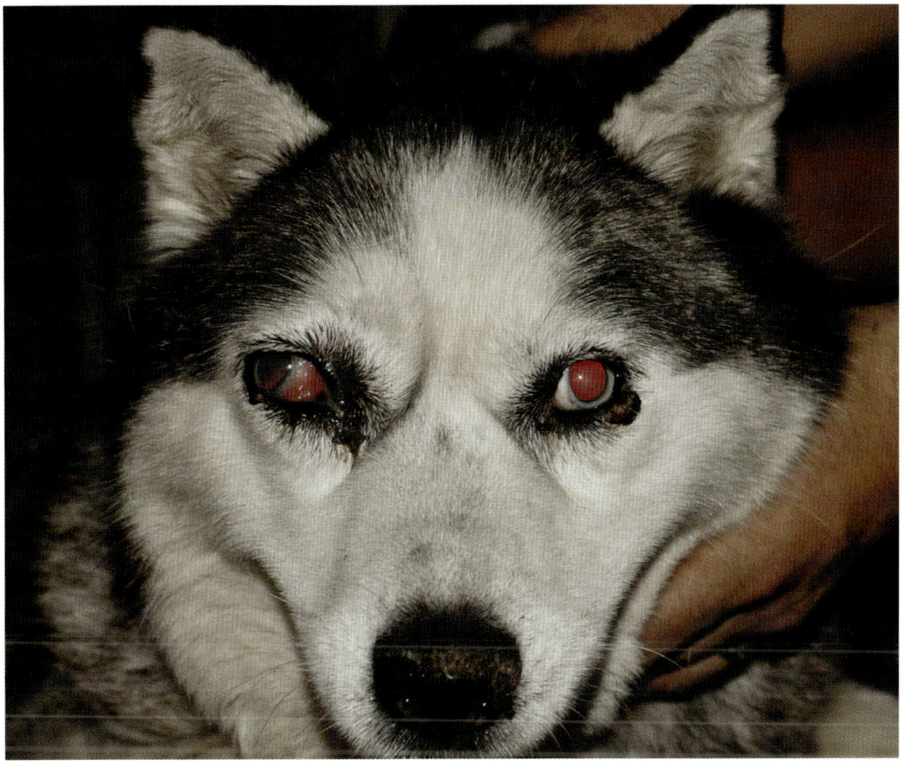

Exophthalmos of the right eye in a Siberian Husky. Time since onset: four days. Retrobulbar abscess.

i

Exophthalmos may also occur in patients with orbital diseases (cellulitis, abscesses, neoplasms, extraocular polymyositis, mucocoeles, etc.) or as a result of trauma.

Important notes

DO NOT CONFUSE exophthalmos with buphthalmos.

Atrophy of the globe

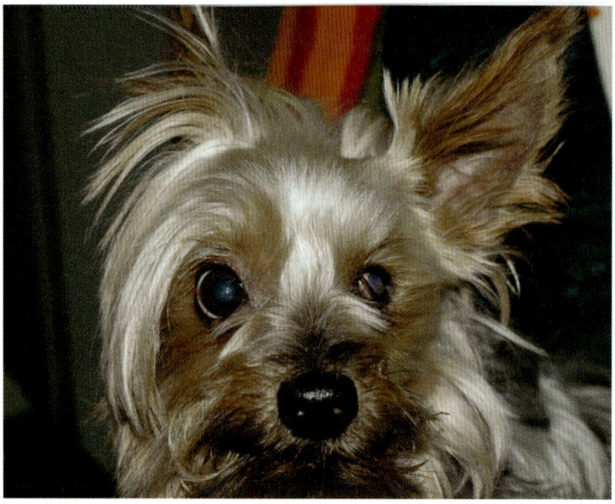

Atrophy of the left globe (phthisis bulbi) in a Yorkshire Terrier who suffered a post-traumatic uveitis eight months earlier. The nictitating membrane protrudes due to a lack of support.

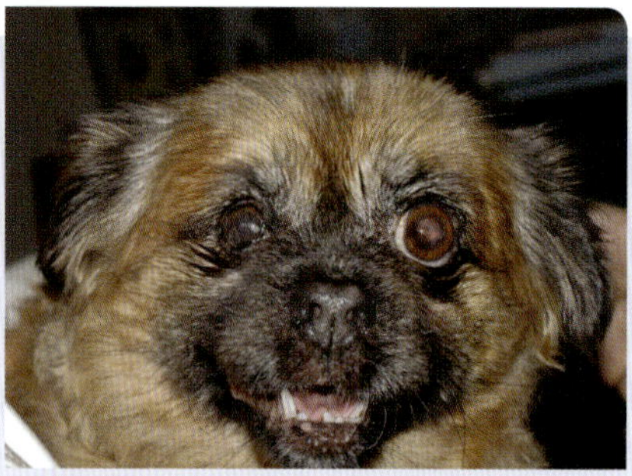

Atrophy of the globe resulting from corneal perforation. The right eye is smaller.

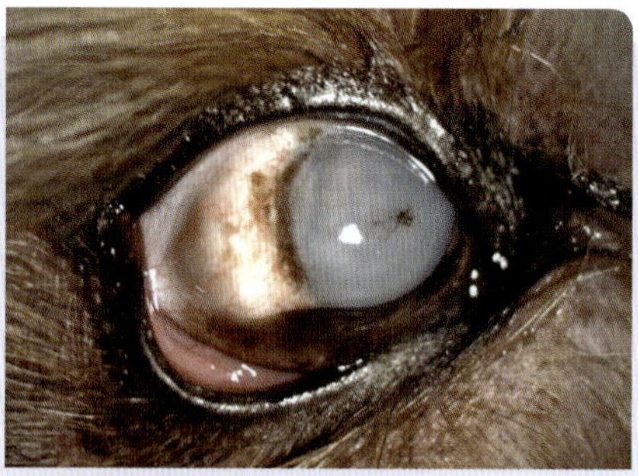

Chronic glaucoma, blind eye.

Interesting notes

- Atrophy of the globe (phthisis bulbi) may result from severe intraocular damage (trauma or penetrating wound) or from anterior uveitis or cyclitis (ciliary body inflammation).
- The intravitreal injection of gentamicin can induce atrophy of the globe in patients with chronic glaucoma (if the eye is blind), by chemically destroying the ciliary body. The patient in the lower right picture may be a candidate.

Buphthalmos

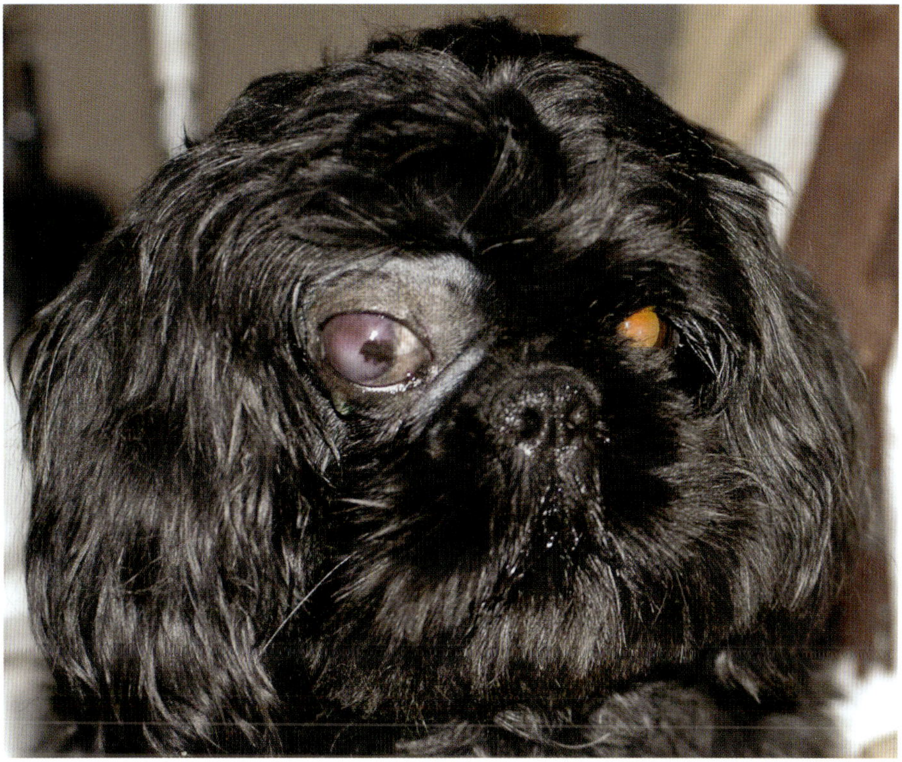

Patient with buphthalmos in the right eye. Close-up of the globe deformity.
Time since onset: six months.
Cause: chronic glaucoma secondary to traumatic uveitis.

i This globe is larger than normal due to distension of the fibrous tunic of the eye (cornea and sclera).

Buphthalmos

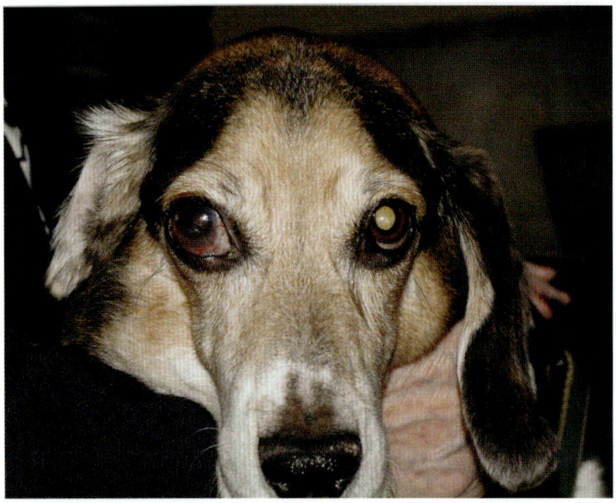

Buphthalmic right eye of a 12-year-old dog.
Time since onset: 45 days.
Intraocular pressure: 41 mmHg.
Cause: glaucoma secondary to an intraocular tumour.

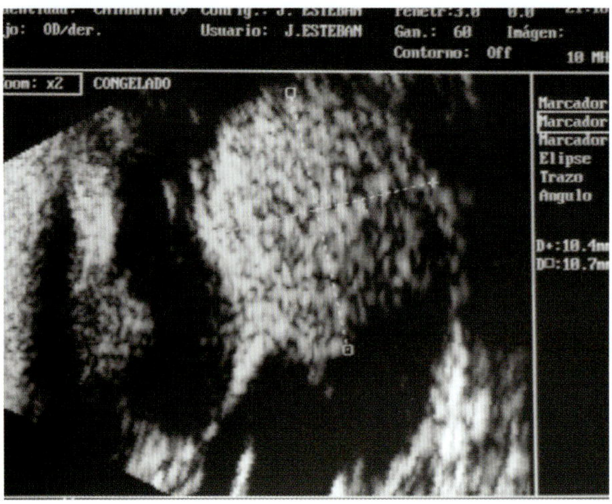

Ocular ultrasound of the patient. Close-up of the intraocular neoplasm.

Important notes

- Chronic glaucoma and intraocular neoplasms are the main causes of buphthalmos.
- THE EYE IS ALWAYS BLIND.

Buphthalmos

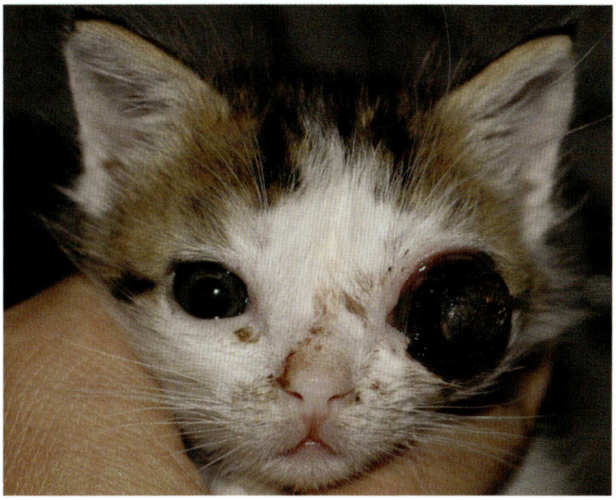

Fourteen-day-old domestic shorthair cat with buphthalmos of the right eye and severe exposure keratitis (crusting).

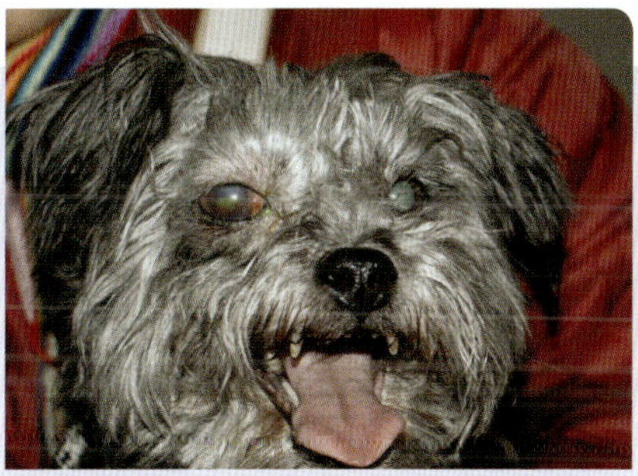

Buphthalmos in a dog after 12 months. Cause: traumatic uveitis and secondary glaucoma following a fight with another dog.

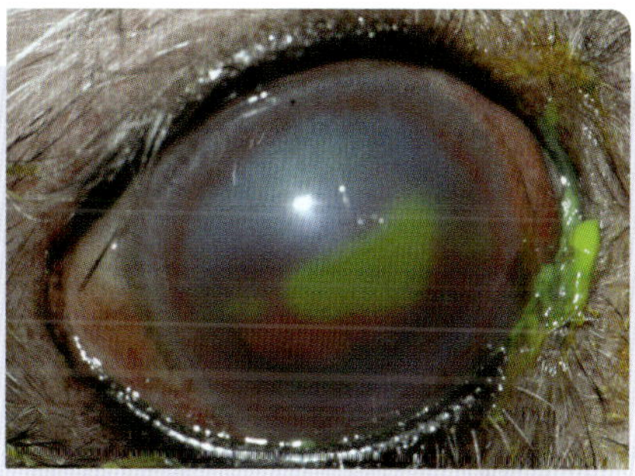

Exposure keratitis from buphthalmos in the same patient as in the previous picture. Central fluorescein uptake.

Treatment

Several surgical options exist:

- Enucleation (if the cornea is damaged).
- Exenteration (in case of an intraocular neoplasm).
- Intrascleral prosthesis (if there is no neoplasm and the cornea is healthy).
- Intravitreal injection of gentamicin (in animals with an anaesthaesic risk or if the owner is financially constrained). Do not perform in cats.

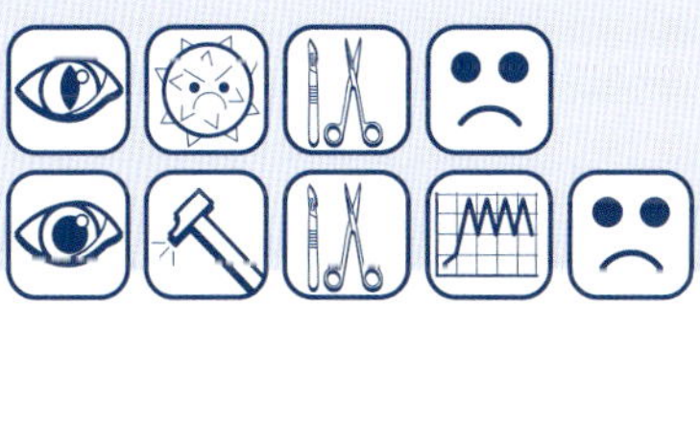

Retrobulbar abscess

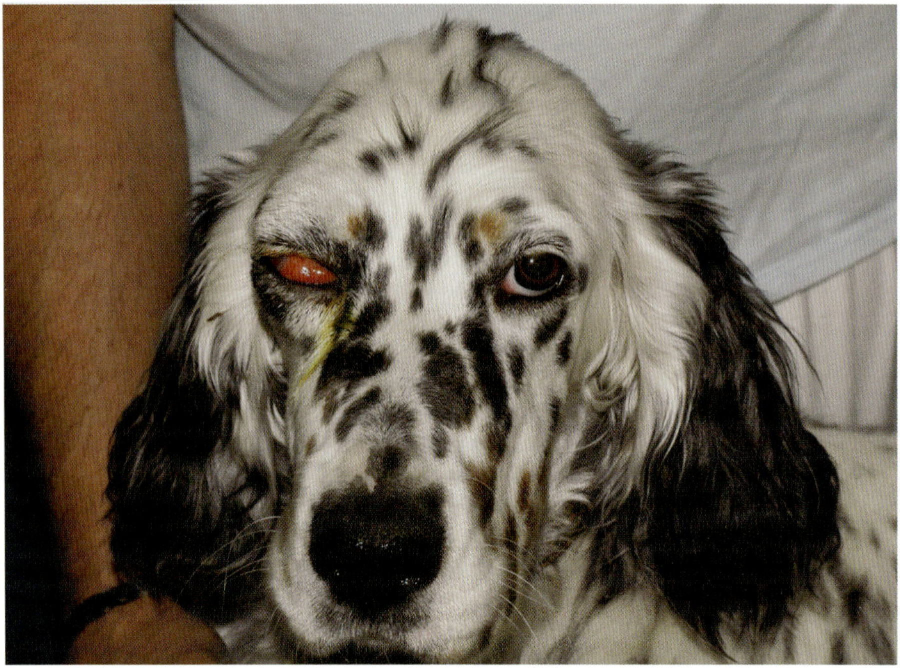

Eight-year-old English Setter with a retrobulbar abscess. Time since onset: three days. Close-up of the exophthalmos and protrusion of the nictitating membrane.

Interesting notes

The most common clinical signs of retrobulbar abscess are the following:

- Exophthalmos.
- Protrusion of the nictitating membrane.
- Pain when opening the mouth.
- Anorexia.
- Depression.
- Fever (often with neutrophilic leukocytosis).
- Resistance to retropulsion of the globe.

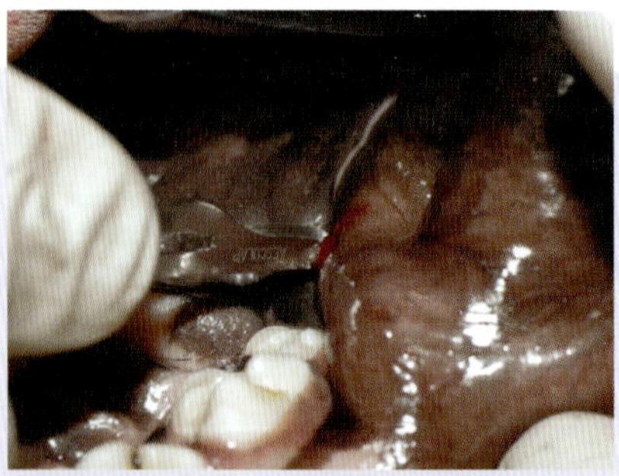

The patient demonstrated severe pain when opening the mouth. The picture shows a bulge in the oral mucosa behind the last molar. Characteristic clinical sign of a retrobulbar abscess.

Retrobulbar abscess

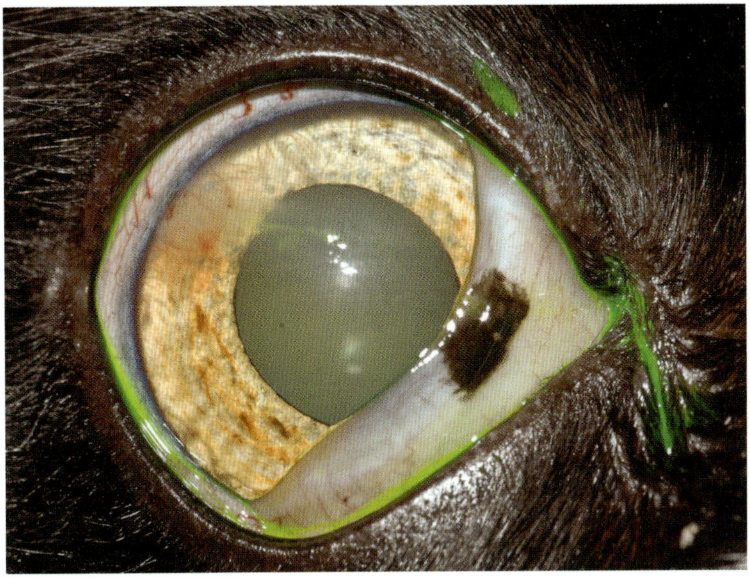

Exophthalmos, exposure keratitis, and protrusion of the nictitating membrane in a cat who presented with a retrobulbar abscess.
Time since onset: 13 days.

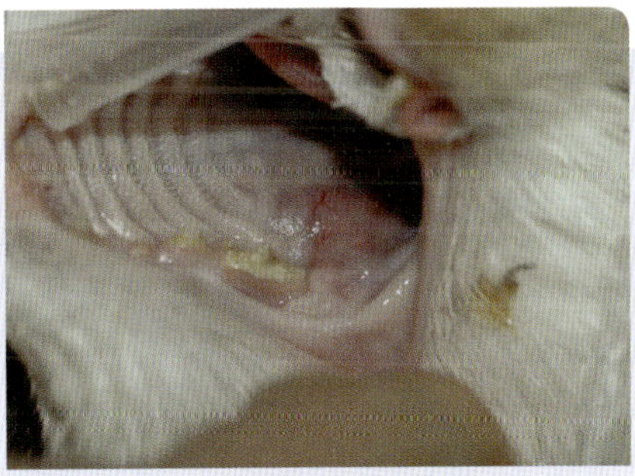

Examination of the patient's oral cavity. The picture shows hyperaemia and a bulge in the oral mucosa caudal to the last molar.

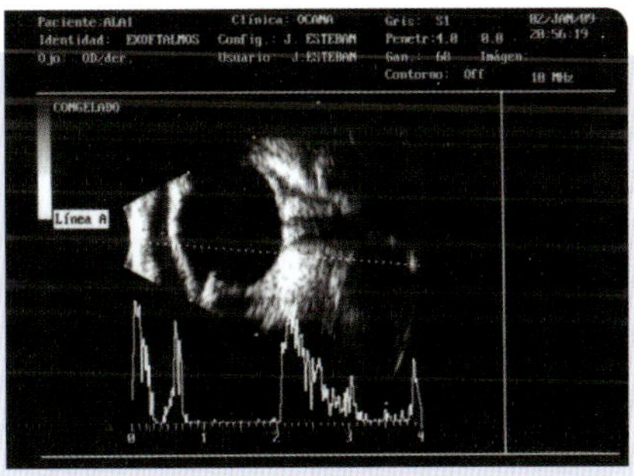

A/B mode orbital ultrasound.
Image of the retrobulbar abscess.

Interesting notes

The most common causes of retrobulbar abscesses are the following:

- Buccal disease (involving tooth roots).
- Foreign bodies.
- Penetrating wounds or bone fractures.
- Haematogenous spread.
- Neoplasms.
- Sinusitis.

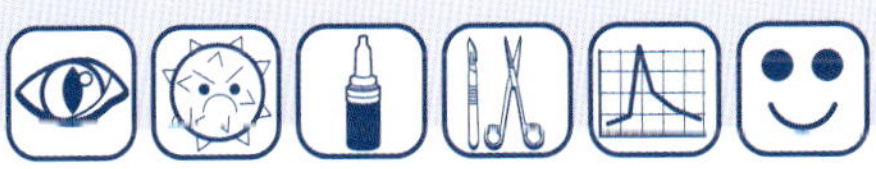

Retrobulbar abscess

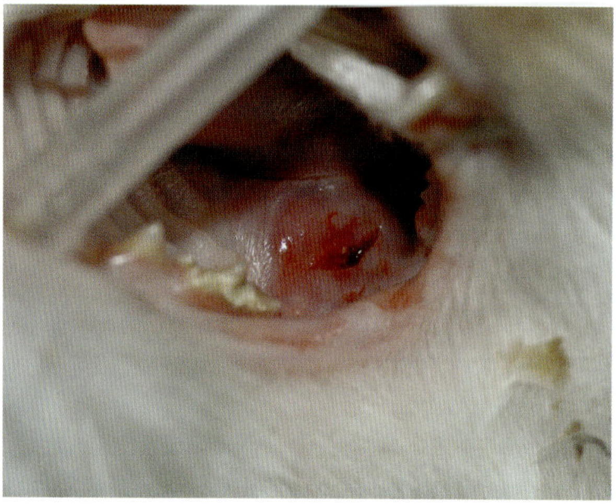

Superficial incision of the oral mucosa with a scalpel blade.

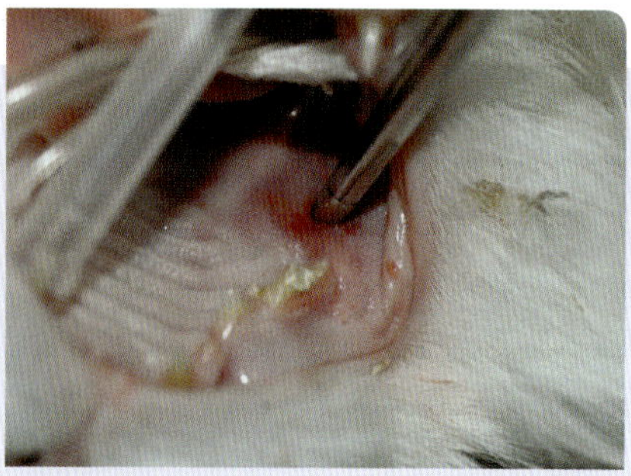

Approach the retrobulbar space with a blunt instrument, and do not open it inside.

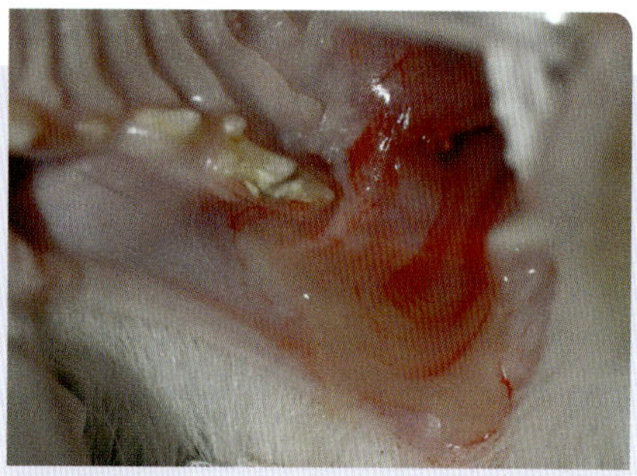

Drainage of the abscess. Release of purulent material.

Contraindicated

- NEVER approach the orbital cavity with a cutting or puncturing instrument: the maxillary artery may be nicked!
- DO NOT EXPLORE TOO DEEPLY inside the cavity: the optic nerve may be damaged or the sclera perforated!

Important notes

- Perform under general anaesthesia with the animal intubated.
- Provide systemic antibiotics and anti-inflammatories with the surgical treatment.
- Apply artificial tears to the cornea.

Orbital cellulitis

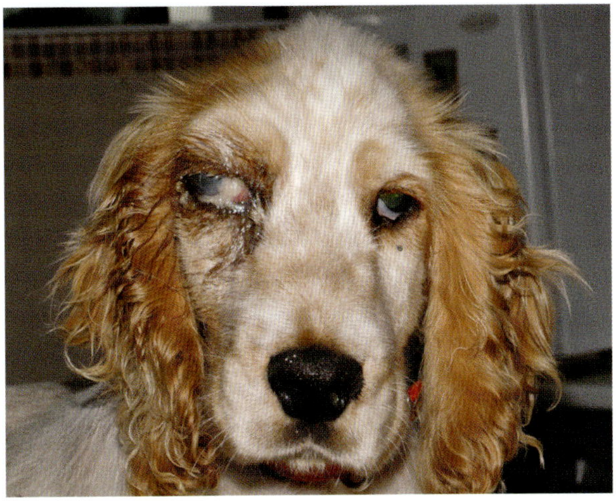

Six-month-old Cocker Spaniel with orbital cellulitis.
Time since onset: 12 hours.
Facial swelling, exophthalmos, and protrusion of the nictitating membrane.

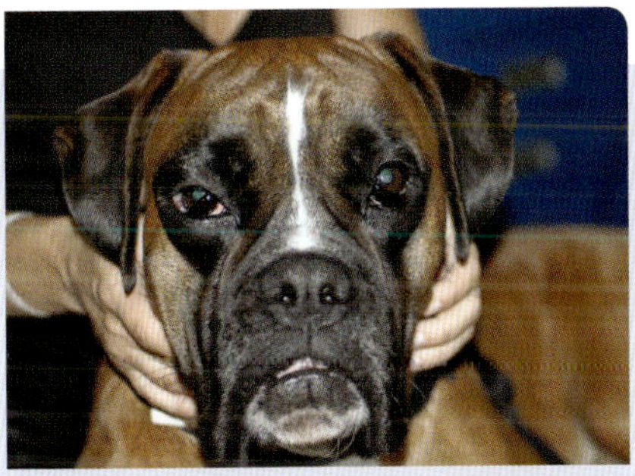

Twelve-month-old Boxer with orbital cellulitis on the right side.

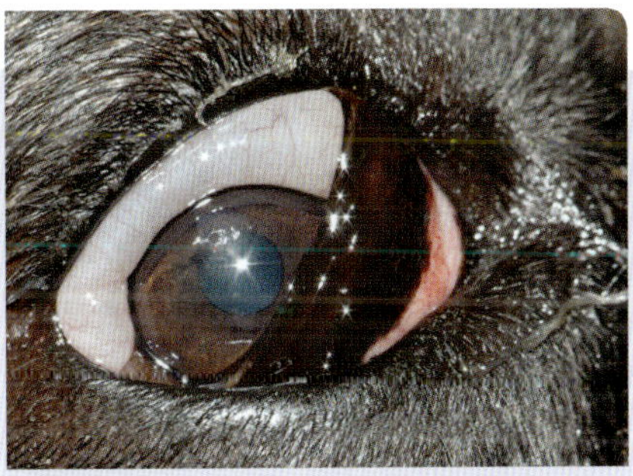

Close-up of the Boxer's eye. Chemosis, protrusion of the nictitating membrane, exophthalmos, and ocular secretions are visible.

Interesting notes

- Orbital cellulitis is a diffuse inflammation of the orbital tissue.
- It presents more acutely than retrobulbar abscess does.
- It tends to affect juvenile animals and may be seasonal.
- The orbital ultrasound (A-mode) peaks are of greater amplitude than in retrobulbar abscesses.

Orbital neoplasms

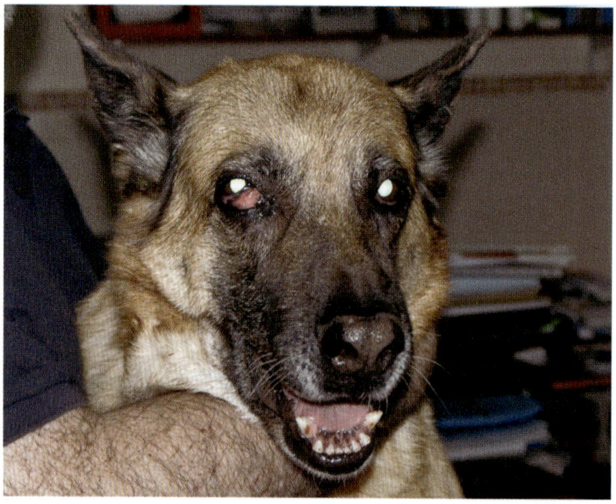

Ten-year-old German Shepherd with signs of orbital disease (protrusion of the nictitating membrane, exophthalmos, strabismus, and epiphora). Duration of progression: six months. No pain when opening the mouth.

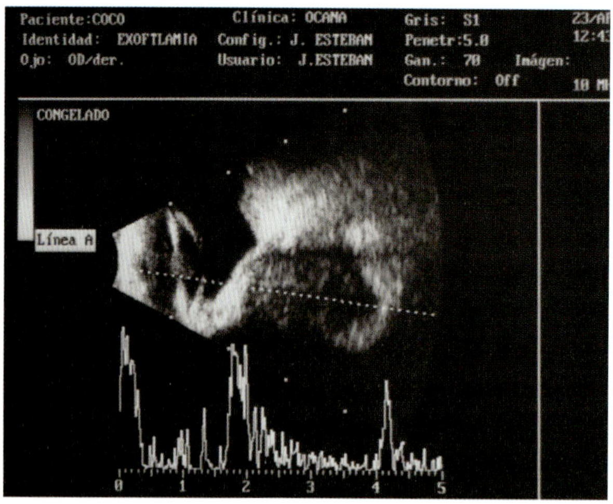

A/B mode ultrasound of the patient. Zygomatic salivary gland adenocarcinoma.

Important notes

- Orbital neoplasms tend to affect older animals.
- Clinical signs may appear slowly and progressively (in contrast to retrobulbar abscess).
- Retropulsion of the globe is often decreased or impossible.
- Ocular ultrasound (mainly A-mode) offers a great deal of information on the size, location, borders, and possible nature (ultrasound-tissue correlation) of the lesion.

Orbital neoplasms

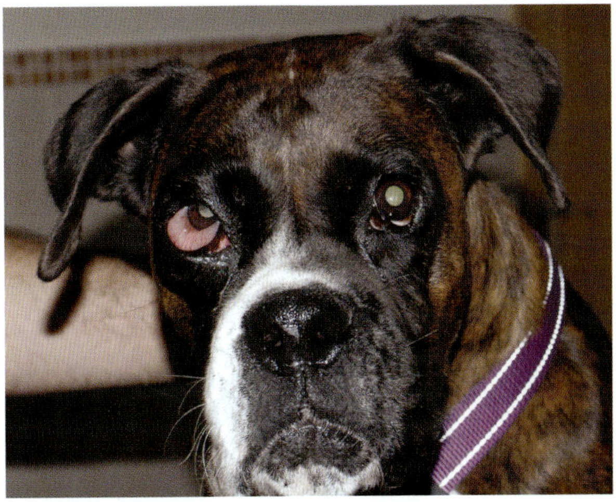

Six-year-old Boxer with orbital disease for the past four months. Inflammation of the periocular tissue, protrusion of the nictitating membrane, and conjunctival chemosis are present.

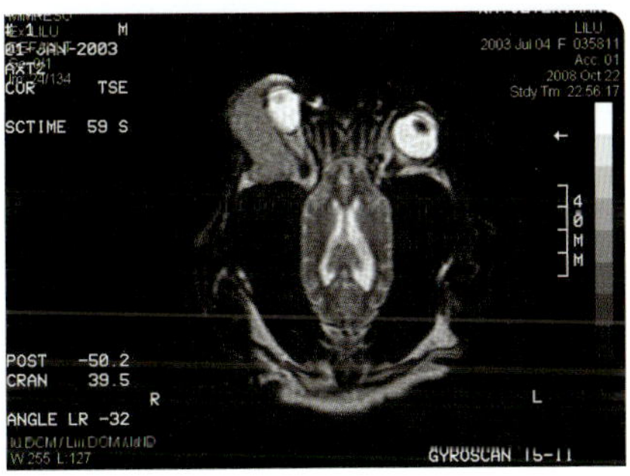

MRI of the patient. T2-weighted dorsal image. Periorbital extraconal neoplasm with infiltration of the zygomatic bone.

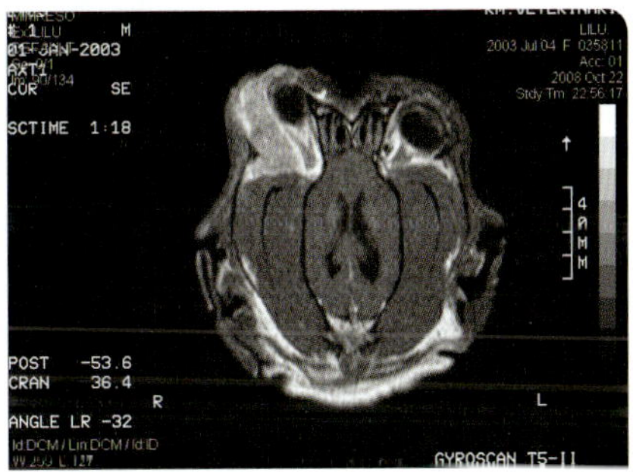

MRI with paramagnetic contrast. Images courtesy of Dr Valentina Lorenzo (Resonancia Magnética Veterinaria).

Interesting notes

- MRI and CT are the most informative diagnostic modalities for orbital neoplasms.
- Orbital neoplasms may be primary or metastatic, and the most common types are fibrosarcomas, lymphosarcomas, adenocarcinomas, meningiomas and squamous cell carcinomas, among others.

Foreign bodies

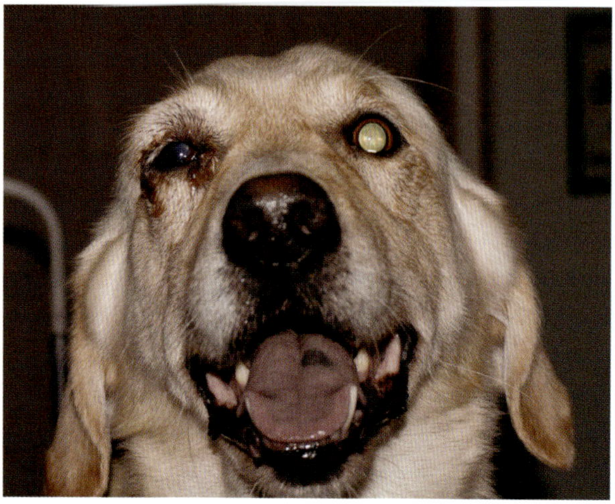

Six-year-old Labrador Retriever with intense blepharospasm and photophobia in the right eye. Copious ocular secretions. Time since onset: 72 hours.

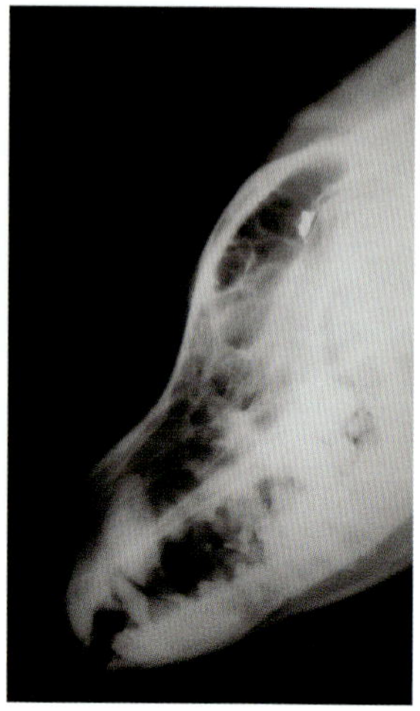

The radiograph shows a pellet lodged in the bone of the orbital cavity. It entered at 12 o'clock and passed through the globe to within 2 mm of the corneoscleral limbus.

Important notes

- When a foreign body is suspected, sedate the animal to perform a detailed examination of the orbit (radiographs, MRI, and/or CT scan) and the intraocular structures (ocular ultrasound).
- The most common foreign bodies in the orbital cavity are shotgun pellets, grass awns, bone fragments (in cases of fracture), and wood splinters (from the oral cavity).

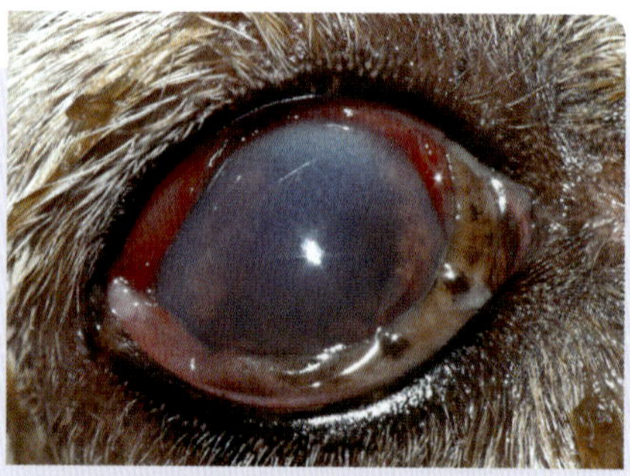

Close-up of the subconjunctival haemorrhage and the intraocular damage (corneal oedema and rubeosis of the iris).

Proptosis

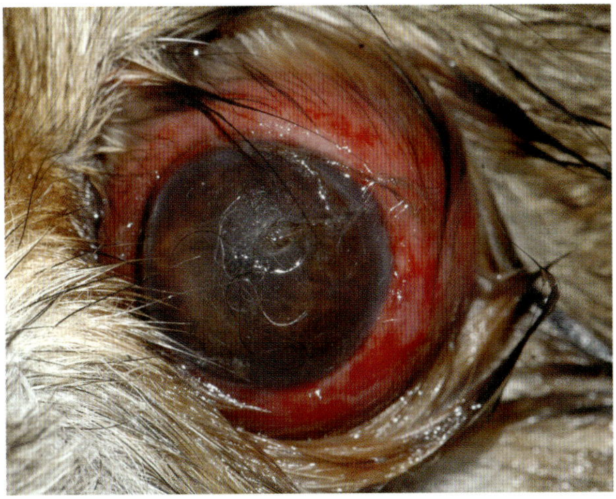

Proptosis of the left eye in a Pomeranian.
Time since onset: 18 hours.
Subconjunctival haemorrhage and exposure keratitis.
Cause: a fight with another dog.

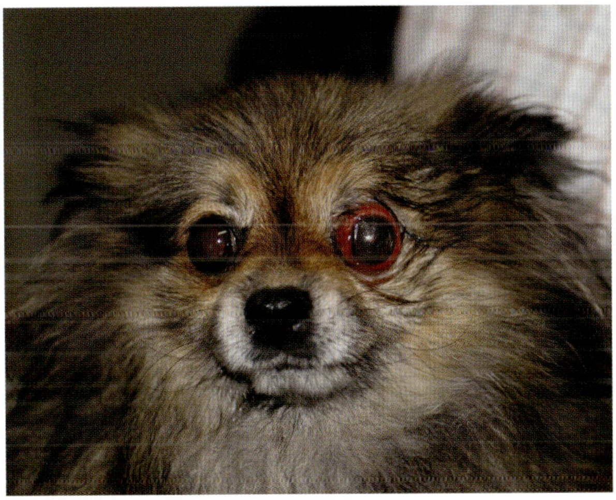

View from a distance.
Close-up of the asymmetric globe positions.

Proptosis is luxation of the globe from the orbital cavity that extends beyond the palpebral margin.

- It is often seen in brachycephalic breeds (Pug, Pekingese, Shih-Tzu, Lhasa Apso, French Bulldog, etc.). Luxation of the globe in these breeds may result from overexcitement, while playing, or while barking (due to their anatomical conformation).
- Dogs of other breeds as well as cats can suffer proptosis following a severe facial trauma.

Proptosis

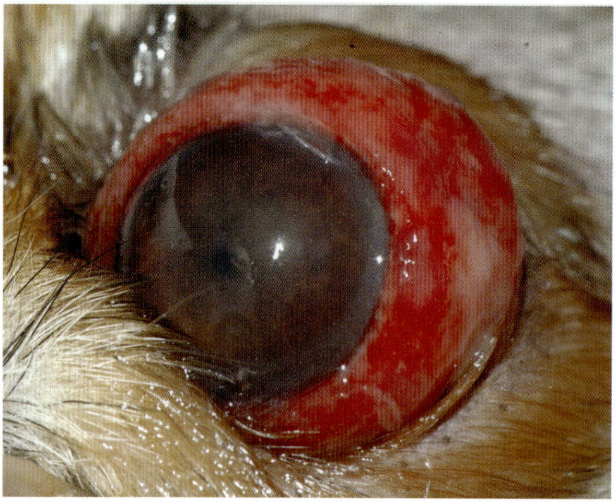

Irrigate and moisten the eye constantly until the globe is returned to the orbital cavity.

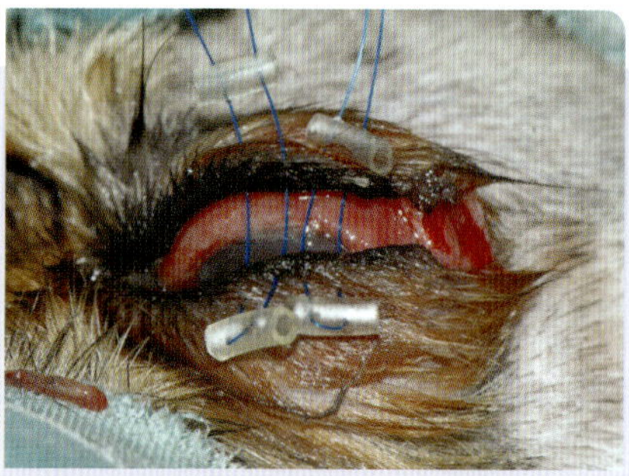

A lateral canthotomy helps to return the globe to its original position. Always cross the palpebral margin through the secretory ducts of the Meibomian glands.

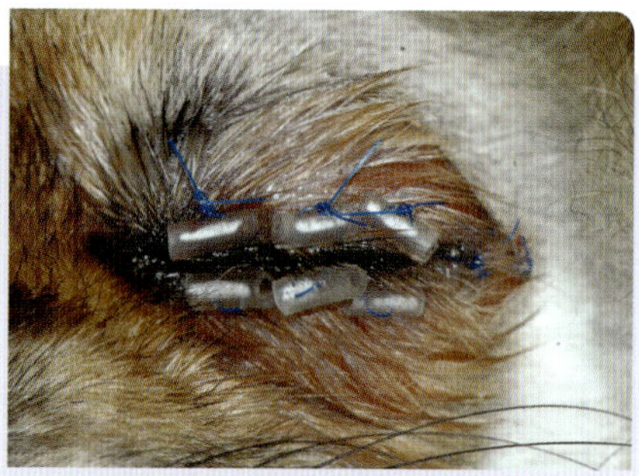

Closure of the lateral canthotomy. Leave the blepharorraphy and/or tarsorraphy in place for at least 20 days.

Important notes

- Following proptosis, preservation of optic nerve function is the main goal. NEUROPROTECTION.
- The viability of the optic nerve will depend on the severity of the proptosis and the time that elapses between the proptosis and the surgery.
- The secondary goal is to treat the exposure keratitis.

Proptosis

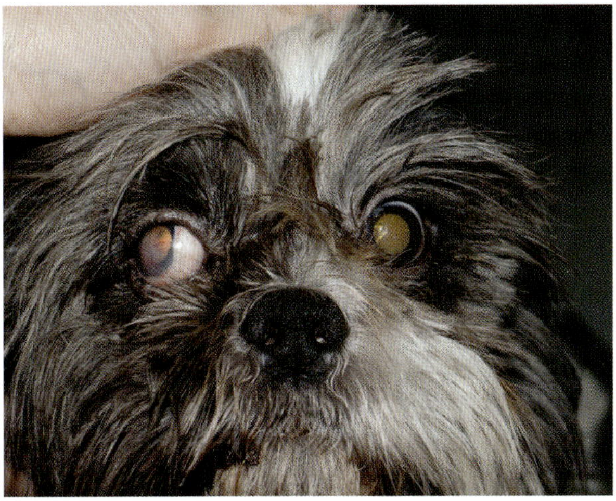

Divergent strabismus (exotropia) in a patient who had proptosis.
Picture taken 35 days after the luxation (the patient was treated).

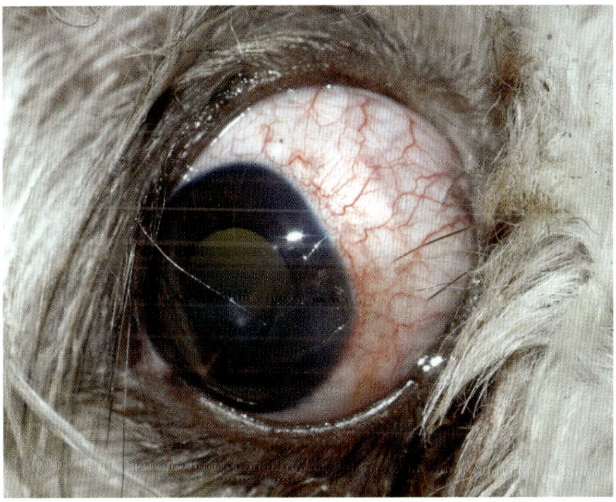

The exotropia is due to rupture of medial rectus muscle at the time of proptosis.

Interesting notes

- Divergent strabismus generally resolves over time (three months).
- The use of botulinum toxin can help correct exotropia in these patients (Morales Fariña, De León Vera, Morales Doreste, 2009).
- Medial canthoplasty protects the cornea after proptosis and prevents subsequent luxation of the globe.

Proptosis

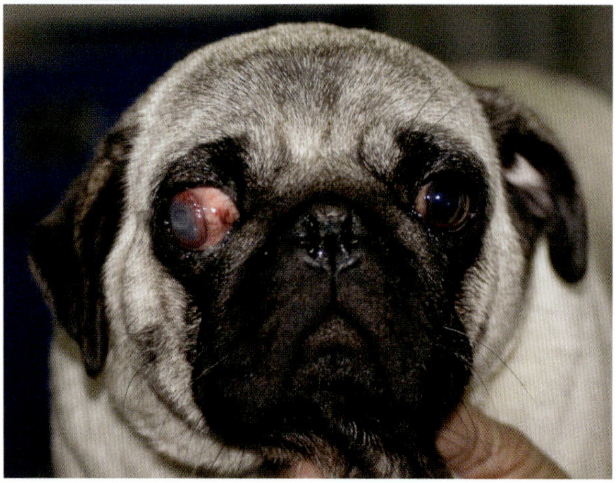

Divergent strabismus and corneal ulcer due to proptosis. Corneal oedema and neovascularisation characteristic of uveitis associated with corneal damage.

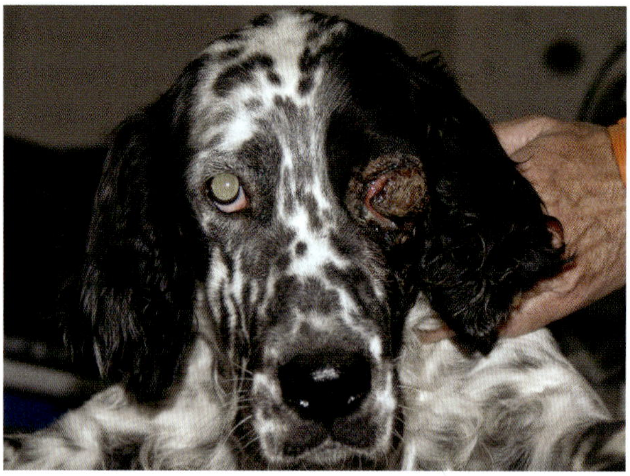

Proptosis of the left eye after six days. Purulent secretions and crusts are present on the cornea.
The right eye is mydriatic.
The patient is blind due to bilateral optic nerve damage.

Important notes

- Always examine the pupillary light reflex in both eyes because neurological damage can be bilateral.
- A luxated globe should be replaced as rapidly as possible.
- Postoperative treatment: systemic anti-inflammatories (corticosteroids), systemic antibiotics (cephalosporins), and topical antibiotics (chloramphenicol).

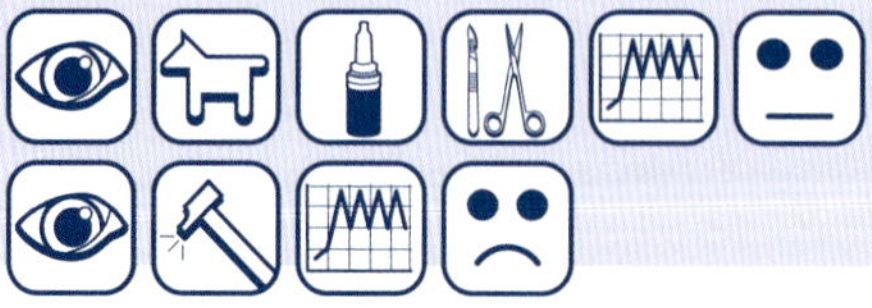

Lacrimal apparatus

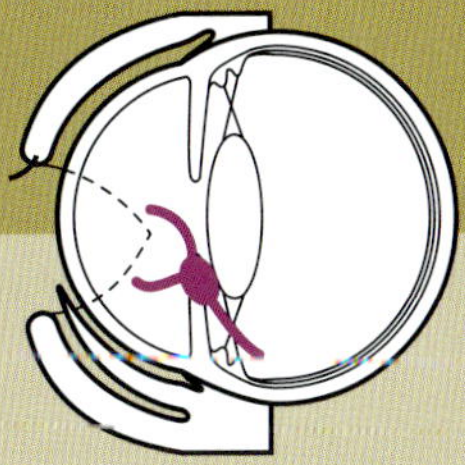

Epiphora

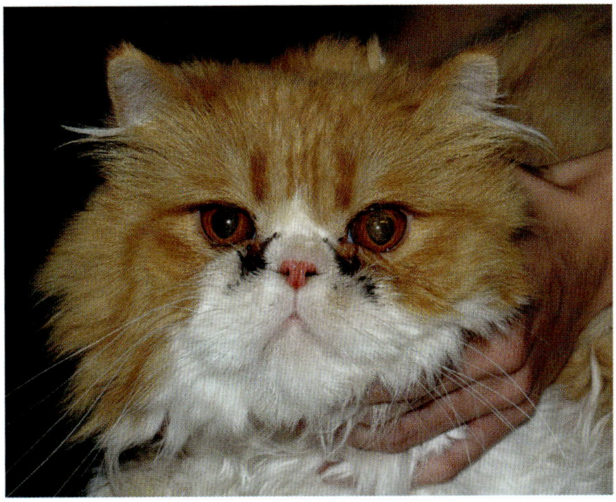

Persian cat with bilateral epiphora.
The dark colour is due to the high concentration of porphyrins in these cats' tears.

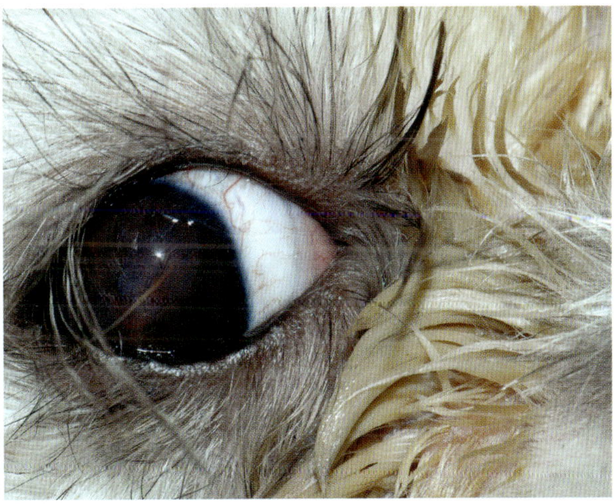

Marked epiphora in a Shih-Tzu. Note the excess moisture in the periocular region.
Cause: distichiasis of several hairs.

i | Epiphora is excessive lacrimation.

The most common causes of epiphora are as follows:

- Ocular irritation or discomfort (entropion, distichiasis, ectopic cilia, corneal ulcers, etc.).
- Obstructed or imperforate lacrimal punctum.
- Very prominent globe.
- Blepharitis.

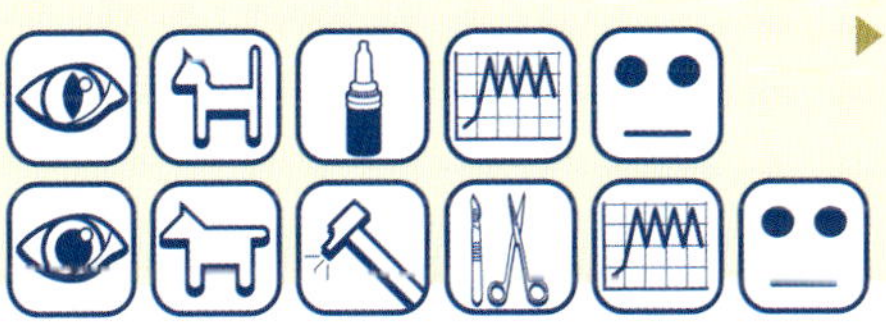

Keratoconjunctivitis sicca

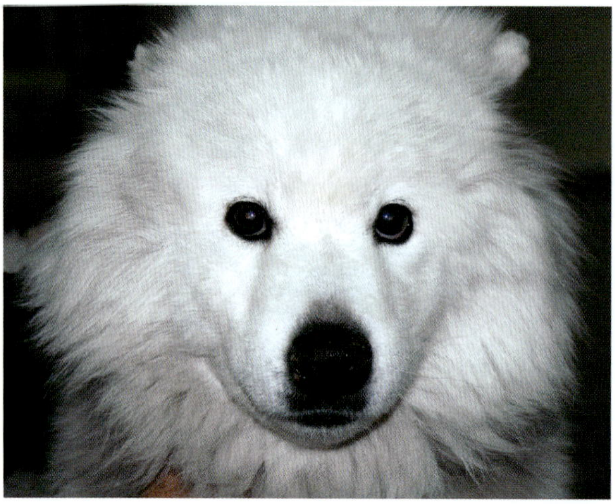

Samoyed with quantitative keratoconjunctivitis sicca (KCS).

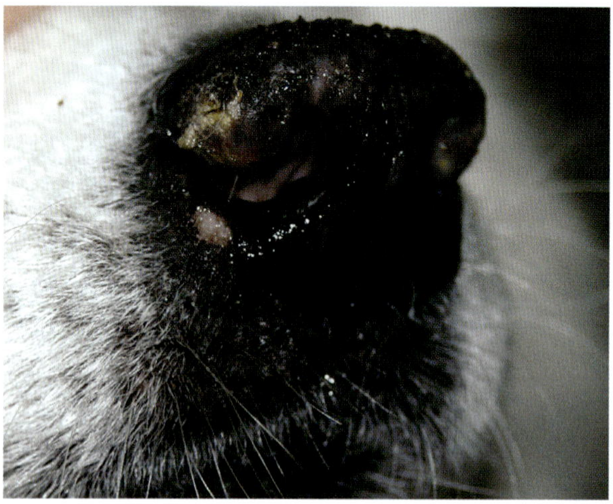

A crusted nose is a common clinical sign of KCS.

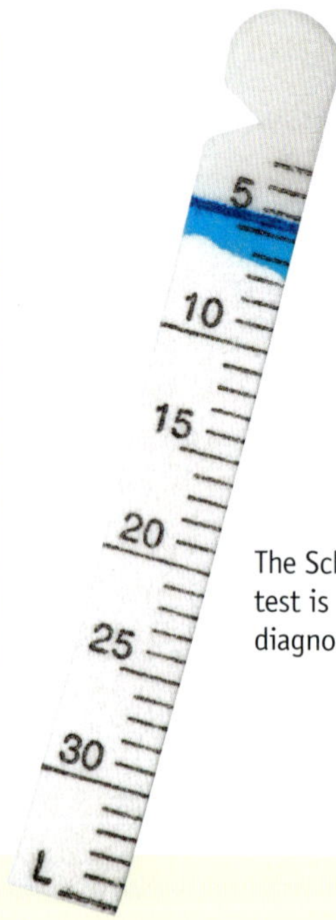

The Schirmer's test is key to diagnosis.

Interesting notes

- KCS is due to a quantitative and/or qualitative deficiency in the precorneal tear film.
- Consult the chapter on the cornea and conjunctiva for the causes of this condition of the lacrimal apparatus, its effects on the surface of the eye, and its impact on animals' vision.

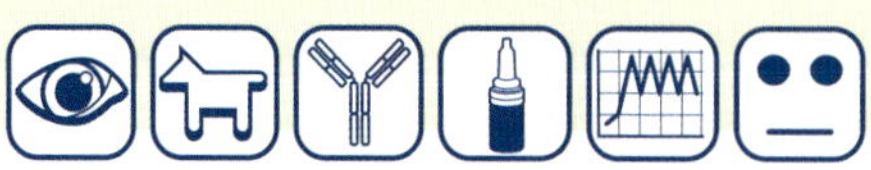

Imperforate lacrimal punctum

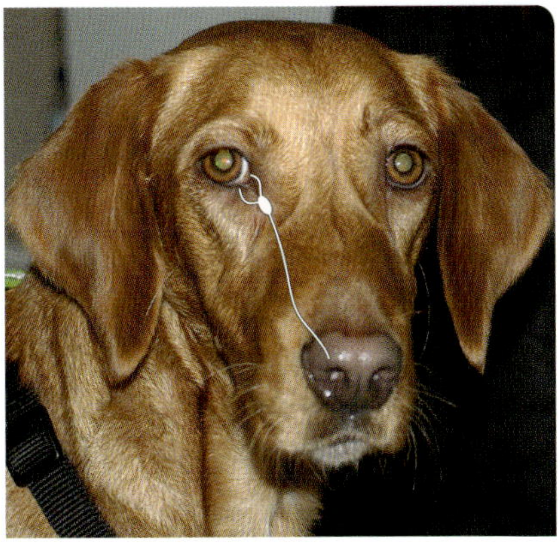

Representation of the nasolacrimal apparatus.

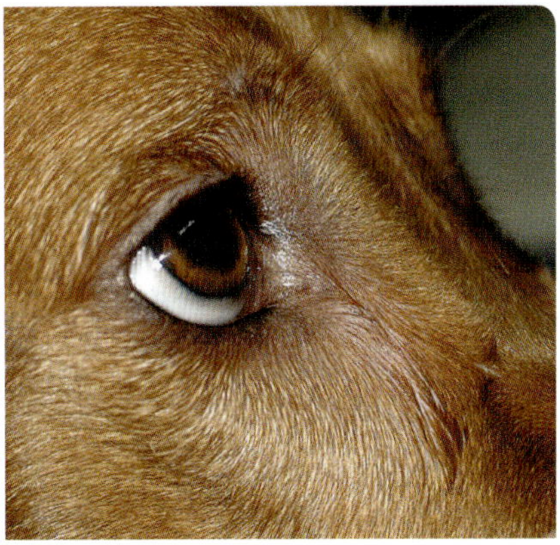

Epiphora is the characteristic clinical sign of an imperforate lacrimal punctum. Ten-month-old mixed-breed dog with agenesis of the lower lacrimal punctum.

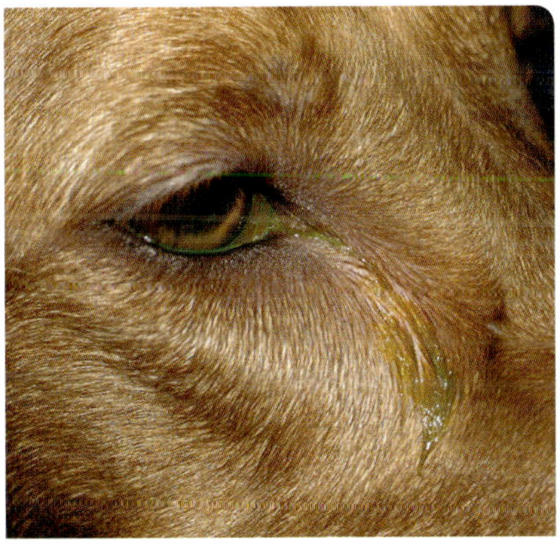

Vital fluorescein stain highlights the epiphora.

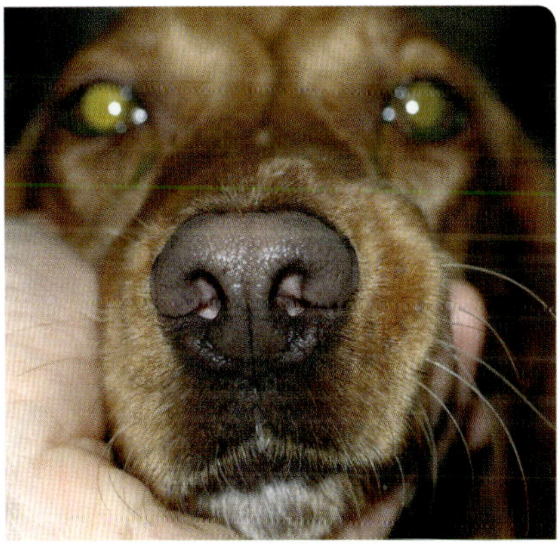

The lack of fluorescein drainage from the nostrils suggests imperforate lacrimal puncta.

Important notes

Recall that an accessory duct runs the length of the nasolacrimal duct and communicates with the posterior nasal cavity. This may explain why in some patients, particularly brachycephalic dogs and Persian cats, fluorescein does not drain from the nose, yet the lacrimal puncta and canaliculi are patent and unobstructed.

Imperforate lacrimal punctum

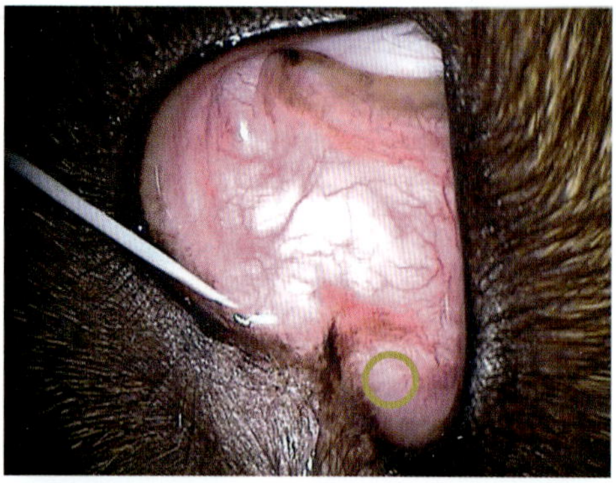

Cannulation of the upper lacrimal punctum. An imperforate lower lacrimal punctum blocks the drainage of normal saline that has been infused through the upper lacrimal punctum.
The conjunctiva bulges when the lower canaliculus is irrigated.

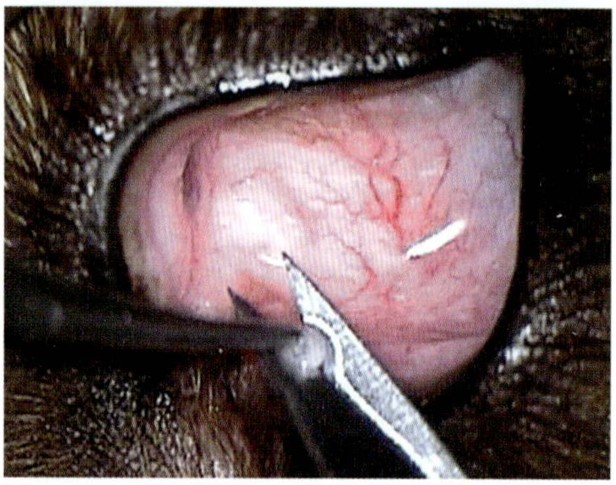

Opening the lower lacrimal punctum.
Cutting the mucosa with Steven's scissors.

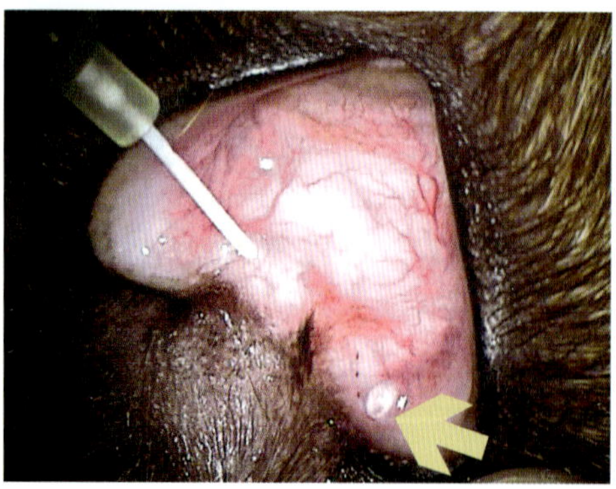

Normal flushing and a functional lower lacrimal punctum.
Close-up of the drainage of normal saline.

Interesting notes

Once the lacrimal punctum is opened, regular flushing and the use of corticosteroid eyedrops can minimise the risk of stenosis or closure due to scarring.

Hypoplasia

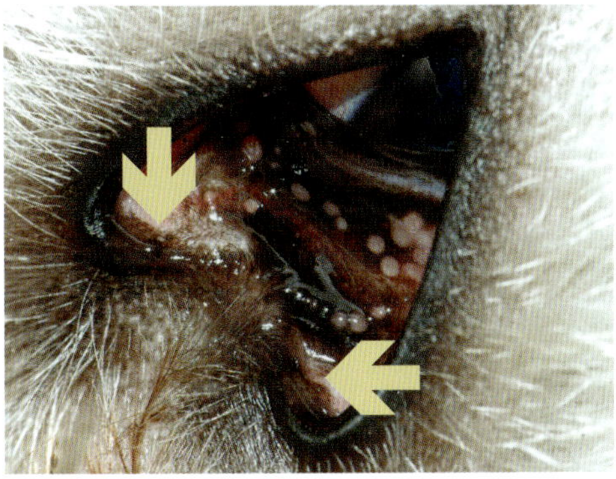

The inability to visualise the lacrimal punctum, along with epiphora, may suggest an imperforate or hypoplastic lacrimal punctum.
Identification of the upper lacrimal punctum but not the lower.

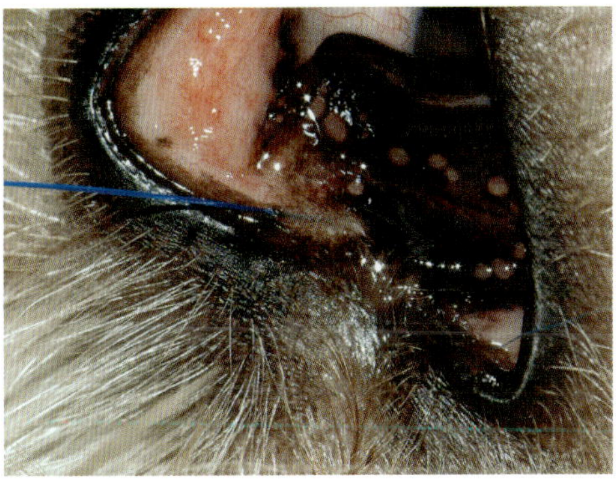

Location of both lacrimal puncta (upper and lower) by probing.
Clear hypoplasia of the lower punctum.
Close-up of the calibre of the suture used to identify it.

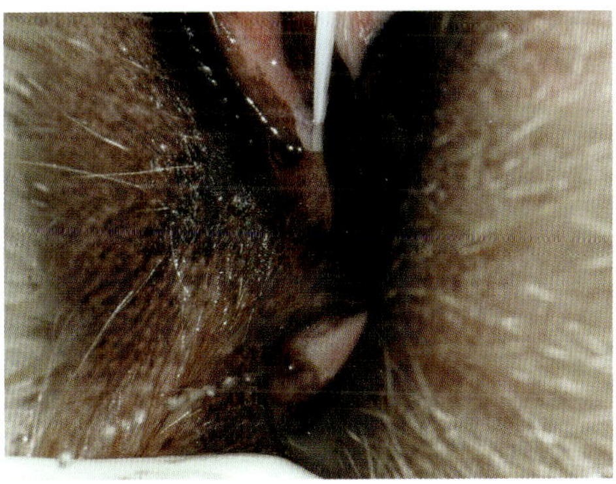

Flushing from the upper lacrimal punctum and decreased fluid drainage from the lower one.

i

Nonpatency (agenesis) and hypoplasia (atresia) mainly affect the lower lacrimal punctum. These may be unilateral or bilateral.

The most predisposed breeds are Retrievers (Golden and Labrador), Cocker Spaniels, and Poodles.

Hypoplasia

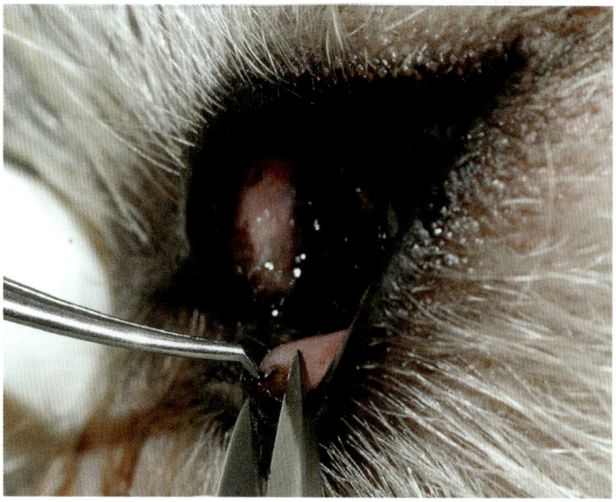

Close-up of a complete opening of the lower lacrimal punctum.

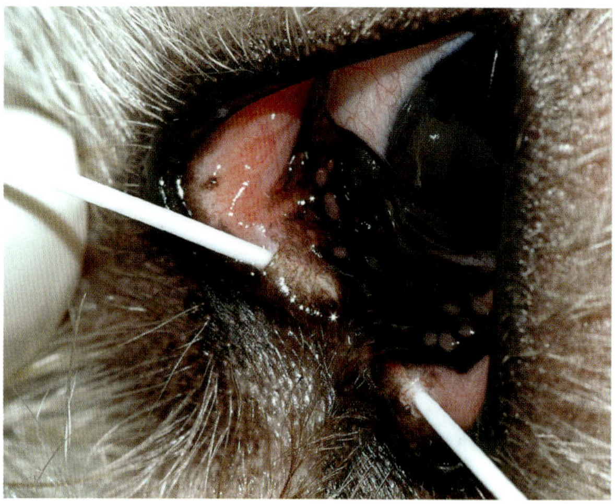

Final diameter of the lacrimal puncta following treatment.

Important notes

- Thoroughly remove the conjunctiva covering the lacrimal punctum to avoid recurrence.
- Insertion of a silicone tube temporarily can help prevent postoperative stenosis. In this case, place an Elizabethan collar.
- Continue topical corticosteroids for 30 days.

Obstruction

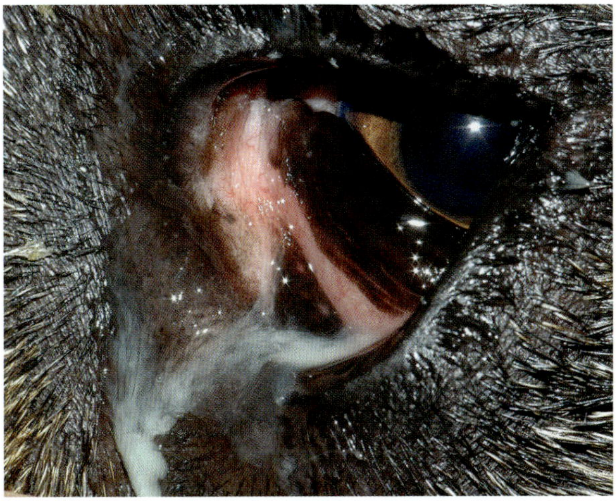

Patient with an obstruction of the lacrimal apparatus.
The animal presented with purulent discharge from the lower lacrimal punctum.
Time since onset: two months.

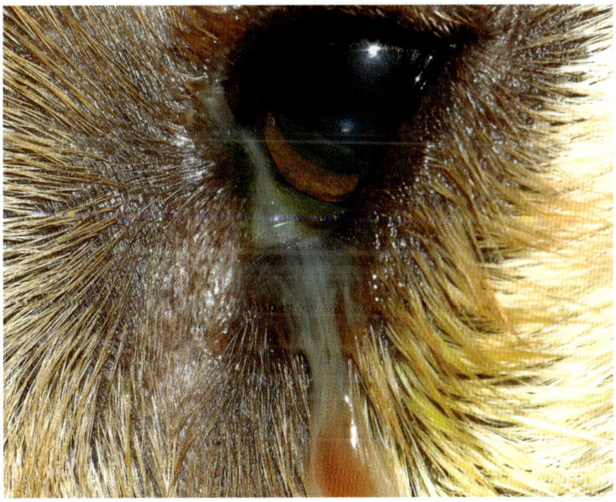

Cannulation from the upper lacrimal punctum often causes mucopurulent material to drain from the lower canaliculus.

The most common causes of obstruction of the lacrimal apparatus are as follows:

- Foreign bodies (plant or small stone) that enter through the lacrimal puncta or the nose.
- Animal bites or trauma to the lacrimal apparatus.
  The secondary scarring reaction can cause stenosis.
- Chronic infections.
- Neoplasms.

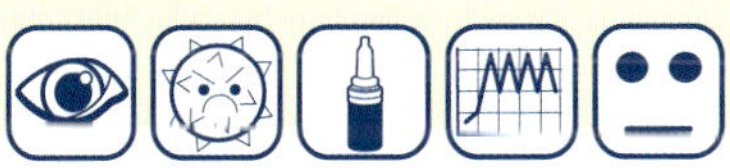

Obstruction

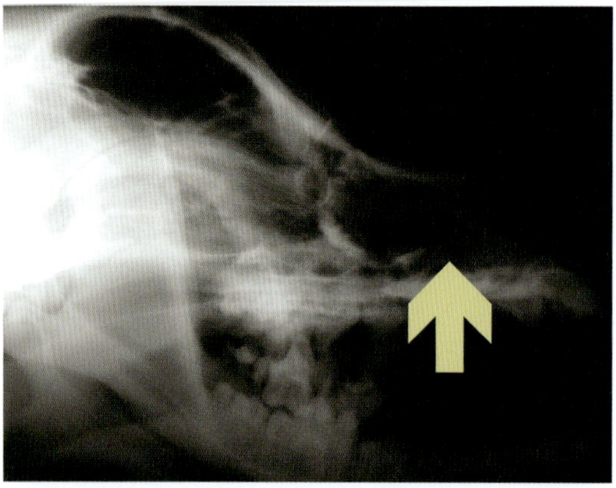

Dacryocystorrhinography of the patient pictured on the previous page (lacrimal apparatus obstruction). The widening of the proximal third of the nasolacrimal duct and the lower concentration of contrast near the nose help to pinpoint the exact location of the obstruction (arrow).

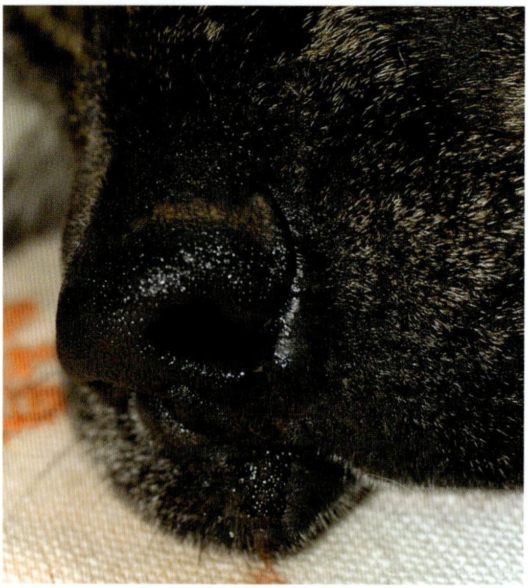

Epistaxis often follows removal of obstructions.

Interesting notes

- Plain and contrast radiographs (dacryocystorrhinography) are essential to diagnose lacrimal apparatus obstructions.
- CT, MRI, or endoscopy may be necessary in complicated cases.

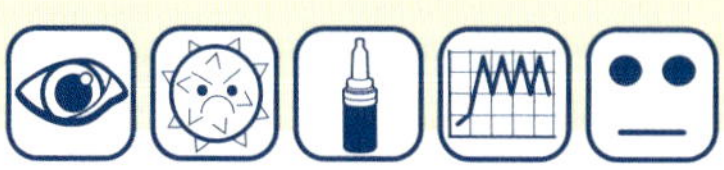

Obstruction

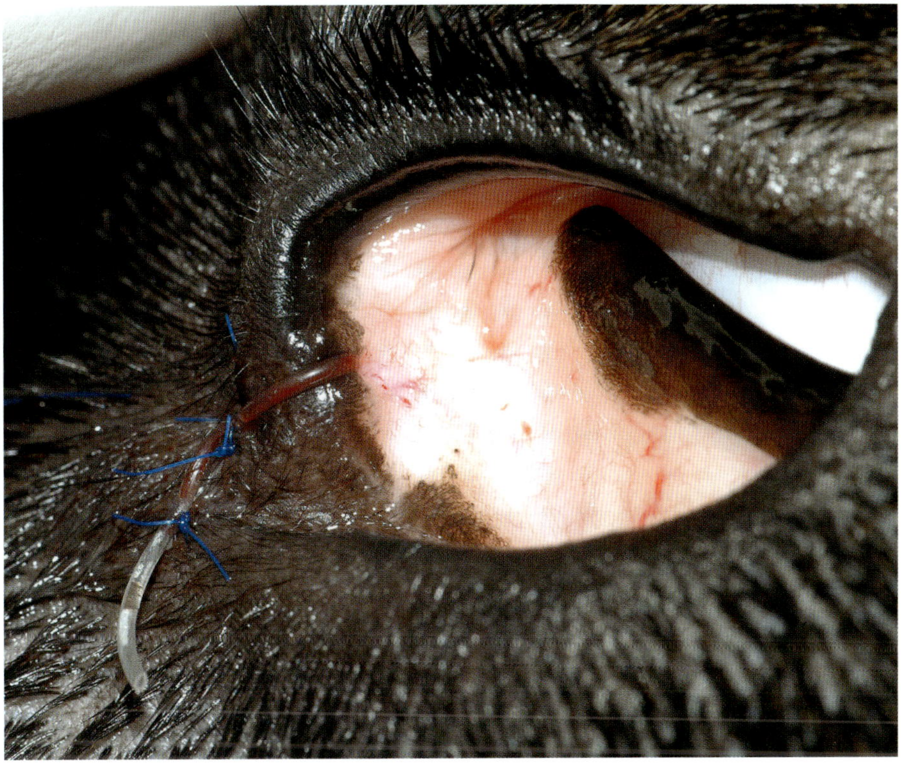

Placement of a silicon tube in a patient's upper canaliculus following extraction of a grass awn. Postinflammatory cicatricial retraction caused the obstruction.
Close-up of the skin fixation.

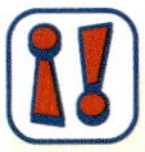

Important notes

Following removal of obstructions:

- Irrigate regularly from the upper lacrimal punctum.
- Continue systemic antibiotic and antiinflammatory therapy for 15 days.
- Continue topical treatments (antibiotics and anti-inflammatories) for at least 30–45 days.
- Leave drainage tubes in place for at least 20 days.
- Reserve conjunctival rhinostomy and conjunctival buccostomy only for severe cases.

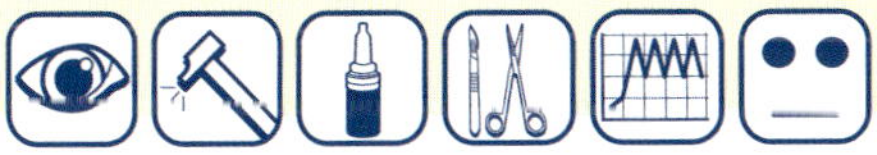

Dacryocystitis

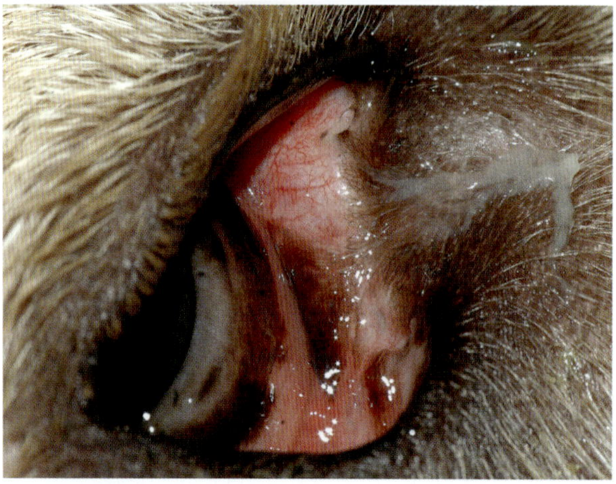

Malodourous mucoid secretions in an eight-month-old Labrador Retriever.
Time since onset: seven days.

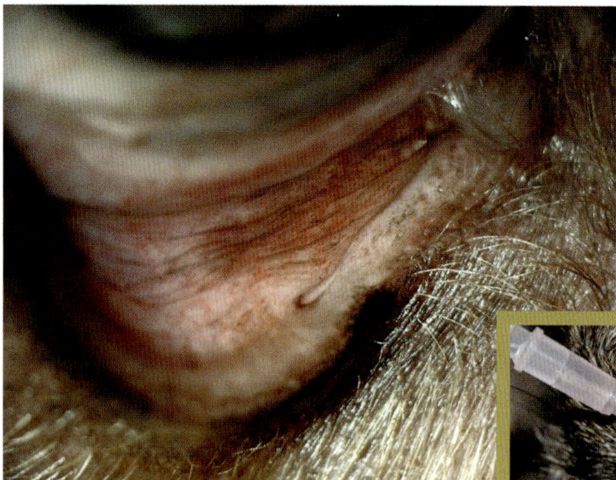

Dilatation of the lower canaliculus in the patient pictured above.

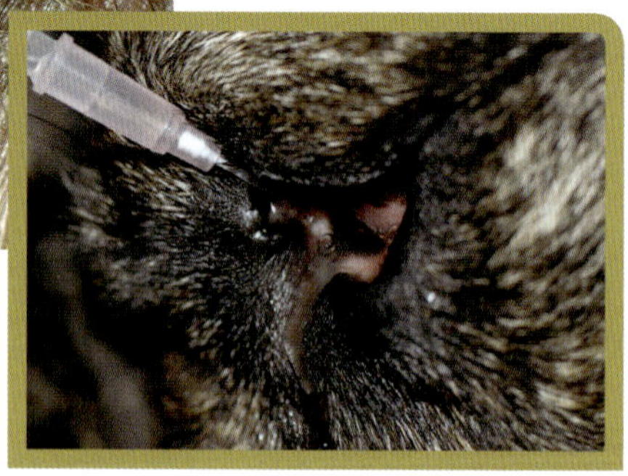

Dacryocystitis in an eight-month-old Presa Canario. Close-up of the mucoid secretions during lavage of the lacrimal apparatus.

Dacryocystitis is an inflammation of the lacrimal sac.

It generally affects younger individuals and presents unilaterally in most cases.

Interesting notes

- Diagnosis tends to take time, and a secondary lesion of the canaliculus or nasolacrimal duct is often present.

Glaucoma

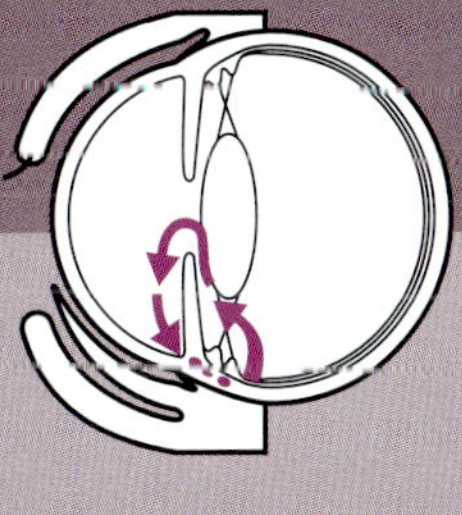

Glaucoma

Diagnosis

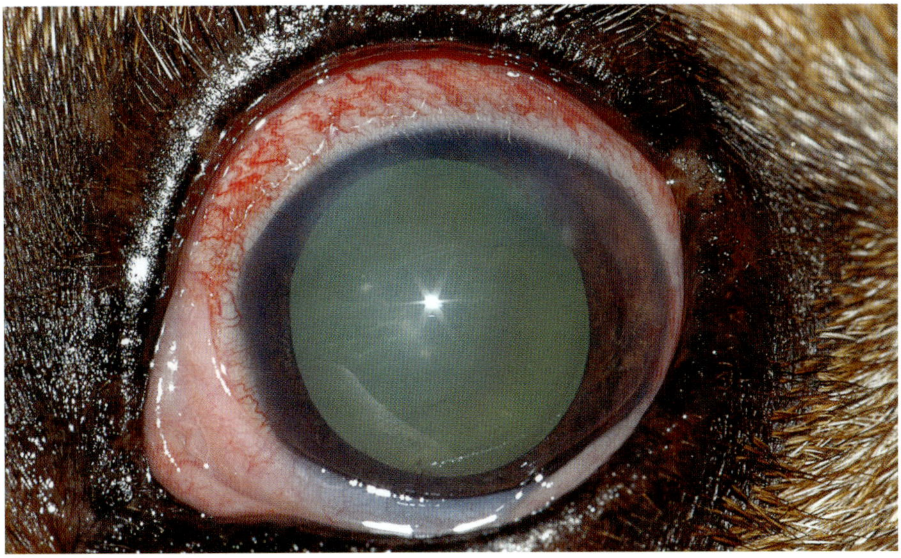

Acute glaucoma in a dog. Time since onset: 24 hours. Mydriasis, episcleral congestion and corneal oedema.

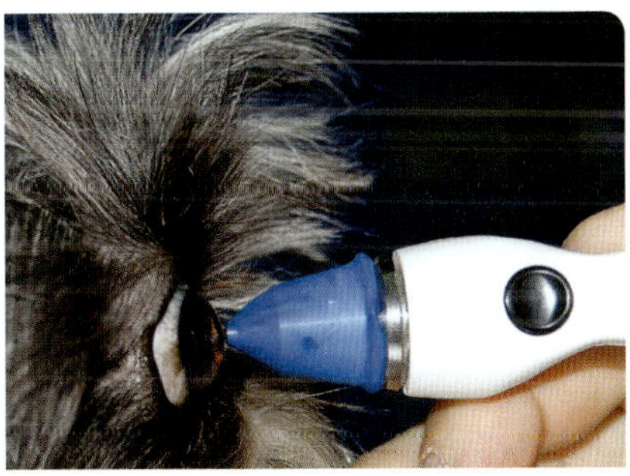

Applanation tonometry (TonoPen XL®).

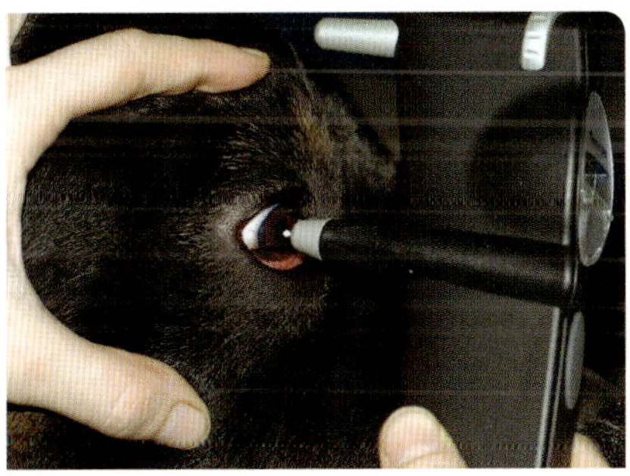

Rebound tonometry (TonoVet®).

i

Optic neuropathy associated with increased intraocular pressure (IOP).

The mechanical compression of the axon and the ensuing effects on the microcirculation lead to the death of retinal nerve cells and potentially irreversible damage to the optic nerve.

Tonometry (IOP measurement) is critical to diagnosis.

Normal IOP is 15–27 mmHg.

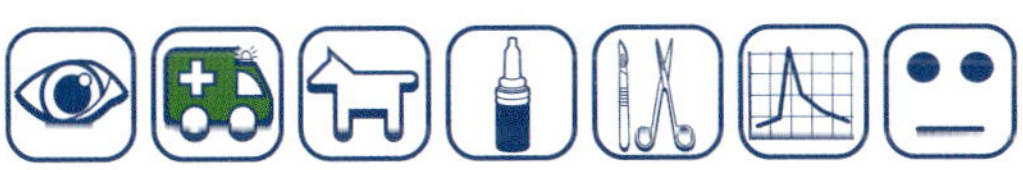

Glaucoma

Diagnosis

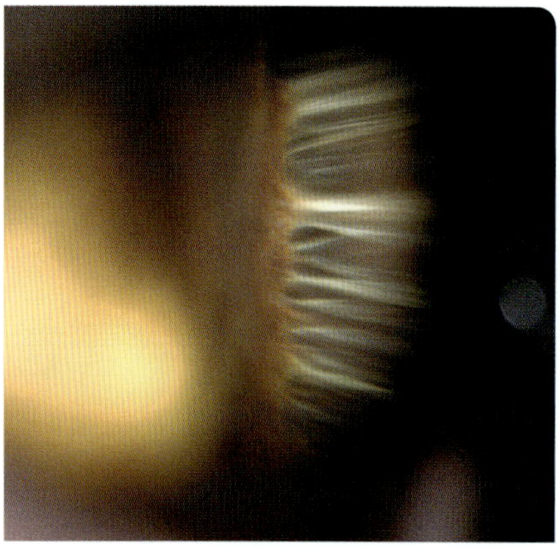

Open iridocorneal angle (ICA) in a domestic shorthair cat. Direct gonioscopy.

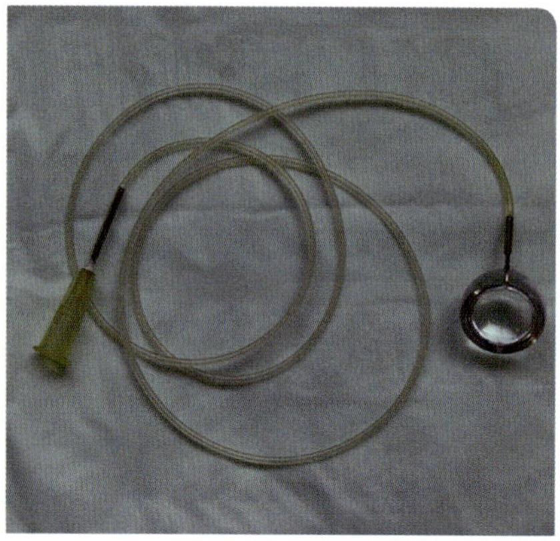

Barkan lens used for indirect gonioscopy.

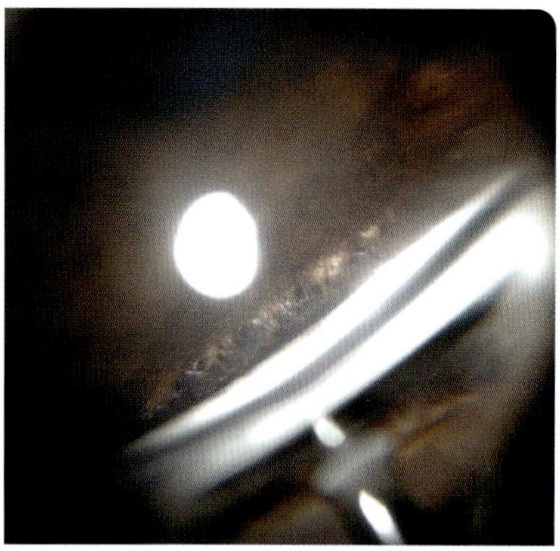

Normal iridocorneal angle examined by indirect gonioscopy.

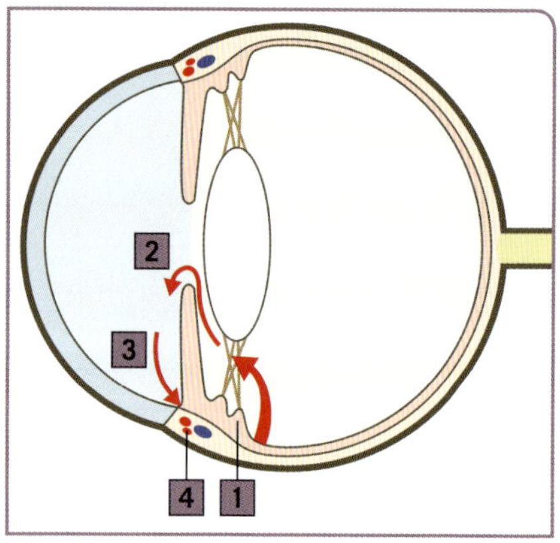

Normal circulation of aqueous humour (AH).

1. Ciliary body epithelium.
2. AH flow from the posterior to the anterior chamber.
3. AH drainage through the ICA.
4. Scleral venous plexus.

i

The lenses most commonly used for gonioscopy are the Barkan lens, Goldman lens, three-mirror lens, and Koeppe lens. A 20 D lens placed directly on the cornea can also be used.

The iridocorneal angle can be examined in detail using gonioscopy.

Use topical anaesthesia of the cornea or sedate the patient.

Glaucoma

Classification

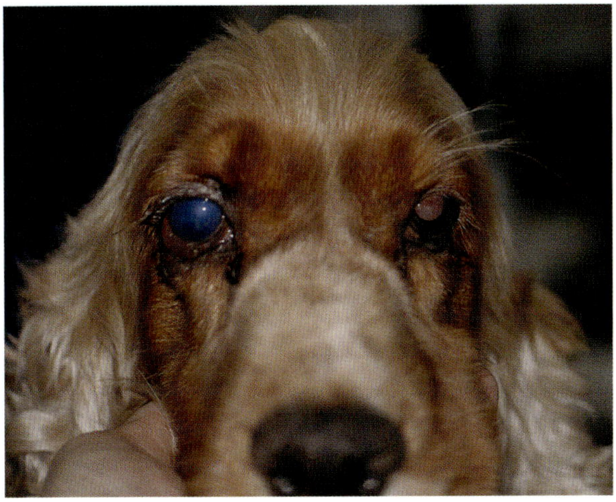

Secondary glaucoma in a 12-year-old English Cocker Spaniel.
Cause: closure of the iridocorneal angle due to an intraocular tumour.
Time since onset: 20 days.
IOP: 52 mmHg (TonoPen XL®).

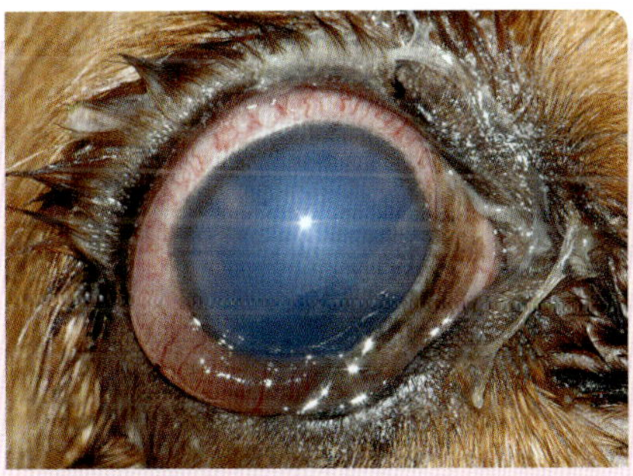

Close-up of the glaucomatous eye of the Cocker Spaniel.
An intraocular neoplasm (melanoma) is visible behind the cornea.

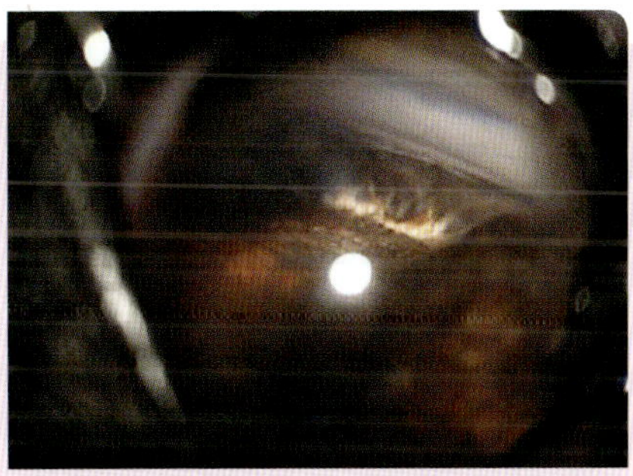

Iris melanoma partly closing the iridocorneal angle. Gonioscopy in a Labrador Retriever.

Important notes

- Glaucoma may be primary (open, narrow, or closed angle) or secondary (due to uveitis, lens luxation, intraocular tumours, or cataracts).
- Breed predispositions for primary glaucoma are the American Cocker Spaniel, Siberian Husky, Basset Hound, Samoyed and Beagle.
- Secondary glaucoma is more common than primary in cats, and the main cause is uveitis.

Glaucoma

Classification

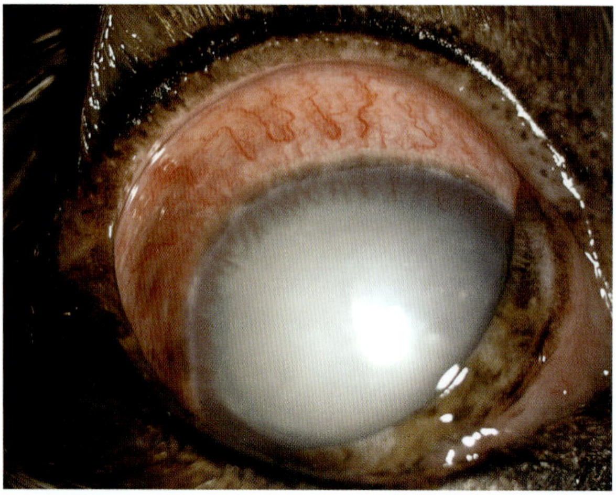

Glaucoma secondary to an anterior lens luxation. Thirteen-year-old dog. Time since onset: four days. Intraocular pressure: 52 mmHg.
Note the episcleral congestion.

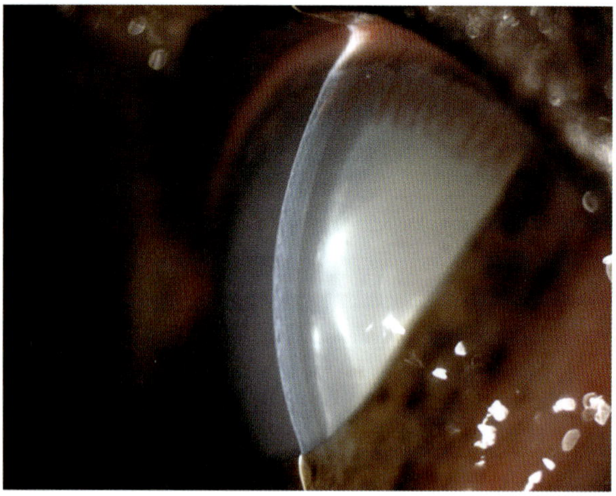

Patient pictured above. The slit-lamp examination reveals the absence of an anterior chamber. The iridocorneal angle is obstructed by the luxated lens.

Important notes

- Glaucoma secondary to an anterior lens luxation is considered a SURGICAL EMERGENCY. Intracapsular lens extraction should be performed.
- The earlier the diagnosis and lens surgery, the better the vision prognosis.
- Persistently high IOP may lead to an irreversible optic neuropathy.

Glaucoma

Clinical signs

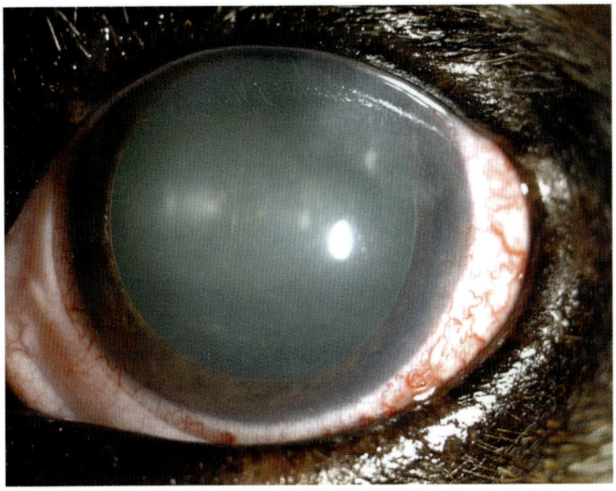

Acute glaucoma in a two-year-old Beagle. Mydriasis and corneal oedema.
IOP: 45 mmHg.
Time since onset: eight hours.

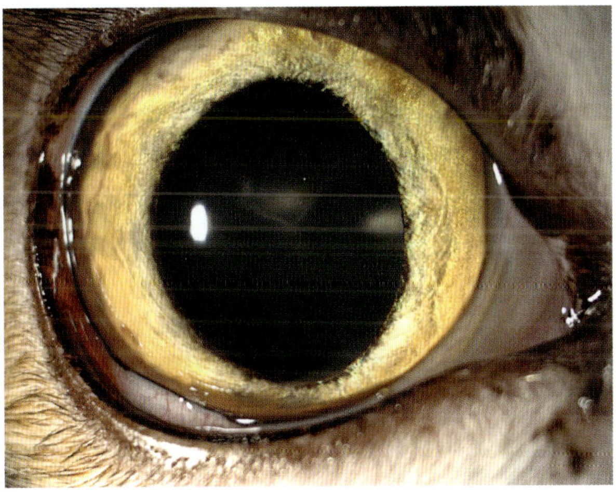

Cat with acute glaucoma in the right eye. IOP 40 mmHg. Mydriasis. Corneal oedema is rare in feline glaucoma.

The main clinical signs of glaucoma are:

- MYDRIASIS (dogs and cats).
- EPISCLERAL CONGESTION (dogs).
- CORNEAL OEDEMA (dogs).
- BLEPHAROSPASM (dogs).
- ANOREXIA (dogs and cats).
- DEPRESSION (dogs and cats).

Glaucoma

Clinical signs

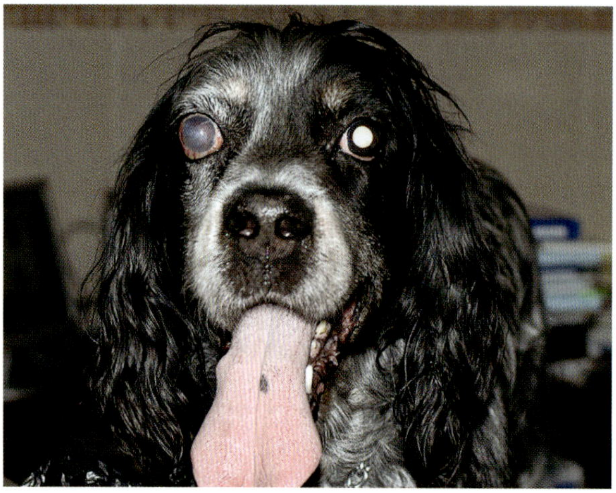

Dog with chronic glaucoma in the right eye.
IOP: 41 mmHg.
Time since onset: two months.

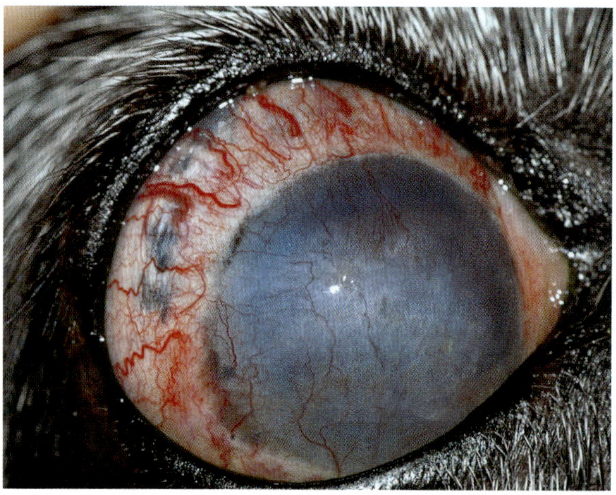

Note the episcleral congestion that is characteristic of glaucoma and the signs of chronicity: distension of the scleral fibrous tunic and exposure keratitis.
IOP: 47 mmHg. Cause: an intraocular tumour.

Interesting notes

- Patients with chronic glaucoma and IOP persistently between 35–45 mmHg generally present with buphthalmos.
- The vision cannot be recovered in these cases, and a medical or surgical palliative treatment with the goal of avoiding pain should be considered.

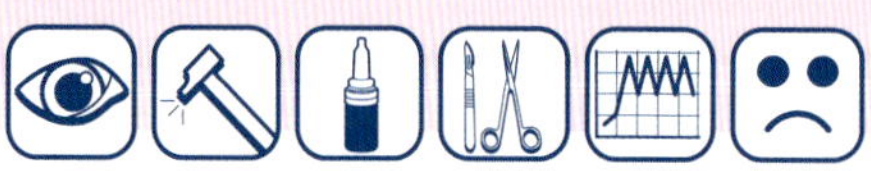

Glaucoma

Clinical signs

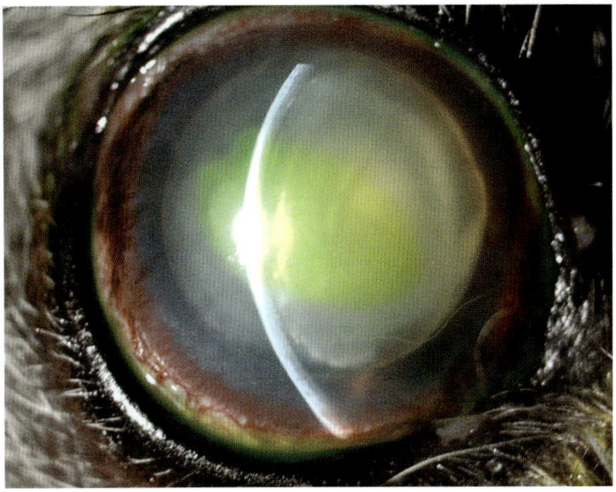

Exposure-induced ulcerative keratitis in a dog with chronic glaucoma.
Close-up of the fluorescein uptake in the central area of the cornea.
Duration of glaucoma: three months.
Cause: anterior lens luxation.

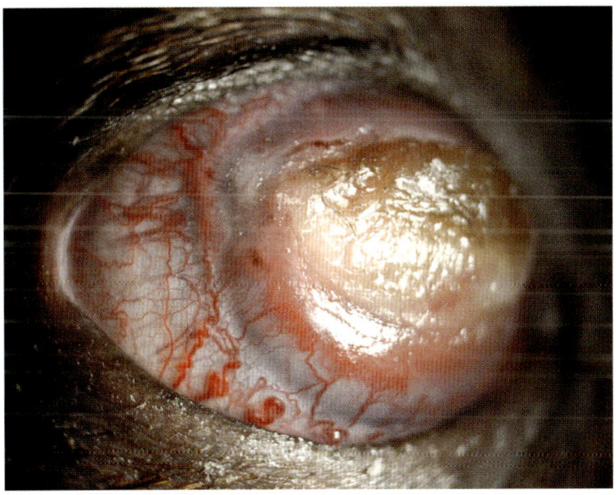

Brachycephalic patient with chronic glaucoma and severe exposure keratitis. Close-up of corneal damage.

Important notes

- One of the most common complications of chronic glaucoma is exposure-induced corneal damage.
- Buphthalmos gives rise to lagophthalmos. The central area of the cornea, which is poorly protected, is continually damaged.
- In very severe cases, ulcerative keratitis can culminate in a corneal perforation.

Glaucoma

Clinical signs

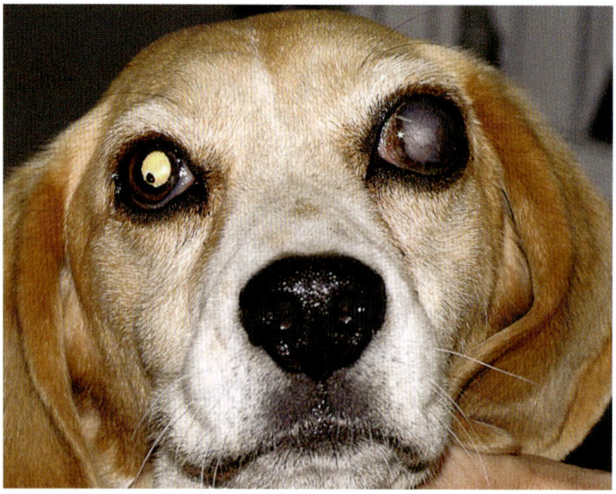

Ten-year-old Beagle with chronic glaucoma.
Note the buphthalmos of the affected eye (left) compared to the normal eye.
IOP: 38 mmHg.
Time since onset: six months.

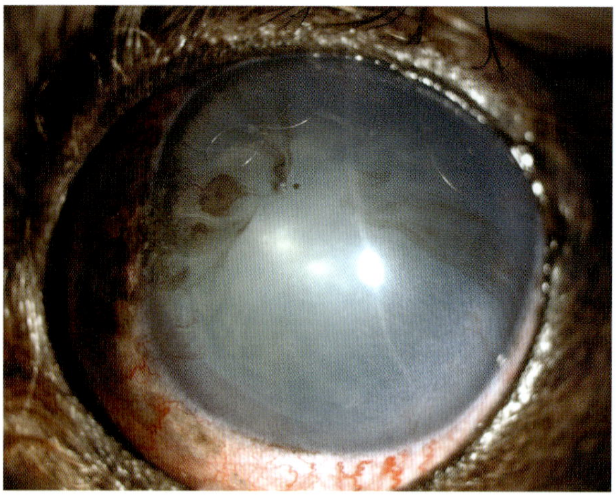

Haab's striae in a patient with chronic glaucoma.

i

Haab's striae (fractures of Descemet's membrane) may appear in patients with chronic glaucoma who have persistently high IOP for a long period.

The fibrous tunic deforms as this corneal condition progresses.

Whitish lines running from one side of the cornea to the other are visible (see picture above).

Glaucoma

Differential diagnosis

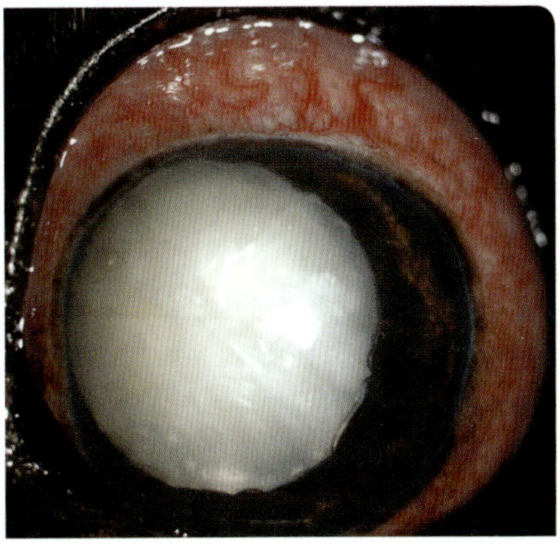

Canine glaucoma, secondary to hypermature cataract.

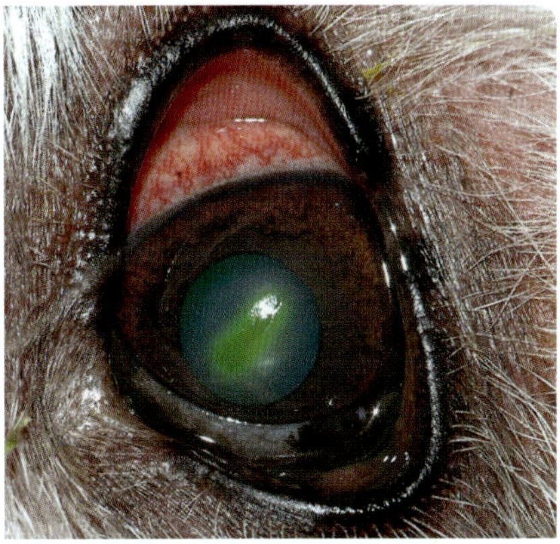

Conjunctival hyperaemia associated with a corneal ulcer.

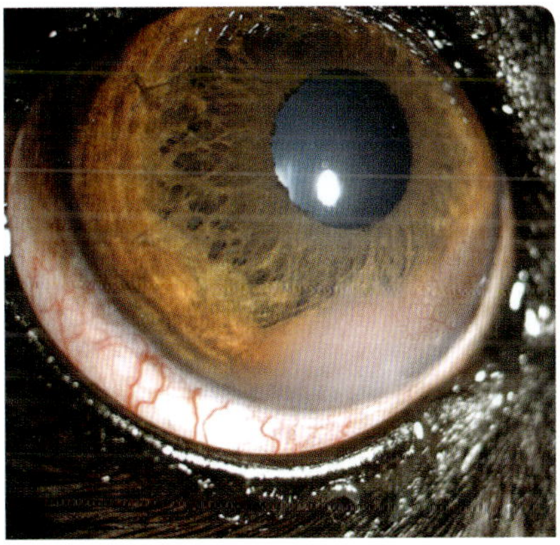

Superficial keratitis in the nasal area of a dog.

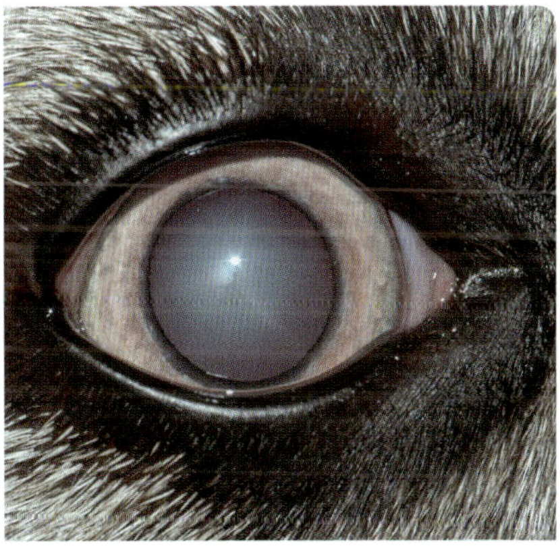

Acute uveitis in a Siberian Husky.

Important notes

In order to avoid confusing glaucoma with uveitis, conjunctivitis, or keratitis, consider the differential diagnosis presented on the following page.

Glaucoma

Differential diagnosis

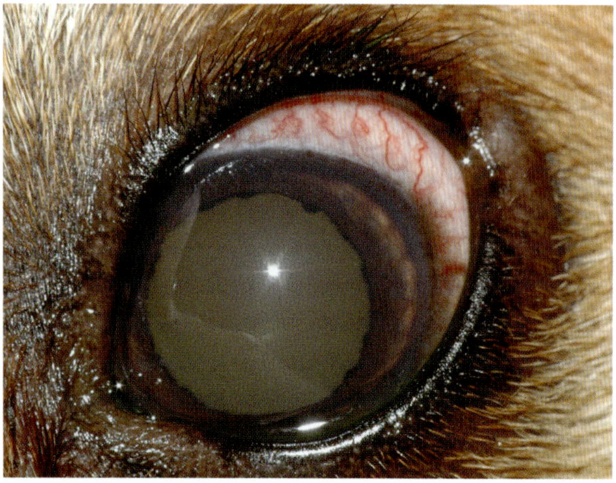

Acute glaucoma.

Differential diagnosis of glaucoma				
	Conjunctivitis	Superficial keratitis	Uveitis	Glaucoma
Conjunctiva	Inflamed, hyperaemic	Not thickened	Normal	Normal
Vascularisation	Superficial, diffuse	Superficial, diffuse	Circumcorneal Straight Fixed	Superficial, diffuse
Pupil	Normal	Normal	Miotic or irregular	Mydriasis
Intraocular pressure	Normal	Normal	Normal Low Sometimes high	High
Pupillary light reflex	Normal	Normal	Weak or nonexistent	Nonexistent
Secretions	Aqueous	Aqueous Serous Mucopurulent	None	None
Vision	Normal	Normal	Decreased	Absent
Photophobia	No	Significant	Moderate	Mild

Glaucoma

Treatment

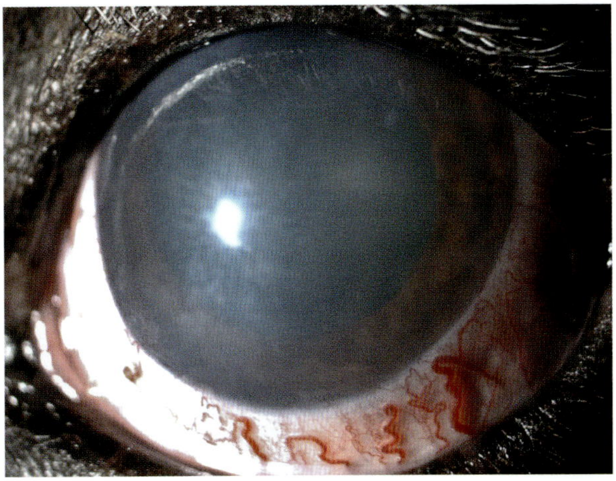

Acute glaucoma.
Corneal oedema, mydriasis, and episcleral congestion.

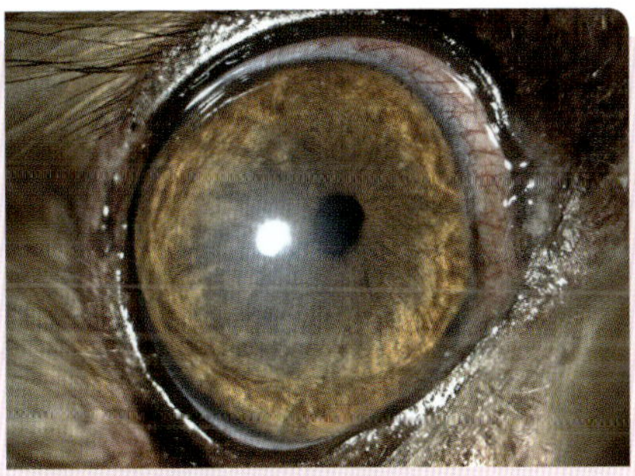

Patient treated with latanoprost (Xalatan®). IOP: 18 mmHg. Drug-induced miosis.

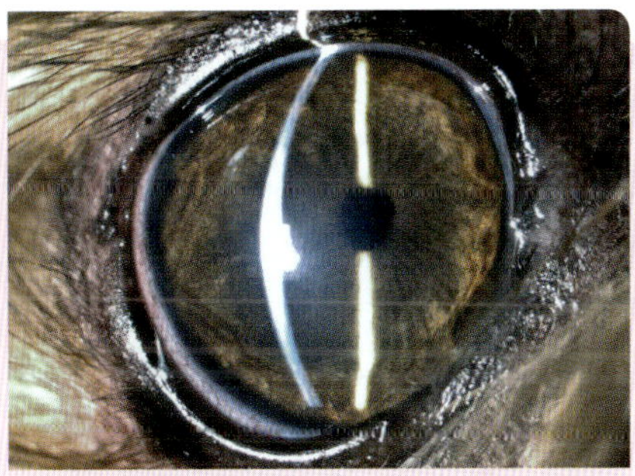

Close-up of the patient's anterior chamber.

Interesting notes

The goal of medical treatment of glaucoma is to favour drainage of aqueous humour and/or inhibit its production. The following medications are used in combination:

- Prostaglandin analogues (latanoprost).
- Carbonic anhydrase inhibitors (dorzolamide, brinzolamide).
- Adrenergic agonists (brimonidine, apraclonidine).
- Cholinergic agents (pilocarpine).
- Hyperosmotics (mannitol).

Contraindicated

NEVER give atropine to patients with glaucoma.

Glaucoma

Treatment

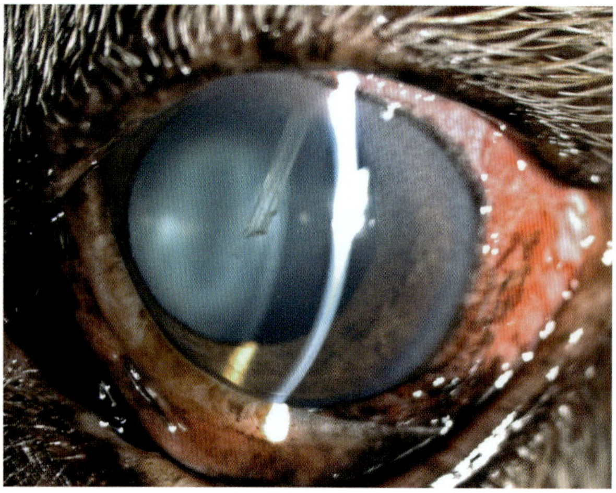

Shunt in the anterior chamber. Close-up of its position using a slit lamp.

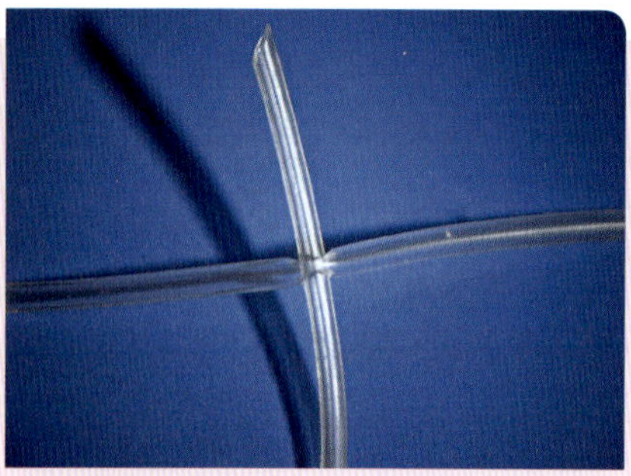

Tube shunt without valves, simple.

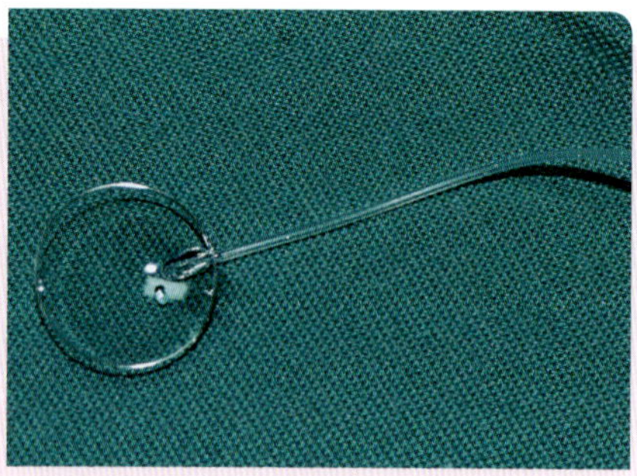

Modified tube shunt without valves.

Important notes

- Glaucoma is considered a surgical disease (medical treatment is only temporary).
- The surgical options for a visual eye with glaucoma:
  - Placement of shunts that divert the aqueous humour to the subconjunctival space (to a filtration bleb).
  - Controlled diode laser cyclodestruction.
- These techniques may be used separately or in combination.

Glaucoma

Treatment

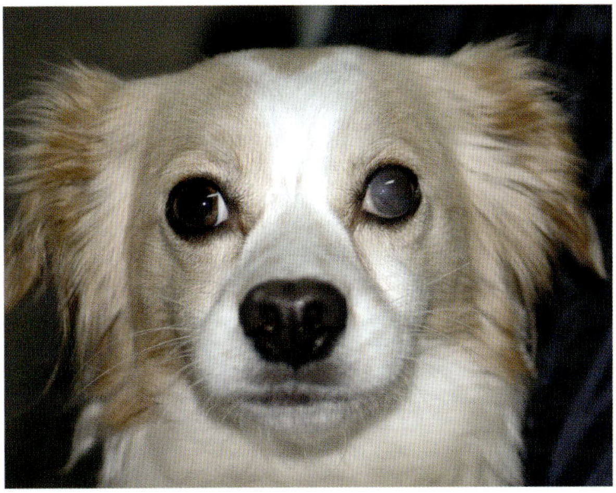

Patient with an intrascleral prosthesis in the left eye. Silicone prostheses are a cosmetic surgical option for patients with glaucoma and blindness.

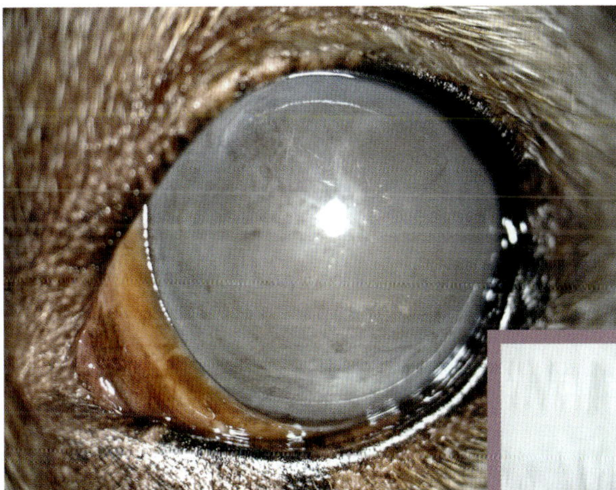

Close-up of an eye with an intrascleral prosthesis. The globe moves normally.

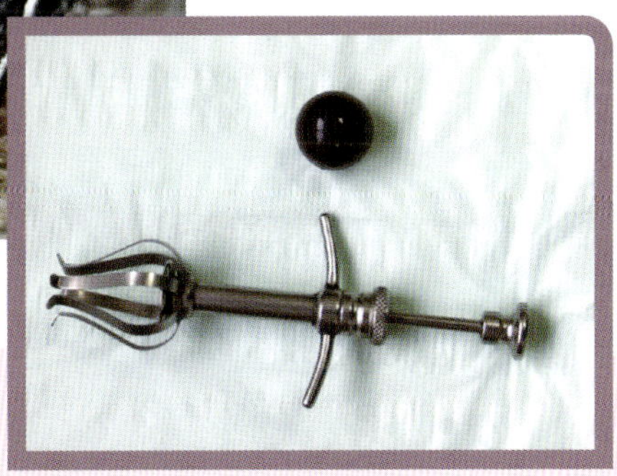

Silicone prosthesis and introducer.

Important notes

- Evisceration followed by silicone prosthesis implantation is an option only if the eye is blind, the cornea is healthy, and no intraocular tumour is suspected.

Contraindicated

- Do not place silicone prostheses in cats due to the risk of sarcoma formation.

Glaucoma

Treatment

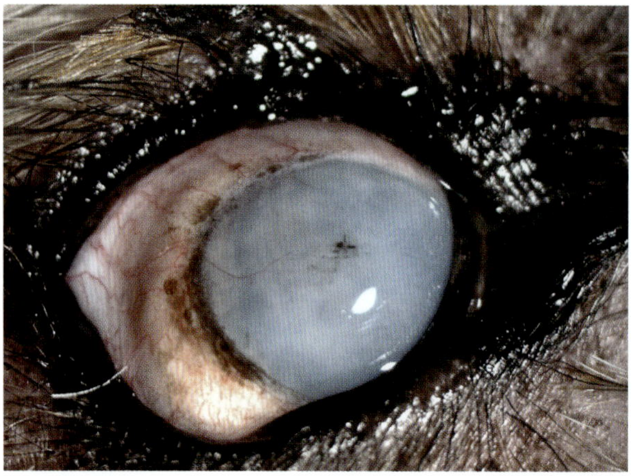

Phthisis bulbi, in a dog, after intravitreal injection of gentamicin.

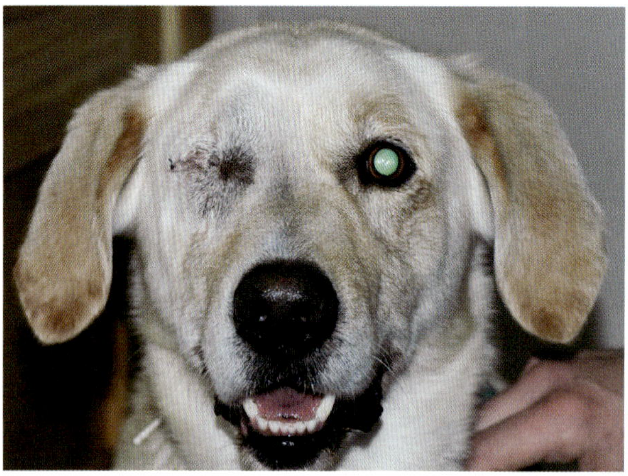

Exenteration in a Labrador Retriever with glaucoma secondary to a neoplasm.

Interesting notes

- Noncosmetic surgical options for glaucoma and blindness are:
  - Drug-induced cyclodestruction (intravitreal injection of gentamicin).
  - Enucleation (excision of the globe and associated structures).
  - Exenteration (excision of the globe, associated structures, and orbital tissue).

Contraindicated

- Intravitreal injection of gentamicin should not be performed in cats (risk of sarcoma) or in the presence of an intraocular neoplasm.

Glaucoma

Sequelae

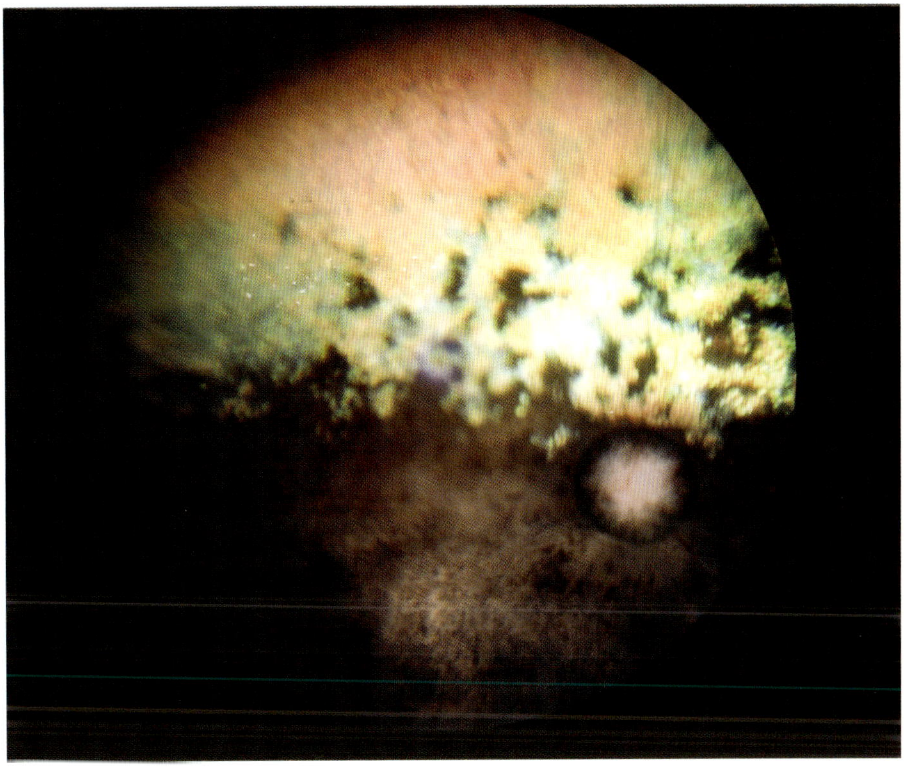

Optic neuropathy in a dog with chronic glaucoma.
Time since onset: 10 months.
Note the excavation and atrophy of the optic nerve.
Retinal degeneration occurs in very late stages.

Important notes

- Glaucoma is an OPTIC NERVE DISEASE.
- Axonal damage to the optic nerve and retinal nerve cell apoptosis may lead to blindness.

Bibliography

American College of Veterinary Ophthalmologists. *Ocular Disorders Presumed to be Inherited in Purebred Dogs*. 3rd edition. Genetics committee of the American College of Veterinary Ophthalmologists, 1999.

Barnett, K.C., Crispin, S. *Oftalmología felina*. Atlas-texto. Buenos Aires: Editorial Inter-médica, 2000.

Barnett, K.C., Sansom, J., Heinrich, C. *Oftalmología canina*. Atlas-texto. Buenos Aires: Editorial Inter-médica, 2003.

Bedford, P. Enfermedades de la retina. In: Herrera, D. *Oftalmología clínica en animales de compañía*. Buenos Aires: Editorial Inter-médica, 2007, pp. 211–238.

Bjerkas, E: Cataract diagnosis and aetiology. *EJCAP*. Oct. 2004, vol. 14(2):187–192.

Chaudieu, G. Eléments díétude simples des affections du fond díoeil chez les carnivores domestiques. *Prat. Med. Chir. Anim. Comp.* 1996, 31:7–32.

Cortadellas, O. Hipertensión arterial sistémica. *Argos*. Apr. 2002, 37:38–39.

Dennos, R. Use of magnetic resonance imaging for the investigation of orbital disease in small animals. *Journal of Small Animal Practice*. Apr. 2000, 41:145–155.

Esteban Martin, J. *Atlas de Oftalmología Clínica del perro y del gato*. Zaragoza: Editorial Servet, 2007.

Esteban Martín, J. Colocación de un gonioimplante no valvulado. *Argos*. 2006, 77, pp. 48–50.

Esteban Martín, J. El cristalino: esclerosis, catarata y luxación. Criterios de diagnóstico y remisión. Oftalmología básica. *Canis et Felis*. Oct. 2008, 94:52–67.

Featherstone, H.J., Sanson, J. Feline corneal sequestra: a review of 64 cases (80 eyes) from 1993 to 2000. *Veterinary Ophthalmology*. 2004, 7(4):213–227.

García Sánchez, G.A. Facoemulsificación ultrasónica como método quirúrgico para la extracción extracapsular de la lente y su reemplazo con lente intraocular. 4th CLOVE congress, Madrid, 2007. *Libro de ponencias*, pp. 119–129.

Gaskell, R., Dawson, S., Radford, A., Thiry, E. Feline herpesvirus. *Vet Res.* 2007, 38(2):337–354.

Gelatt, K.N. *Veterinary Ophthalmology*, vol. 1, 4th edition. Ames, Iowa: Blackwell Publishing, 2007.

Gilger, B.C., Whitley, R.D. Surgery of the cornea and sclera. In: Gelatt, K.N. *Veterinary Ophthalmology*, 3rd edition. Philadelphia: Lippincott Williams and Wilkins, 1999, pp. 675–689.

Herrera, D. Avances en el tratamiento del glaucoma canino. *Argos*. Apr. 2002, 37:36–37.

Herrera, D. *Oftalmología clínica en animales de compañía*. Buenos Aires: Editorial Inter-médica, 2007.

Lackner, P.A. Techniques for surgical correction of adnexal disease. *Clin. Tech. Smal. Anim. Pract.* 2001, vol. 16:40–50.

López Murcia, M., García Sánchez, G.A., Piñón Cabrera, A. Glaucoma, alteraciones de la lente y del fondo ocular. *Consulta Difusión Veterinaria*. 2005; 119:65–72.

Martin, C.L. *Ophthalmic Disease in Veterinary Medicine*. London: Manson Publishing, 2005.

Matoon, J.S., Nyland, T.G. Ocular Ultrasonography. *Veterinary diagnostic ultrasound*. Philadelphia: Saunders, 1990, pp. 178–197.

Petersen-Jones, S.M., Forcier, J., Mentzer, A.L. Ocular melanosis in the Cairn Terrier: clinical description and investigation of mode of inheritance. *Vet Ophthalmology*. 2007, 10:63–69.

Rodríguez Alvaro, A., González Alonso-Alegre, E. Tumores oculares en el perro y en el gato. *Consulta Difusión Veterinaria*. 2002; 93:71–82.

Sagredo, P, Miro, G. *Atlas de dermatología del perro y del gato*. Tomo I y II. Madrid: Luzán Ediciones, 2004.

Sapienza, J. Feline Disorders. *Clin. Tech. Smal. Anim. Pract.* May 2005, 20(2):102–107.

Simon, M. Les uvéites chez les carnivores domestiques. *Recueil de médicine vétérinaire*. 1989, 3:257–262.

Slatter, D. *Fundamentos de Oftalmología Veterinaria*. 3ª edición. Buenos Aires: Editorial Inter-médica, 2004.

Stades, F.C., Gelatt, K.N. Diseases and surgery of the canine eyelid. In: Gelatt, K.N. *Veterinary Ophthalmology*, 4th edition. Ames, Iowa : Blackwell Publishing, 2007, pp. 563–614.

Syme, H.M. Diagnóstico y tratamiento de la hipertensión felina. *Waltham Focus*, 2005, I, vol. 15.

Tovar, M.C. Enfoque clínico del glaucoma: ¿cómo reconocerlo? Oftalmología básica. *Canis et Felis*. Oct. 2008, 94:68–80.

Tovar, M.C. Queratitis ulcerativas. *Consulta Difusión Veterinaria*. 2003; 106:53–60.

Villagrasa, M. Ecografía ocular. In *Oftalmología clínica en animales de compañía*. Daniel Herrera. Buenos Aires: Editorial Inter-médica, 2007, pp. 51–62.

Ward, D.A. Diseases and Surgery of the Canine Nictitating Membrane. In: Gelatt, K.N. *Veterinary Ophthalmology*, 3rd edition. Philadelphia: Lippincott Williams-Wilkins, 1999, pp. 609–618.

Wilkie, D.A., Whittaker, C. Surgery of the cornea. *Vet. Clin. North Am. Small Anim. Pract.* 1997, 27:1067–1107.

Willis, A.M., Wilkie, D.A. Ocular Oncology Clinical Techniques. *Small Animal Practice*. 2001, 16(1):77–85.

Woods, M. Corneal ulceration. *Irish Veterinary Journal*. Oct. 2004, 14(2):179–185.

Alphabetical index

A

B

C

D

E

F

G

H

I

K

L

M

N

O

P

Q

R

S

T

U

V

W